CELLULAR AND MOLECULAR BIOLOGY OF ERYTHROCYTES

CELLULAR AND MOLECULAR BIOLOGY OF ERYTHROCYTES

Edited by

Haruhisa YOSHIKAWA

Samuel M. RAPOPORT

UNIVERSITY PARK PRESS

Baltimore • London • Tokyo

UNIVERSITY PARK PRESS
Baltimore • London • Tokyo

Library of Congress Cataloging in Publication Data

Yoshikawa, Haruhisa, 1909–
Cellular and molecular biology of erythrocytes.

1. Erythrocytes. I. Rapoport, Samuel Mitja, joint author.
II. Title. [DNLM: 1. Erythrocytes. 2. Erythrocytes—Cytology.
3. Molecular biology. WH150 Y65c 1974]
QP96.Y67 612′.111 74–3500
ISBN 0–8391–0688–2

UTP 3047–67961–5149

Printed in Japan.

Originally published by
UNIVERSITY OF TOKYO PRESS

PREFACE

The red cell has been an object of research since the beginning of modern science. There has been no waning of interest in this simple biological system; on the contrary, the red cell continues to be in the focus of multidisciplinary research on a steadily expanding scale. In the study of this system the interests of the molecular biologists who are concerned with differentiation and maturation, protein synthesis or membrane processes with those of the clinical hematologists, pathologists and specialists in blood preservation meet. Corresponding to the diversity of disciplines, research results are published in a variety of journals with different groups of readers. Thus pertinent information is widely scattered and an accumulation of it is not easily available to any single group or individual. This circumstance, combined with the rapidity of progress, constitute the main reasons for the recurring pressing need for authoritative reviews by leaders in the field, in which scientific advances are summarized and digested for the benefit of the scientific community as a whole. While there have been in the last years a multitude of international symposia on various aspects of the red cell, no comprehensive collection of reviews has appeared in which the molecular and cellular biology of the red cell has been the main subject. For this reason the editors have approached a number of international experts with the request to contribute to such an enterprise. The response to the proposal was most gratifying, and those who responded spent much time and effort preparing their contributions. It is sincerely hoped that the monograph will fulfill its purpose to present an up-to-date account of the most significant areas of research on red cells, and will find wide readership.

From the beginning to the end of the preparation of the monograph the editors have been helped greatly by their colleagues Makoto Nakao and Shigeki Minakami, whom they wish to express their sincere thanks. They are also very grateful to the publishers, the University of Tokyo Press, for their understanding and patience and their willingness to permit additions and alterations even at a very late stage of publication in order to make the monograph as useful as possible.

The fact that this monograph appears in Japan and includes a large share of contributions by Japanese researchers reflects the importance of the work of Prof. H. Yoshikawa, his pupils and his colleagues. It is a fitting tribute to the life's work of a dedicated resourceful and highly original scientist of great modesty and generosity.

January 1974

S. M. Rapoport

CONTENTS

CONTENTS

ABBREVIATIONS

Enzymes

HK	hexokinase
PHI	hexosephosphate isomerase
PFK	phosphofructokinase
TIM	triosephosphate isomerase
GAPD	glyceraldehyde-3-phosphate dehydrogenase
PGK	phosphoglycerate kinase
PGM	phosphoglyceromutase
PK	pyruvate kinase
LDH	lactate dehydrogenase
DPGM	diphosphoglycerate mutase
2,3-DPGase	2,3-diphosphoglyceratephosphatase
G-6-PD	glucose-6-phosphate dehydrogenase
TA	transaldolase
TK	transketolase
PGI	phosphoglucoisomerase
RNase	ribonuclease
DNase	deoxyribonuclease
GK	glucokinase
PPase	pyrophosphatase
ATPase	adenosinetriphosphatase
AK	adenylate kinase
SDH	succinade hydrogenase
ICDH	isocitrate dehydrogenase

Substrates and Others

DHAP	dihydroxyacetone phosphate
GAP	glyceraldehyde-3-phosphate
1,3-DPG	1,3-diphosphoglycerate
2,3-DPG	2,3-diphosphoglycerate
2-PG	2-phosphoglycerate
3-PG	3-phosphoglycerate
PEP	phosphoenolpyruvate
Pi	inorganic phosphate
ATP	adenosine triphosphate
ADP	adenosine diphosphate
GlcNAc	N-acetylglucosamine
NANA	N-acetylneuraminic acid
NGNA	N-glycolylneuraminic acid
CMH	ceramide monohexoside
CDH	ceramide dihexoside
CTH	ceramide trihexoside
F antigen	Forssman antigen
GNT	globo-N-tetraose
UTP	uridine triphosphate
XTP	xanthosine triphosphate
CTP	cytosine triphosphate
PRPP	phosphoribosyl pyrophosphate
GTP	guanosine triphosphate
IHP	inositol hexaphosphate
2,4-DNP	2,4-dinitrophenol
GSH	reduced glutathione
GSSG	oxidized glutathione
3-AT	3-amino-1,2,4-triazole
ALA	aminolevulinic acid
dsRNA	double-stranded ribonucleic acid

DCIP	2,6-dichlorophenol-indophenol
ACD	acid-citrate-dextrose solution
CPD	citrate-phosphate-dextrose solution
mRNA	messenger ribonucleic acid
tRNA	transfer ribonucleic acid
DOPA	dihydroxyphenylalanine
FAD	flavin adenine dinucleotide
FH_4	tetrahydrofolic acid
IU	international unit(s)
HADH	nicotinamide adenine dinucleotide (reduced)
NADPH	nicotinamide adenine dinucleotide phosphate (reduced)
PCMB	*p*-mercuribenzoic acid
deoxy-Hb	deoxyhemoglobin
Met-Hb	methemoglobin
DNA	deoxyribonucleic acid
cyt c	cytochrome c
Co A	coenzyme A
OPP	oxidative pentose phosphate pathway
EM	Embden-Meyerhof pathway
REF	renal erythropoietic factor
EDTA	ethylenediaminetetraacetic acid

CELLULAR AND MOLECULAR BIOLOGY OF ERYTHROCYTES

Introduction

H. Yoshikawa

Department of Physiological Chemistry and Nutrition, Faculty of Medicine, The University of Tokyo, Tokyo, Japan

INTRODUCTION

While blood has been regarded as the seat of "vital spirit" since ancient times, there were no serious scientific inquiries on circulation and on the red cell until the sixteenth century. The publication of William Harvey's monograph, "Motion of the Heart and Blood" in 1628 was an epoch-making event in the progress of medical knowledge. In 1658, one year after Harvey's death, Jan Swammerdam noted an immense number of "ruddy globules" in the blood of frogs. Shortly thereafter, in 1665, Malpighi, the discoverer of capillary circulation, also observed corpuscles "looking like a rosary of red coral" in a blood vessel of a hedgehog, but he mistook them for fat globules.

It was in 1674 that the first accurate description of the erythrocyte was given by Leeuwenhoek. He showed that the corpuscles were circular in mammals, but oval in birds and fishes, and that the red color of the blood was due to the corpuscles and not to the fluid. He established the size of erythrocytes at about 8 microns in diameter by comparing them with the known size of a grain of sand. A century later, William Hewson showed that these red particles were not globules, as they were called, but biconcave discs, and that if they were put in water, they swelled and ruptured, whereas they shrank in hypertonic saline.

The recognition of the principal physiological function of the red cell, the transport of oxygen and carbon dioxide, had to wait for nearly two centuries after the discovery of the blood circulation. In 1777 Antoine Laurant Lavoisier identified respiration with the process of oxidation, and showed that venous blood became bright by absorbing "Oxygine", as he called it, from the air and that bright blood turned dark on absorbing "Aeriform calcic acid" which was carbon dioxide.

It was Menghini who first showed the presence of iron in the ash of red blood cells in 1747. Justus von Liebig proposed in 1852 the idea that red cells contained a compound of iron which could combine with oxygen or carbon dioxide in a reversible process, but he did not clarify the real nature of the iron compound. Hemoglobin was isolated in a crystalline form from the blood of guinea pig by Reichert in 1849, and Hoppe-Seyler demonstrated the unique property of this pigment in absorbing and discharging oxygen in 1862. It was then that the functional significance of hemoglobin and of the red cells in which it is carried became clear.

Another problem was the origin of the red cells. The question remained unresolved until 1868, when Ernst Neumann demonstrated that mammalian red corpuscles were derived, throughout life, from colorless nucleated cells in the bone marrow. With the introduction of the aniline dyes by Ehrlich, morphological studies of the blood and bone marrow received much attention and remarkable progress in the understanding of hematopoiesis was attained. On morphological grounds, a number of stages in the development of the erythrocyte have been identified. The stem cells give rise to proerythroblasts which divide to form basophilic erythroblasts. Successive cell divisions yield polychromatophilic erythroblasts and orthochromatophilic erythroblasts, which mature into normoblasts and reticulocytes without further cell division. The reticulocyte has been so named because these cells can be stained with supravital dyes such as brilliant cresyl blue, revealing a reticulum. Final maturation takes place both in the bone marrow and the peripheral circulation.

Recent studies on the structure and metabolism of the red blood cell reflect the development of cellular biochemistry in many directions, such as the molecular structure and function of proteins, the biosynthesis of cell constituents and its general control, the mechanism of metabolic regulation, the active transport of cations across cell membranes, and the process of differentiation and aging in individual cells.

Hemoglobin, as readily available protein, has been the subject of intensive investigations. It is widely distributed in nature and possesses heme as the prosthetic group, which is attached to the colorless basic protein, globin. Hemoglobins of different species differ in their physical, chemical and biological properties. Further, different hemoglobins have been found within a single species and even in the same individual. Thus, human hemoglobin formed in fetal red cells differs from that formed after birth as regards the oxygen-dissociation curves,[1] the resistance to denaturation by alkali,[2] and electrophoretic mobility.[3] It is now established that all these differences are entirely due to the different primary structures of the globin moieties since the heme structure is the same.

Teichmann, in 1853, was the first to observe the formation of hemin crystals, known as Teichmann's crystals, by reacting blood with glacial acetic acid and sodium chloride. The task of elucidating the chemical structure of hemin, which is the chloride of the prosthetic group, and related porphyrins engaged some of the most brilliant minds in organic chemistry: Willstätter, Nenck, Piloty and Küster. Finally in 1929, Hans Fischer[4)] achieved the triumph of synthesizing hemin identical in every respect with that obtained from hemoglobin.

Information about the molecular structure of hemoglobin remained scanty until the advent of modern techniques of protein chemistry. It is known that the smallest possible molecular weight of hemoglobin, which contains 1 gram atom of iron, is around 17,000. In 1925, Adair[5)] estimated the molecular weight to be about 700,000 by measurements of the osmotic pressure, and later, in 1926, Svedberg[6)] obtained the same figure by employing an ultracentrifuge devised by himself. This corresponds to the tetramer.

Further investigations have shown that all mammalian hemoglobins consist of 4 polypeptide chains, usually in pairs. Two kinds of chains in hemoglobin A have been termed α and β, and those in hemoglobin F, α and γ. The complete amino acid sequences of these 3 chains have been established by the concurrent efforts of 3 groups, Braunitzer *et al.*,[7)] Konigsberg and Hill,[8)] and Schroeder *et al.*[9)] The secondary, tertiary and quaternary structures of horse hemoglobin was determined X-ray crystallographically by Perutz and his collaborators.[10)] In a hemoglobin molecule, 4 subunits are arranged in a tetrahedral array, the 4 heme groups lying in separate crevices on the surface. Of particular importance is the finding that tertiary structure of the chains of hemoglobin is very similar to that of myoglobin, as demonstrated by Kendrew *et al.*,[11)] and that oxygenation of hemoglobin results in a decrease in the distance between the β chains.[12)]

In 1910 Herrik discovered sickle-cell anemia in a Negro, and suggested that the abnormality in shape might be related to some unrecognized change in the corpuscle itself. In 1949, Pauling, Itano, Singer and Wells[13)] showed that the red cells from sickle-cell anemia contained an unusual form of hemoglobin. This discovery introduced into medicine the concept of "molecular disease", which implies that disease may result from a genetically determined fault in protein synthesis. They found that this form was different from normal hemoglobin not only in its lower solubility of the reduced form but also in its reduced electrophoretic mobility. Later, in 1956, Ingram[14] demonstrated that in sickle-cell hemoglobin, the glutamic acid residue at position 6 in the normal β chain is replaced by a valine residue. To date, a large number of abnormal haemoglobins have been discovered, and characterized by abnormalities in the amino acid sequence of one of the polypeptide chains. The occurrence of such a change in the protein is explained as due to a mutation in the gene that controls the synthesis of the polypeptide chains.

Much investigative work on hemoglobin biosynthesis has employed the reticulocyte, largely because this denucleated cell, which can be obtained in high concentrations in the peripheral blood, still possesses the mitochondria, endoplasmic reticulum and ribosomes required for the biosynthesis. The nucleated nonmammalian erythrocyte is also suitable for this purpose, as indicated by its active metabolic processes.

Application of isotope tracer techniques demonstrated that the complicated protoporphyrin molecule is synthesized from 2 simple precursors, glycine and acetate. Deuterioacetic acid was fed to rats, and the isolated hemin was found to contain excess deuterium (Bloch and Rittenberg, 1945).[15] The next step was the demonstration that the feeding of glycine labeled with ^{15}N resulted in the presence of excess isotope in hemin.[16] Most of the later experiments have been carried out by means of *in vitro* techniques, using nucleated red cells of the duck[17] as well as mammalian reticulocytes.[18] The pathway of heme synthesis has been elucidated by the work of Shemin, Rittenberg, London, Granick, Neuberger, Rimington and others, as outlined below.[19] Acetate is utilized as succinyl coenzyme A, which combines with glycine to form δ-aminolevulinic acid. Two molecules of δ-aminolevulinic acid condense under the influence of a specific enzyme to yield porphobilinogen, identical with the chromogen excreted in acute porphyria. Four molecules of porphobilinogen undergo enzymatic condensation to form uroporphyrinogen, type III plus some type I. Uroporphyrinogen III is converted to coproporphyrinogen by decarboxylation, and this is oxidized and decarboxylated to yield protoporphyrin IX. Mitochondria are required for the formation of succinyl coenzyme A via the tricarboxylic acid cycle. δ-Aminolevulinic acid synthetase and coproporphyrinogen III oxidase are bound to mitochondria, while the enzymes responsible for the pathway from δ-aminolevulinic acid to coproporphyrinogen are contained in the cytosol.

The final step in heme synthesis involves the incorporation of ferrous iron into protoporphyrin by heme synthetase or ferrochelatase bound to mitochondria. This reaction was investigated initially by studying the incorporation of radioactive iron *in vitro* into mammalian reticulocytes[20] and avian erythrocytes.[21] The enzyme was solubilized by treating cellular particles with surface-active agents,[22,23] and the properties of the partially purified enzyme were investigated.[24,25]

The formation of peptide bonds in red-cell protein *in vitro* was first observed by Shemin and co-workers in 1950[26] with intact duck erythrocytes. Subsequent studies on the biosynthesis of globin have been conducted effectively with mammalian reticulocytes. Incorporation of radioactive amino acids into the protein was followed both in the intact cell[27] and in cell-free systems.[28] Schweet and his associates[29] and Dintzis[30] demonstrated that the formation of peptide chains starts at the N-terminal amino acid, valine, and continues by steady sequential addition of amino acids until elongation of the chain terminates at the C-terminal end. Electron microscopic observations of reticulocyte microsomes indicated that protein synthesis occurs in aggregations of ribosomes, the so-called polysomes, which are strung along a messenger RNA strand.[31]

Newly synthesized heme is accepted by globin, apparently by a nonenzymatic process, to yield hemoglobin.[32] Earlier studies on the synthesis of heme and globin have indicated a parallelism in the rates of the 2 synthetic processes.[27,33,34] London and his associates[35] reported that on the addition of hemin to rabbit reticulocytes *in vitro*, there was marked inhibition of heme synthesis at the step of δ-aminolevulinic acid synthetase, together with stimulation of incorporation of valine into newly formed hemoglobin.[36] The claim by Schwartz and others[37] that the insertion of iron into protoporphyrin was enhanced in the presence of globin could not be confirmed by subsequent investigations.[32] Details of the mechanism by which the syntheses of heme and of globin are normally coordinated must await further investigation.

The reticulocyte possesses functioning glycolytic and hexose monophosphate shunt pathways, tricarboxylic acid cycle, and an intact electron transfer and oxidative phosphorylation systems. Besides the biosynthesis of hemoglobin, the reticulocyte also has the capability to carry out *de novo* synthesis of purine nucleotides from low molecular precursors to some extent.[38]

In contrast to the reticulocyte, the mature mammalian erythrocyte lacks mitochondria and ribosomes. Hence the electron transfer and oxidative phosphorylation systems are absent, the tricarboxylic cycle is not functioning although some of its enzymes are present, and synthesis of hemoglobin does not occur. It was natural that, for many years, the nonnucleated mature erythrocyte was thought to be an inert membranaceous bag containing a concentrated solution of hemoglobin, and was therefore called a red corpuscle. But by now it is clear that the erythrocyte is metabolically quite active: in fact, pure human red cells utilize about 2 μmoles glucose per ml per hour, producing nearly an equivalent amount of lactic acid.

The gradual disappearance of sugar from the blood *in vitro* was first demonstrated by Bernard in 1876. This phenomenon was later extensively investigated, and Evans[39)] showed that the breakdown of glucose was paralleled by the formation of lactic acid. It occurred only in the presence of blood cells, and especially of white blood cells, and some investigators believed that the glycolytic activity of normal blood resided predominantly, or even exclusively, in leucocytes. However, quantitative studies[40)] revealed that the glycolysis of blood was attributable mostly to the red blood cells. By 1930, acid-soluble phosphorus compounds such as hexose phosphate, adenosine triphosphate (ATP), and 2,3-diphosphoglycerate (2,3-DPG) had been found in whole blood, and the significance of these compounds in the glycolytic process was recognized. The existence of hexose phosphate was reported by Lawaczek[41)] and by Goodwin and Robison.[42)] "Adenylic acid" separated from whole human blood by Jackson[43)] appears to be identical with ATP which was isolated from muscle by Embden and Zimmermann[44)] and given the correct chemical formula by Lohmann[45)] later. 2,3-DPG was discovered in red blood cells by Greenwald[46)] in large amounts. The importance of phosphorylation in blood glycolysis was suggested by Rona and Iwasaki[47)] and hexose phosphate was regarded as an intermediate of glycolysis by Roche and Roche.[48)] Subsequent studies yielded evidence that the maintenance of a normal level of phosphoric esters in the blood was a consequence of their continuous synthesis and decomposition during glycolysis.[49,50)]

The breakdown of sugars is carried out almost exclusively via the well-known Embden-Meyerhof pathway, which comprises 11 sequentical reactions catalyzed by specific enzymes. For each molecule of glucose metabolized, 2 molecules of ATP are consumed and 4 molecules of ATP are produced, thus generating 2 molecules of ATP per molecule of glucose. One function of the glycolytic system of the erythrocyte is to provide an easily available supply of energy in the form of ATP. ATP is decomposed to adenosine diphosphate (ADP) and inorganic phosphate by adenosinetriphosphatase. The energy released by this hydrolysing process is utilized for the active transport of cations across the erythrocyte membrane. It has been demonstrated that ATP is also essential for the maintenance of the normal biconcave discoidal shape of the cell. While in the circulation, the energy-rich terminal phosphate groups of ATP undergo rapid turnover and each of the glycolytic intermediates, as well as the nucleotides, is in a dynamic equilibrium, generally kept at a constant level under continuous supply of glucose and removal of lactic acid.

In addition to ATP formation, glycolysis plays an important role in preventing hemoglobin from autoxidation to methemoglobin. The existence of an enzyme which catalyses the reduction of methemoglobin by NADH in human red blood cells was suggested by Gibson.[51]

The hexose monophosphate shunt, or pentose phosphate cycle, has been detected in erythrocytes.[52] This pathway diverges from glycolysis at the level of glucose-6-phosphate and produces pentose phosphates after dehydrogenation and decarboxylation.[53,54] The pentose phosphates are finally converted to fructose-6-phosphate and glyceraldehyde phosphate, and so return to the glycolytic pathway. The metabolic flow through this pathway is estimated at only 10% of the total glucose metabolism.[55] When inosine is added to erythrocytes, a nucleoside phosphorylase splits the nucleoside to give hypoxanthine and ribose-1-phosphate and the latter is converted to ribose-5-phosphate and disposed of by the same cycle.[56] More recently, it has been demonstrated that there is another pathway which metabolizes xylitol via xylulose and its phosphate, leading to the pentose phosphate cycle.[57] In a normal state, however, this enzyme system seems to be dormant because of a lack of substrate in the erythrocyte.

Characteristic of the human erythrocyte is the existence of a bypass, called the Rapoport-Luebering cycle, via a large pool of 2,3-DPG. 1,3-DPG, which is produced by a phosphorylating dehydrogenase from triose phosphate, is converted to a low-energy 2,3-diester by diphosphoglycerate mutase[58] and this in turn is hydrolysed to give 3-phosphoglycerate (3-PG) by a specific phosphatase.[59] 2,3-DPG combines with hemoglobin, causing a decrease in its affinity for oxygen and a displacement of the oxyhemoglobin dissociation curve to the right.[60,61] Thus, its presence in the erythrocyte assists oxyhemoglobin to unload oxygen.

Although the red blood cell has neither a respiratory chain nor an active tricarboxylic acid cycle, the cell contains isocitrate dehydrogenase, fumarase and malate dehydrogenase, but their significance is not clear.[62]

In the erythrocytes of most mammals, the concentration of potassium inside the cells is much higher than in plasma while that of sodium is much lower. This uneven distribution of ions was formerly thought to arise during the formation of erythrocytes and to be maintained in mature cells because their membranes were impermeable to both Na^+ and K^+. Around 1940, the idea of impermeability was abandoned because experiments with radioactive tracers indicated that the cell membranes were permeable to both cations.[63,64] It was also found that red cells stored in the cold were able to reverse the changes in cation concentrations produced by storage, when the temperature was raised to 37°C, and that this phenomenon required the presence of glucose and was inhibited by fluoride or iodoacetate,[65] thus indicating the involvement of active transport across the cell membrane, against the concentration gradient. Cardiac glycosides such as ouabain prevented the uptake of K^+.[66]

It was speculated that active transport is accomplished in the presence of high-energy phosphate bonds. This view was confirmed when Gardós invented ingenious methods for introducing ATP into erythrocyte ghosts.[67] By means of this technique, he was able to show that ghosts which had lost glycolytic activity, were still able to accumulate potassium, provided ATP was introduced into the cells. Post and his co-workers[68] reported the existence of an ATPase in the membranes of erythrocytes that required the presence of Na^+, K^+ and Mg^{2+} for maximal activity and was inhibited by cardiac glucosides. On the basis of further studies with membrane ATPase preparations it has been supposed that the overall hydrolysis of ATP proceeds in at least 2 stages. The first step is the formation of an intermediary phosphorylated compound, which is dependent on the presence of sodium ions. The second step of the reaction is the subsequent hydrolysis of the intermediate with the release of inorganic phosphate; the latter reaction is dependent on potassium ions and is inhibited by low concentrations of cardiac glycosides. Whittam[69] postulated that the operation of the ion pump in moving Na^+ outwards and K^+ inwards is linked to a rotation of the enzyme in the membrane or a part of it, so that the active center of the enzyme is alternately exposed to the outside and the inside.

The problem of how the cell membrane directs the passage of ions from one side to the other is difficult to solve by traditional methods of biochemistry such as purification and characterization of enzymes. In approaching the problem, experiments with intact erythrocytes or ghosts are very convenient, because of their simple membrane structure.

The mechanism by which erythrocytes maintain their biconcave shape remained unclear for a long time. Furchgot and Ponder[70)] once proposed the existence of an antisphering factor in blood plasma, but later Ponder himself[71)] was in considerable doubt about this. More recently, Nakao and his collaborators[72)] demonstrated an intimate relationship between the shape of a red cell and the concentration of ATP within it. They observed that fresh human erythrocytes were transformed through crenated forms to spherocytes as the intracellular ATP level was lowered by inhibiting glycolysis with fluoride, followed by regeneration of discs as the ATP level was increased to normal by removing the inhibitor and subsequently incubating the erythrocytes with adenine and inosine. This finding afforded experimental support for Prankerd's suggestion[73)] that the erythrocyte envelope might possess contractile properties dependent upon continuous regeneration of ATP.

One of the most striking examples of the importance of the evolutionary process is found in the mammalian erythrocyte. The development of hemoglobin makes possible the transport of 100 times as much oxygen as could be carried by the plasma alone. The biconcave shape of the erythrocyte has been shown to be the best shape for the effective exchange of gases across the cell boundary. Another source of efficiency is the absence of a nucleus. Neither mitochondria nor endoplasmic reticulum occur in the mature erythrocyte, so that the only metabolic process which remains intact is the utilization of glucose via glycolysis and partly via hexose monophosphate shunt pathway.

To sum up, the red corpuscle is no longer regarded as being a completely inert protoplasmic particle. It is a highly specialized cell with the characteristic features that, with increased specialization, the cellular structure and the metabolic system have become extremely simplified. These simple features help us, in turn, to understand the life processes occurring in cells in general.

REFERENCES

1 Barcroft, J., *Physiol. Rev.*, **16**, 103 (1936).
2 Haurowitz, F., *Z. Physiol. Chem.*, **232**, 125 (1935).
3 Hoch, H., *Biochem. J.*, **46**, 199 (1950).
4 Fischer, H. and Zeile, K., *Ann. Chem.*, **468**, 98 (1929).
5 Adair, G. S., *Proc. Roy. Soc. London*, A, **109**, 292 (1925).
6 Svedberg, T. and Nichols, J. B., *J. Amer. Chem. Soc.*, **49**, 2920 (1927).
7 Braunitzer, G., Gehring-Müller, G., Hilschmann, N., Hilse, K., Hobom, G., Rudloff, V. and Wittam-Liebold, B., *Z. Physiol. Chem.*, **325**, 283 (1961).
8 Konigsberg, W. and Hill, R. J., *J. Biol.*, **237**, 2547 (1962).
9 Schroeder, W. A., Shelton, J. R., Shelton, J. B. and Cormick, J., *Proc. Natl. Acad. Sci. U. S.*, **48**, 284 (1962).
10 Perutz, M. F., Rossman, M. G., Cullis, A. F., Muirhead, H., Will, G. and North, A. C. T., *Nature*, **185**, 416 (1960).
11 Kendrew, J. C., Dickerson, R. E., Strandberg, B. E., Hart, R. G., Davies, D. R., Phillips, D. C. and Shore, V. C., *Nature*, **185**, 422 (1960).
12 Muirhead, H. and Perutz, M. F., *Cold Spring Harbor Symp. Quant. Biology*, **28**, 451 (1963).
13 Pauling, L., Itano, H. A., Singer, S. J. and Wells, T. C., *Science*, **110**, 543 (1949).
14 Ingram, V. M., *Nature*, **178**, 792 (1956).
15 Bloch, K. and Rittenberg, D., *J. Biol. Chem.*, **159**, 45 (1945).
16 Shemin, D. and Rittenberg, D., *J. Biol. Chem.*, **166**, 621 (1946).
17 Shemin, D., London, I. M. and Rittenberg, D., *J. Biol. Chem.*, **173**, 799 (1948).
18 London, I. M., Shemin, D. and Rittenberg, D., *J. Biol. Chem.*, **183**, 749 (1950).
19 London, I. M., *Harvey Lectures*, **56**, 151 (1961).
20 Walsh, R. J., Thomas, E. D., Chow, S. K., Fluharty, R. G. and Finch, C. A., *Science*, **110**, 396 (1949).
21 Jensen, W. N., Ashenbrucker, H., Cartwright, G. E. and Wintrobe, M. M., *J. Lab. Clin. Med.*, **42**, 833 (1953).
22 Krueger, R. C., Melnick, I. and Klein, J. R., *Arch. Biochem. Biophys.*, **64**, 302 (1956).
23 Kagawa, Y., Minakami, S. and Yoneyama, Y., *J. Biochem.*, **46**, 771 (1959).
24 Yoneyama, Y., Ohyama, H., Sugita, Y. and Yoshikawa, H., *Biochim. Biophys. Acta*, **62**, 261 (1962).
25 Yoshikawa, H. and Yoneyama, Y., Iron Metabolism, an International Symposium (Springer-Verlag, Berlin, 1964), p. 24.

26 Shemin, D., London, I. M. and Rittenberg, D., *J. Biol. Chem.*, **183**, 757 (1950).
27 Kruh, J. and Borsook, H., *J. Biol. Chem.*, **220**, 905 (1956).
28 Schweet, R., Lamfrom, H. and Allen, E., *Proc. Natl. Acad. Sci. U. S.*, **44**, 1029 (1958).
29 Bishop, J., Leahy, J. and Schweet, R., *Proc. Natl. Acad. Sci. U. S.*, **46**, 1030 (1960).
30 Dintzis, H. M., *Proc. Natl. Acad. Sci. U. S.*, **47**, 247 (1961).
31 Warner, J. R., Knopf, P. M. and Rich, A., *Proc. Natl. Acad. Sci. U. S.*, **49**, 122 (1963).
32 Yoneyama, Y., Ohyama, H., Sugita, Y. and Yoshikawa, H., *Biochim. Biophys. Acta*, **74**, 635 (1963).
33 Nizet, A., *Bull. Soc. Chim. Biol.*, **39**, 265 (1957).
34 Morell, H., Savoie, J.-C. and London, I. M., *J. Biol. Chem.*, **233**, 923 (1958).
35 Karibian, D. and London, I. M., *Biochem. Biophys. Res. Comm.*, **18**, 243 (1965).
36 Bruns, G. P. and London, I. M., *Biochem. Biophys. Res. Comm.*, **18**, 236 (1965).
37 Schwartz, H. C., Hill, R. L., Cartwright, G. E. and Wintrobe, M. M., *Biochim. Biophys. Acta*, **36**, 567 (1959).
38 Lowy, B. A., Cook, J. L. and London, I. M., *J. Biol. Chem.*, **236**, 1442 (1961).
39 Evans, C. L., *J. Physiol.*, **56**, 146 (1922).
40 Lundsgaard, E., *Ergebn. Enzymforsch.*, **2**, 179 (1933).
41 Lawaczek, H., *Biochem. Z.*, **145**, 351 (1924).
42 Goodwin, H. W. and Robison, R., *Biochem. J.*, **18**, 1161 (1924).
43 Jackson, H., *J. Biol. Chem.*, **59**, 529 (1924).
44 Embden, G. and Zimmermann, M., *Z. Physiol. Chem.*, **167**, 114, 137 (1937).
45 Lohmann, K., *Biochem. Z.*, **282**, 120 (1935).
46 Greenwald, I., *J. Biol. Chem.*, **63**, 339 (1925).
47 Rona, P. and Iwasaki, K., *Biochem. A.*, **184**, 318 (1927).
48 Roche, A. and Roche, J., *C. R. Soc. Biol.*, **97**, 802, 804 (1927).
49 Meyerhof, O., *Biochem. Z.*, **246**, 249 (1932).
50 Guest, G. M. and Rapoport, S., *Physiol. Rev.*, **21**, 410 (1941).
51 Gibson, Q. H., *Biochem. J.*, **42**, 13 (1948).
52 Dische, Z., Phosphorus Metabolism, Vol. 1 (Johns Hopkins Press, Baltimore, 1951), p. 171.
53 Warburg, O., Christian, W. and Griese, A., *Biochem. Z.*, **282**, 159 (1935).
54 Warburg, O. and Christian, W., *Biochem. Z.*, **287**, 440 (1936).
55 Brin, M. and Yonemoto, R. H., *J. Biol. Chem.*, **230**, 307 (1958).

56 Gabrio, B. W., Donohue, D. M., Huennekens, F. M. and Finch, C. A., *J. Clin. Invest.*, **35**, 657 (1956).
57 Asakura, T., Adachi, K., Minakami, S. and Yoshikawa, H., *J. Biochem.*, **62**, 184 (1967).
58 Rapoport, S. and Luebering, J., *J. Biol. Chem.*, **183**, 507 (1950).
59 Rapoport, S. and Luebering, J., *J. Biol. Chem.*, **189**, 683 (1951).
60 Chanutin, A. and Curnish, R., *Arch. Biochem. Biophys.*, **121**, 96 (1967).
61 Benesch, R., Benesch, R. E. and Yu, C. I., *Proc. Natl. Acad. Sci. U. S.*, **59**, 526 (1968).
62 Rubinstein, D., Ottolenghi, P. and Denstedt, O. F., *Canad. J. Biochem. Physiol.*, **34**, 222 (1956).
63 Cohn, W. E. and Cohn, E. T., *Proc. Soc. Exp. Biol. Med.*, **41**, 445 (1939).
64 Mullins, L. J., Fenn, W. O., Noonan, T. R. and Haege, L. F., *Amer. J. Physiol.*, **135**, 93 (1941).
65 Harris, J. E., *J. Biol. Chem.*, **141**, 579 (1941).
66 Schatzmann, H. J., *Helv. Physiol. Acta*, **11**, 346 (1953).
67 Gardós, G., *Acta Physiol. Acad. Sci. Hung.*, **6**, 191 (1954).
68 Post, R. L., Merritt, C. R., Kinsolving, C. R. and Albright, C. D., *J. Biol. Chem.*, **235**, 1796 (1960).
69 Whittam, R., *Biochem. J.*, **84**, 110 (1962).
70 Furchgott, R. F. and Ponder, E., *J. Exp. Biol.*, **17**, 117 (1940).
71 Ponder, E., *Blood*, **9**, 227 (1954).
72 Nakao, M., Nakao, T., Yamazoe, S. and Yoshikawa, H., *J. Biochem.*, **49**, 487 (1961).
73 Prankerd, T. A. J., Altmann, K. I. and Young, L. E., *J. Clin. Invest.*, **34**, 1268 (1955).

Glycolipids from Erythrocyte Membranes as Cell Antigens

T. Yamakawa

Department of Biochemistry, Faculty of Medicine, University of Tokyo, Tokyo, Japan

In studies of animal-cell membranes, red cells are frequently used as the experimental material since they are readily available.

The ghost or stroma obtained by hemolyzing red blood cells is a very good model for medical and biological research. Moreover, intact erythrocytes are especially important in the field of practical medicine as sensitive reagents for immune seroreactions such as hemagglutination or hemolysis. The functional groups which can be called the cell antigens are considered to exist in the cell-surface membrane. The stroma or vesicle containing large quantities of hemoglobin is chemically not a single protein, carbohydrate or lipid, but consists of a so called heteropolymer, such as glycoprotein, glycolipid or lipoprotein.

EARLY STUDIES

In 1951, Yamakawa and Suzuki[1)] isolated a large amount of erythrocytes from horse blood coagula which had been abandoned in the process of antiserum production. After hemolyzing the cells by the addition of 5 volumes of 0.3% acetic acid in water followed by centrifugation, stroma were obtained. The lipids were extracted from the stroma with a methanol-ether mixture. This fraction contained cholesterol and phospholipids. When the residue was extracted with hot chloroform-methanol, a dark brown extract was obtained, from which a type of glycolipid was obtained after concentration and precipitation with acetone from a chloroform solution. This glycolipid was named 'hematoside'. When hematoside was further purified and methanolyzed, long-chain fatty acids (mostly lignoceric acid), sphingosine, galactose and glucose, as well as an N-containing hydroxy acid called 'hemataminic acid' was obtained.

The term 'gangliosides' was not widely known in those days, though in 1942 Klenk[2)] had obtained peculiar glycolipids called gangliosides from brain. These contained a material called 'neuraminic acid' besides ceramide, glucose and galactose.

Although hemataminic acid was later proved to be identical with neuraminic acid, the name, hematoside, has been adopted for the glycolipid class containing neuraminic acid but not hexosamine, though the term is more often used as a synonym for G_{M3}, a kind of ganglioside.

In 1952, Klenk and Wolter[3] confirmed the above results. Furthermore Klenk and Lauenstein[4] succeeded in isolating a kind of glycolipid from human erythrocytes which contained galactosamine but no neuraminic acid. Subsequently, Yamakawa and Suzuki[5] obtained such a glycolipid from human blood stroma and confirmed their results. On that occasion, we named the glycolipid 'globoside'. Our interest was focused upon the difference between the glycolipid components of horse and human blood cells, since they both belonged to the mammalia. We collected glycolipids from blood cells of various animals and analyzed them for hexosamine and sialic acids (acylated neuraminic acid). The results are indicated in Table I.[6,7]

Glycolipids from human, pig, guinea pig, rabbit and sheep samples contained galactosamine or glucosamine, but no sialic acid (globoside type). Glycolipids from horse, dog and cat samples contained sialic acid, but not hexosamines (hematoside type). In glycolipids from cow, some types contained both, and were considered to be gangliosides, a mixed type.

Since then, many experimental results have accumulated and it has been shown that horse glycolipids also contain a small amount of

TABLE I. Nature of hexosamines and sialic acids in erythrocyte mucolipid of various mammals.

Animal	Glucosamine	Galactosamine	Sialic acid
Globosides			
Man	−	++	−
Pig	−	++	−
Guinea pig	−	++	−
Rabbit	++	−	−
Ox	++	−	+ or −
Sheep	+	++	−
Goat	+	++	−
Hematosides			
Horse	−	−	++ (NGNA)
Dog	−	−	++ (NANA>NGNA)
Cat	−	−	++ (NGNA)

Abb.: NGNA, N-glycolylneuraminic acid; NANA, N-acetylneuraminic acid.

globoside, and that a very small amount of hematoside was present in human glycolipid fraction. Nevertheless, this classification and nomenclature are used because it is generally valid and is very convenient.

It was more or less by chance that Yamakawa and Iida,[8] in 1953, found ABO blood-group activity in the globoside from human erythrocytes. Yamakawa, Matsumoto, Suzuki and Iida[9] isolated globoside from blood cells of groups A, B, O and AB, respectively, and confirmed that the inhibition was group-specific and was not a nonspecific reaction due to the lipid nature of the material. However, materials in those days were still crude and efforts to prepare purer material have continued up to present, as will be mentioned later.

Until the 1950's, solubility differences in various organic solvents were used to isolate and purify the lipid. It was in the late 1950's that the application of column chromatography to lipid chemistry became familiar, but it was not until 1960 that thin-layer chromatography (TLC) and gas chromatography (GLC) became widely available. When silicic acid of high quality became available, column chromatography also became an important tool for the purification of lipids and the glycolipids and products which had been thought to be single materials were often separated into several components. In this way, the molecular differences of red-cell glycolipids of various animals, as shown in Table I, became visible as different patterns on the column chromatogram.[10,11]

The test sample, loaded on a column packed with silicic acid, was eluted with stepwise increases in concentration of methanol in chloroform. When the effluent was measured for hexose content, each glycolipid fraction gave a characteristic pattern. Thus, the membranes of blood cells do not consist of a single material but of an assembly of various glycolipids in an particular ratio. For instance, the chromatographic pattern of human erythrocyte glycolipids (Fig. 1) shows that the main constituent is Globoside I, thought to be a ceramide tetrasaccharide, but a group of simpler glycolipids, ceramide monohexoside (CMH), ceramide dihexoside (CDH) and ceramide trihexoside (CTH) were eluted before Globoside I and more complicated minor glycolipids followed Globoside I. They were named Globosides II and III.[12] Blood-group activities were present in these minor components.

DETERMINATION OF CHEMICAL STRUCTURES

After purification of the glycolipids, the next step was to deter-

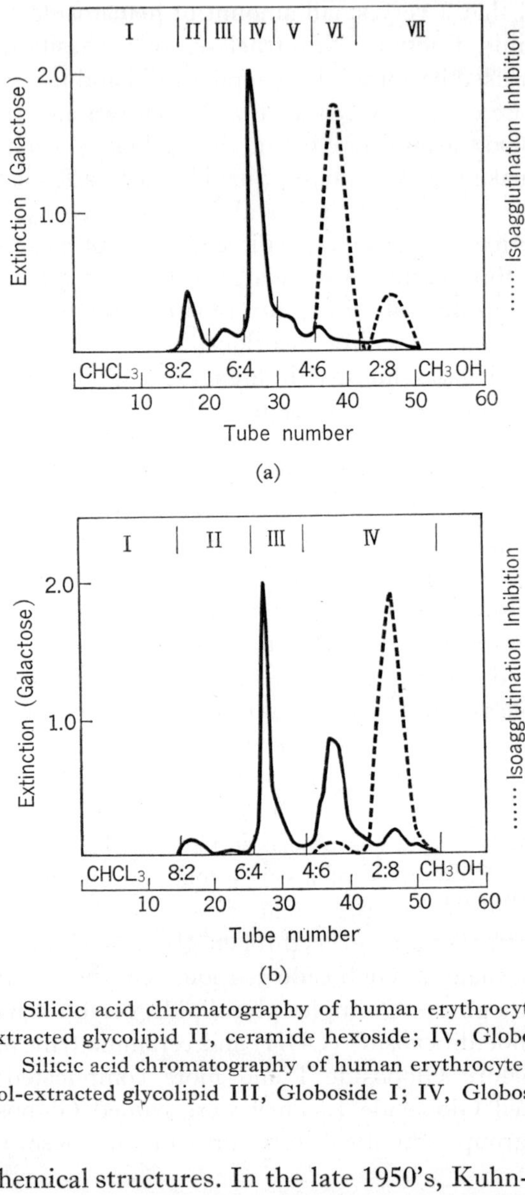

Fig. 1(a). Silicic acid chromatography of human erythrocyte methanol-ether-extracted glycolipid II, ceramide hexoside; IV, Globoside I.

(b). Silicic acid chromatography of human erythrocyte chloroform-methanol-extracted glycolipid III, Globoside I; IV, Globosides II and III.

mine their chemical structures. In the late 1950's, Kuhn-Wiegandt and Klenk-Gielen in Germany, and Svennerholm in Sweden engaged in the purification of brain gangliosides and found that the glycolipid could be fractionated into several components. The chemical structures proposed for ganglioside up to were thus meaningless, since they had been applied to mixtures. From 1960 to 1963, the gangliosides were classified and the chemical structures were determined, especially by the Kuhn-Wiegandt group (Fig. 2).

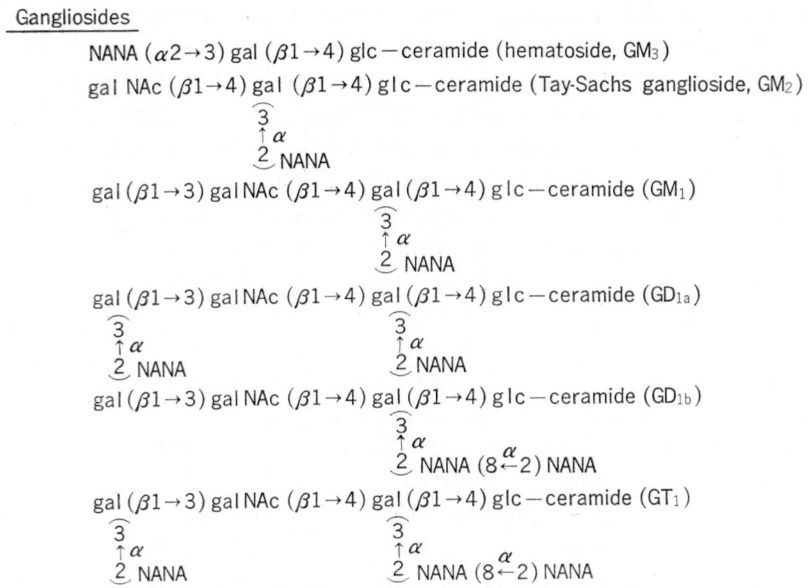

Fig. 2.

They had been working on N-containing oligosaccharides from human milk in previous years. On that basis, they compared the oligosaccharide moieties of gangliosides with their materials from milk.

On the other hand, the structure of hematoside, the simplest ganglioside, was determined by Klenk and Padberg[13] as;

$$\mathrm{NGNA(2\to3)Gal(1\to4)Glc\text{-}ceramide.}$$

Handa and Yamakawa[14] and Handa and Handa[15] determined the structures of hematosides from blood cells of horse, dog and cat by the technique of permethylation, methanolysis and gas chromatography, as will be mentioned later.

Glycolipids from human erythrocytes were separated into several fractions, as indicated in Fig. 1. Globoside I, the principal component, consisted of 4 moles of monosaccharides, so it was rather difficult to determine the structure. The component sugars were identified by gas chromatography after trimethylsilylation as 1 glucose, 2 galactose and 1 N-acetylgalactosamine. The glycolipid was hydrolysed with dilute HCl and the carbohydrate fragments were obtained by dialysis through a cellophane bag. A disaccharide was separated by charcoal column chromatography, and was shown to be GalNAc (β 1→3)Gal from its periodate consumption and infrared absorption spectrum.[16]

Until that time, gas chromatography had not been considered as a useful tool for the determination of carbohydrate structure. In 1960, a prediction was made by Jones[17]: 'These and other new techniques indicate that we are entering a new phase in the determination of structures of polysaccharides and oligosaccharides. It will soon be possible to determine their structures on a very, very small amount indeed of polysaccharide, perhaps of the order of 10 mg or less, without any ambiguity'. In fact permethylation of carbohydrate material in amounts as small as several milligrams became possible after the discovery of an improved reagent, using dimethylformamide as a solvent by Kuhn, Trischmann and Löw[18] and together with clear-cut identification of partially methylated sugars by gas chromatography this has lead to great progress in structural studies of carbohydrates.

Prior to the application of this method to Globoside I, simpler ceramide dihexosides of human erythrocytes and brain sulfatide were examined by this technique.[19] The structure of CDH or 'Cytolipin H' was reported by Rapport *et al.*[20] to be lactosyl ceramide, in an immunological inhibition study. The identification of methyl 2,3,4,6-tetramethylgalactoside and methyl 2,3,6-trimethylglucoside by GLC confirmed their result. Quite unexpectedly, the structure of brain sulfatide, which had been believed to be cerebroside-5'-sulfate since its discovery by Blix in 1932, proved to be cerebroside-3'-sulfate, because distinct peaks of an anomeric mixture of methyl 2,4,6-trimethylgalactoside were identified by GLC of the methanolysate of permethylated sulfatide.

After a similar procedure, Globoside I gave peaks corresponding to methyl 2,3,6-trimethylglucoside, methyl 2,3,6-trimethylgalactoside and methyl 2,4,6-trimethylgalactoside. From these results, the structure;

GalNAc(1→3)Gal(1→4)Gal(1→4)Glc-ceramide

was proposed for Globoside I.[16,12] A material similar to Globoside I was obtained from human kidney[21,22] and a chemical structure was proposed which was the same as that of Globoside I.[23] Rapport[22] named this glycolipid Cytolipin K. Later, globoside from pig erythrocytes proved to have the same structure.[24]

At that time, the anomeric configurations of each sugar linkage were not exactly determined, except for the galactosidic linkage in CDH and the N-acetylgalactosaminidic linkage of Globoside I, based on the infrared absorption spectra, and it had been considered that all of the glycosidic bonds in these glycolipids were in the β configuration as in brain gangliosides, through without any special evidence. Recently, since the finding that Fabry's disease is caused by α-galactosidase deficiency by Kint in 1970,[25] a number of papers have reported the terminal galactosidic linkages of CTH and ceramide digalactoside, the accumulated glycolipids in this disease, to be α[26–28] by NMR analysis, though this was first suggested by Kawanami in 1967.[29] The configuration of Globoside I is now established as follows;

GalNAc(β1→3)Gal(α 1→4)Gal(β 1→4)Glc(β 1→1)ceramide

The terminal N-acetylgalactosamine unit of Globoside I was liberated by β-N-acetylhexosaminidase from hog epididymis.[30a]

As for hematoside, Hakomori and Saito[30b] obtained another hematoside with a higher migration rate on TLC from equine erythrocyte membrane. The sialosyl residue of this glycolipid was not hydrolysed by neuraminidase. The sialic acid isolated from the acid hydrolysate, was identified as a new sialic acid. O-acetyl(N-glycolyl)neuraminic acid. On the other hand, McCluer and Evans considered it to be an intramolecular ester.[30c] Up to now, the structures of the following erythrocyte glycolipids have been determined or suggested:

CMH Glc-ceramide
CDH Gal(β1→4)Glc-ceramide
CTH Gal(α1→4)Gal(β1→4)Glc-ceramide

Hematoside: Horse: NGNA(α2→3)Gal(β1→4)Glc-ceramide
Dog:
{NGNA(α2→3)Gal(β1→4)Glc-ceramide (27%)
{NANA(α2→3)Gal(β1→4)Glc-ceramide (73%)
Cat: NGNA(α2→8)NGNA(α2→3)Gal(β1→4)Glc-ceramide

Globosides: Pig, Human: GalNAc(β1→3)Gal(α1→4)Gal(β1→4)Glc-ceramide
Guinea pig: GalNAc(β1→4)Gal(β1→4)Glc-ceramide[60]
Rabbit: Galα(1→3)Gal(1→3)GlcNAc(1→3)Gal(1→4)Glc-ceramide[31]

$$\left.\begin{array}{l}\text{Sheep}\\\text{Goat}\end{array}\right\}: \begin{array}{l}\text{GalNAc}(\alpha 1\rightarrow 3)\text{GalNAc}(\beta 1\rightarrow 3)\\\qquad\text{Gal}(\alpha 1\rightarrow 4)\text{Gal}(\beta 1\rightarrow 4)\text{Glc-ceramide}\end{array}$$

QUANTITATIVE DETERMINATION

As previously mentioned, human erythrocytes contain various glycolipids in addition to Globoside I, which accounted for about 70% of the total glycolipid content. Simpler neutral glycolipids were eluted prior to Globoside I by silica gel column chromatography: CMH, CDH and CTH were present. These neutral glycolipids were also usual components in the red cells of other animal species, in the visceral organs such as spleen and kidney and also in the blood plasma.

Recently variations in the amounts of these glycolipids as well as of hematosides on the surface membranes of cultured cells have attracted the interest of many researchers in relation to malignant cell transformation. Thus, a microanalytical method for the quantification of these lipids has become necessary. Vance and Sweeley[32,33] reported a procedure to determine the content of each glycolipid. They extracted lipids from 50 ml of packed red cells and obtained the glycolipid fraction after Unisil column chromatography. The glycolipids were separated by silica gel TLC and the individual glycolipids were scraped off the plate and their carbohydrate contents were determined by GLC after methanolysis and trimethylsilylation with mannitol as an internal standard, as indicated in Table II.

TABLE II. The concentration of the major glycosphingolipids in freshly drawn normal human erythrocytes.[33]

Sample	μ mole/100 ml. erythrocytes			
	(CMH)	(CDH)	(CTH)	(Globoside I)
DV	0.50	1.12	1.42	8.64
JN	0.40	1.30	1.40	8.40
JG	0.38	1.44	1.14	7.50
PS	0.40	1.24	1.06	7.00
JN	0.38	0.98	1.42	6.82
—	0.58	1.23	1.62	6.55
—	0.57	1.39	1.41	6.55
—	0.57	1.39	1.12	6.23
—	0.49	1.77	1.07	6.86
—	0.71	1.47	1.04	5.95
mean	0.50	1.43	1.27	7.05

Eberlein and Gercken[34] reported on the different TLC patterns of various animal red-cell glycolipids. However, the quantitative separation of these glycolipids is rather difficult and the procedure required to prepare the glycolipid samples somewhat tedious, so Ohashi and Yamakawa[35] recently devised a new procedure.

The principle of the method consists of the isolation of oligosaccharides by ozonolysis and alkaline fragmentation according to Wiegandt and Baschang.[36] The oligosaccharide obtained was reduced with sodium borohydride and the material was trimethylsilylated and

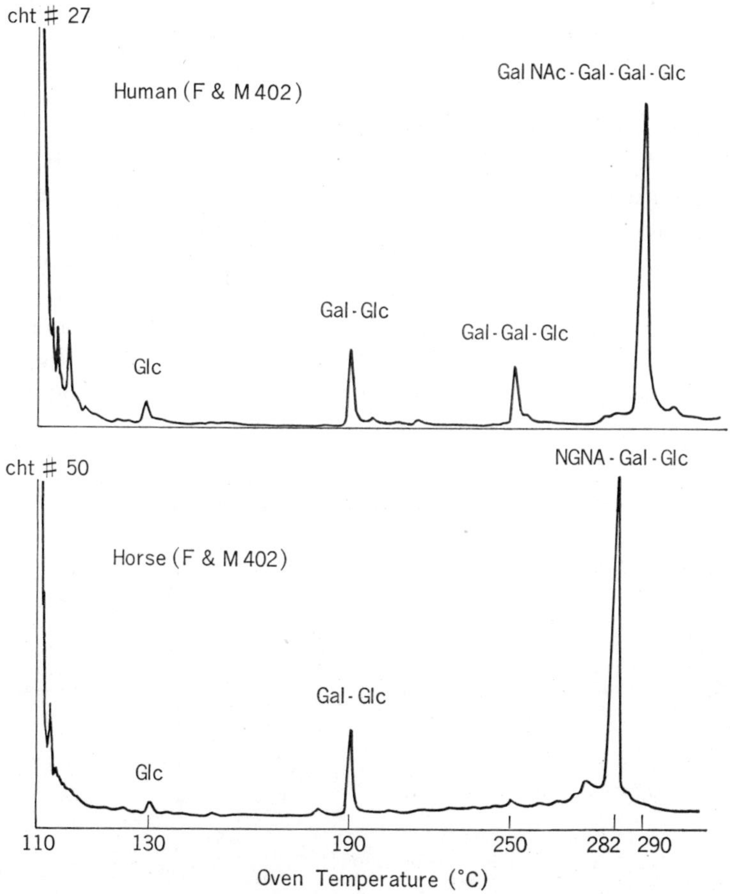

Fig. 3. Gas chromatography of reduced oligosaccharide from glycolipids of human and horse erythrocytes after trimethylsilylation; Column 1% OV-1 on Anakrom SD(3 mm × 30 cm).

applied to a GLC apparatus equipped with a glass column as short as 30 cm in length. In the column, 1% OV-1 on Anakrom SD was packed and the column temperature was programmed from 100° to 350°C at an increment of 10°C per minute. In the gas chromatogram shown in Fig. 3, sugar moieties derived from CMH, CDH, CTH and Globoside I or hematoside were clearly separated in about 30 minutes. The recovery was fairly good. On the other hand, Evans and McCluer[37] recently reported the separation of these glycolipids by high-speed liquid chromatography using benzoylated samples, the amount being determined by ultraviolet absorption, and this may become popular in the future.

IMMUNOLOGICAL PROPERTIES

1) *ABO Blood-Group Antigen*

Since Landsteiner discovered ABO blood groups at the beginning of this century, the materials which determine these specificities had been considered to exist on the blood cell surface. Various attempts had been made to isolate these materials and to determine their chemical structures. There were some papers reporting that extracts of erythrocytes in hot ethanol contained the activity, and the material was heat-stable, giving a positive sugar reaction. In the 1940's, the blood-group substances were isolated in a fairly good yield from body fluids

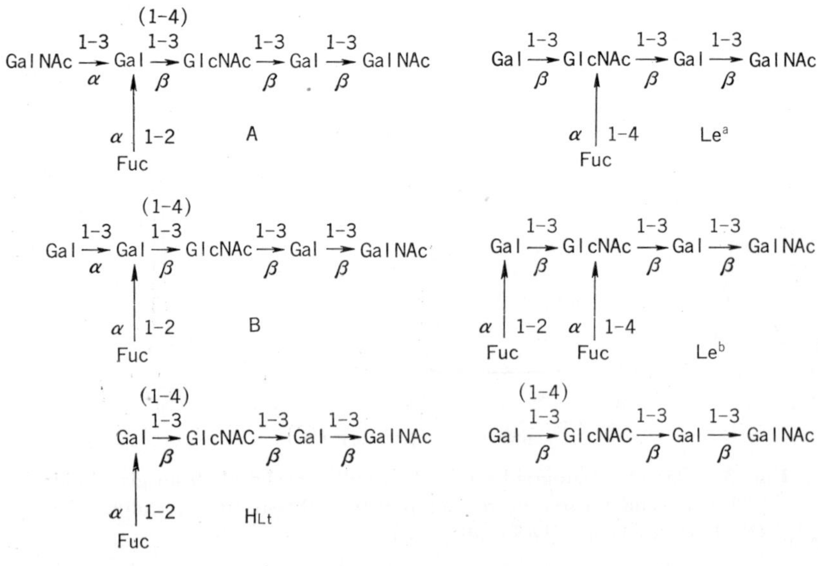

or secretions such as gastric juice, saliva and ovarian cyst fluid, and Morgan in England, Kabat in the U.S.A. and Masamune in Japan began to work on the structures of the antigens which determine the specificity with materials of a mucoid nature. However, it gradually appeared that studying the group substances by using red blood cells was not the best approach. Today, the structures determining each blood-group activity are determined as follows by studying the mucoid substances from body fluids.

ABO antigens from red cells were reported to be carbohydrates by Hallauer in 1934,[38] whereas Hamasato in Masamune's laboratory suggested them to be lipids in 1950.[39] As mentioned previously, Yamakawa and Iida (1953) reported that the globoside of human erythrocytes had the capacity to inhibit the hemagglutination of red cells by its corresponding iso-antibody. Globosides isolated from human A, B, O and AB erythrocytes, respectively, were examined and their group activities were compared with that of the group substance from gastric mucin.[9] However, the materials studied at that time proved to be a mixture, and the active fractions were eluted after Globoside I as minor components by silicic acid chromatography.[10,11] Kabat[40] commented on these results in his monograph "Blood Group Substances", saying that the group substances of erythrocytes were also polysaccharides and suggesting that our glycolipid antigen might contain a small amount of carbohydrate, though there was no positive evidence for this. Following this dispute we prepared immune-specific precipitates by the addition of a potent anti-A agglutinin to aqueous globoside solution. The material recovered from these precipitates with chloroform-methanol, gave an even stronger inhibitory reaction and also showed a typical glycolipid pattern in the infrared absorption spectrum.[41] The results of many workers[42–47] supported our view and today the glycolipid antigen theory is generally accepted. That is to say, group substances contained in the secretory fluids are polysaccharides complexed with peptides and the group antigen on the red cell surface is composed of glycolipid. The chemical structure of the oligosaccharide part of this glycolipid is similar to that of the determinant carbohydrate of group mucoid, both giving a specific antigen-antibody reaction. The presence of antigenic glycolipids on the cell surface is analogous to the fact that the type-specific properties of Gram-negative bacteria are manifested by lipopolysaccharide on the cell wall. It is likely that the coexistence of lipids is necessary for the determinant carbohydrate structure to define the cell-membrane architecture. It is noteworthy that the poly-

TABLE III. Analytical values for Globosides.

	Globoside I	Globoside II	Globoside III
R_f (TLC on Kieselgel G, $CHCl_3$: MeOH : H_2O=60 : 35 : 8)	1	0.81	0.65
Hexose (Anthrone, as galactose	50	38.5	36.7
Glucosamine	0	8.2	5.3
Galactosamine	18	7.4	2.2
Sialic acid	0	2.1	6.1
Fucose : glucose : galactose	0 : 1 : 2	ca. 1 : 2 : 3	ca. 1 : 2 : 4
Isoagglutination inhibition against 4 units antibody	0	1.39 μg	4.4 μg

saccharide-peptide complex containing sialic acid obtained by phenol extraction of thoroughly delipidized blood cell membranes gave MN blood-group activities[48)] and, furthermore, strongly inhibited hemagglutination by influenza virus,[49)] though it had no ABO-group activity at all.

As mentioned above, the group-specific glycolipid was present only in small amounts in blood cells. Handa[47)] analysed this glycolipid after storage for a number of years, and found that the activity of this material remained relatively stable against alkali, and that the antigens recovered from specific precipitates with antibody were also glycolipid, consisting of glucose, galactose, glucosamine, galactosamine, fucose and sialic acid, besides ceramide. Our earlier reports were confirmed by these results. He further showed the immunochemical similarity of this material to mucoid material by a quantitative precipitin reaction, the Ouchterlony technique and immunoelectrophoresis. Yamakawa, Nishimura and Kamimura[12)] named the glycolipids eluted after Globoside I as Globosides II and III (Fig. 1b). Several runs of preparative TLC were carried out on Globoside II until a single spot was obtained. The same procedure was repeated with Globoside III, but the chromatogram continued to show 2 spots. The chemical characteristics of the 3 Globosides are shown in Table III. Purification was not complete at this stage of research, however.

Recently, Hakomori and Strycharz[50)] purified these minor components by silicic acid chromatography after acetylation. The fractions were deacetylated and finally gave a single spot on TLC. The molar ratio of the constituent carbohydrates was determined by GLC. The group A-active fraction or 'Component I' contained glucose, galactose, glucosamine, galactosamine and fucose in a ratio of 1: 2: 1: 1: 1. More

TABLE IV.

	Fuc	Glc	Gal	Glc NAc	Gal NAc	NANA	Sphing-osines
A-30-III	—	1	1.93	1.11	—	—	1.14
A-40-VI	0.82	1	2.24	0.92	0.97	—	
A-Hematoside	—	1	1.13	—	—	1.18	0.98
A-60-III	—	1	2.09	0.83	—	1.13	1.12

recently, Ando and Yamakawa[51)] isolated and purified the minor glycolipids eluted after Globoside I, starting from 1 kg of dry stroma of group A red cells, solely by repeating carefully conducted column chromatography with silicic acid of high quality. So far, at least 4 glycolipids have been obtained in pure state. They were named A-30-III, A-40-VI, A-60-III and hematoside, and the yields were 17.5 mg, 12.4 mg, 42.6 mg and 35.5 mg, respectively, from 10 *l* of packed red cells. The molar ratios of sugar components, as determined by GLC, are listed in Table IV.

Of these glycolipids, only A-40-VI strongly inhibited the hemagglutination of group A red cells by its corresponding antibody, and this probably corresponded to the 'Component I' of Hakomori and Strycharz.[50)] Earlier preparations containing a small amount of sialic acid must be still impure, and the chemical structure of this group-active glycolipid may be as follows;

GalNAc(α1→3)Gal(β1→4)GlcNAc(β1→3)Gal(β1→4)Glc-ceramide
2
↑ α
1
Fuc

The minor glycolipid, A-30-III, which was present to the extent of 2% of Globoside I, proved to have the structure Gal-GlcNAc-Gal-Glc-ceramide, so it may possibly act as a precursor of group-active A-40-VI. The recent finding of Marchesi (1971) that a glycoprotein fraction obtained from erythrocytes by diiodosalicylate treatment is particularly interesting.[52)] Whether the glycoprotein fraction contains the glycolipid antigen, or whether the activity is present in both fractions, will be examined in future.

2) Forssman Hapten

Early in this century, Forssman discovered that the antiserum produced by injecting an emulsion or ethanol extract of guinea pig kidney into rabbit, hemolyzed sheep erythrocytes in the presence of complement. It has been considered that this hemolysis was due to the presence of a common antigen in both kidney and sheep red cells. The antigen was called Forssman antigen (F-antigen) or heterophile antigen. Immunological studies revealed that F-antigen was distributed ubiquitously in some living organisms, and was especially potent in

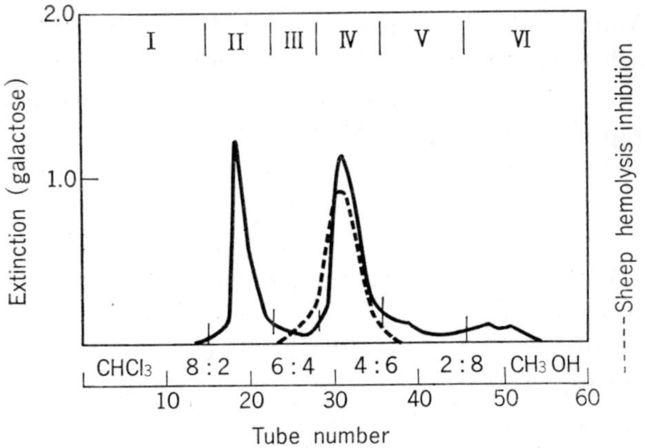

(a)

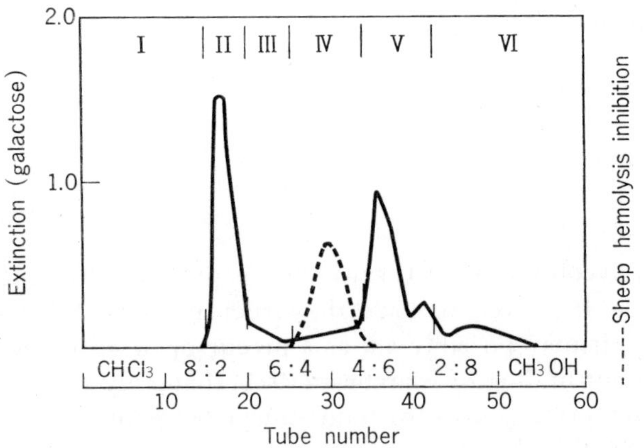

(b)

Fig. 4(a). Silicic acid chromatography of sheep erythrocyte methanol-ether-extracted glycolipid.

(b). Silicic acid chromatography of cat erythrocyte methanol-ether-extracted glycolipid II, ceramide hexoside IV, Forssman-active mucolipid V, hematoside. (disialo)

the red blood cells of sheep, goat and cat, in the visceral organs of guinea pig and horse, and in several microorganisms.

The paper of Brunius (1936) was probably the first to mention that the activity resided in glycolipid, as he reported the F-antigen isolated from horse kidney possessed lipid and also carbohydrate characteristics.[53] However, it was Papirmeister and Mallette[54] in 1955 who pointed out that the F-hapten isolated from sheep blood cells was a glycolipid similar to globoside from human erythrocytes. Makita and Yamakawa[55] observed F-activity in the glycolipid fraction of horse spleen and kidney. Prior to this, Yamakawa, Irie and Iwanaga (1960) found that F-activities were easily and thoroughly extracted from sheep and cat red cells by methanol-ether, whereas ABO activity was partially released by methanol-ether and completely extracted by hot chloroform-methanol from human red cells, indicating that the F-antigen was linked rather loosely to the cell architecture.[11] The F-activities of horse spleen and kidney, and of red blood cells of sheep and cat, were all eluted at the same locus on the chromatogram, and the active materials from various sources were considered to be the same (Fig. 4).

Fraction IV from sheep erythrocytes (Fig. 4) was considered to contain 1 mole of glucose and galactosamine and 2 moles of galactose, besides ceramide, *i.e*, the same as Globoside I from human erythrocytes. The specific rotation in pyridine was, however, $+45°$ which was much more dextrorotatory than Globoside I, $+19°$. As Cheese and Morgan[56] pointed out that the structure of the non-reducing terminal of the F-activity was GalNAc (α1→3)Gal, it was thought that the terminal disaccharide must have that structure. Makita, Suzuki and Yosizawa[57] came to the same conclusion, and proposed the structure, GalNAc (α1→3)Gal(1→4)Gal(1→4)Glc-ceramide, for the F-glycolipid from horse kidney. Abe, Handa and Yamakawa[30] also suggested the presence of a terminal α linkage, as β-N-acetylhexosaminidase from pig epididymis released the terminal hexosamine of Globoside I, but did not act on the F-hapten from horse kidney and sheep red cells.

Furthermore, Ando and Yamakawa[58] isolated an oligosaccharide from sheep F-glycolipid by ozonolysis and separated it into 2 fractions, FHS_1 and FHS_2, by charcoal chromatography. However, their *Rf* values on PPC were identical. The *Rf* value of globo-N-tetraose (GNT), obtained by the same procedure from Globoside I, was slightly higher than those of above 2 fractions. The oligosaccharides were reduced with sodium borohydride and subjected to NMR analysis. The NMR signals of the anomeric proton appeared in general at lower magnetic

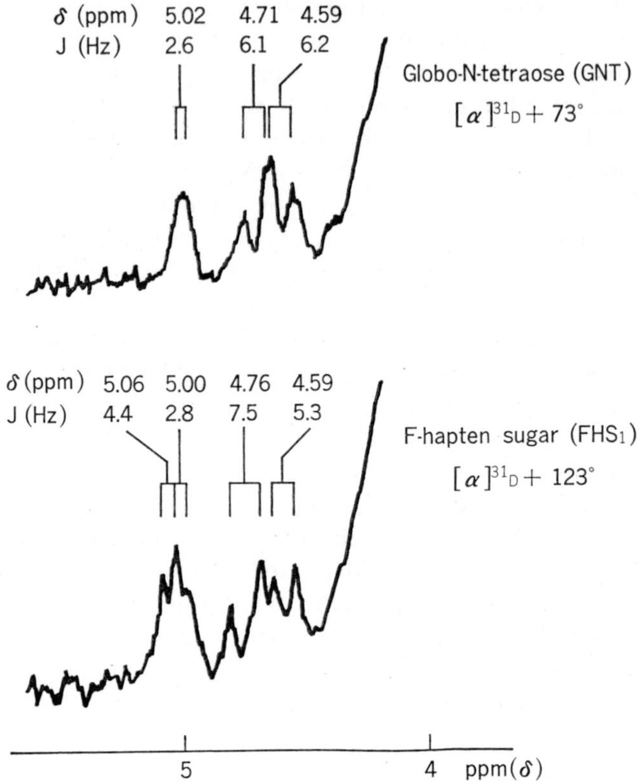

Fig. 5. Proton magnetic resonance spectra of reduced oligosaccharides from Globoside I and Forssman hapten. Determinations were made in heavy water at 100°C and 60 MHz. Assignments in original paper[58] are modified.

field than those of the ring protons, and so can be determined easily even in some quite complex oligosaccharides. In the reduced FHS_1, 2 β-anomeric protons at 4.59 and 4.76 ppm and 2 α-anomeric protons at 5.00 and 5.06 ppm were found. In a similar way, the presence of an α-anomeric proton with a coupling constant of 2.6 Hz at 5.02 ppm was clearly indicated in GNT (Fig. 5). Thus, the presence of an α linkage in both glycolipids was again confirmed.

The *Rf* value of F-glycolipid on TLC was slightly lower than that of Globoside I and this difference had been thought to be due to the different configuration of the terminal N-acetylgalactosaminidic linkage, since both substances were thought to be ceramide tetrasaccharide, with the same sugar sequence at that time.

On the other hand, Siddiqui and Hakomori[59] reported in 1971 that F-active glycolipid from horse spleen was found to be a ceramide pentasaccharide, containing 2 moles of N-acetylgalactosamine, 2 moles of galactose and 1 mole of glucose per ceramide. An α-N-acetylgalactosaminidase from hog liver hydrolyzed the terminal α-N-acetylgalactosaminyl residue with simultaneous loss of F-activity. The resultant compound was identified as Globoside I. Hence, they proposed the structure of F-hapten to be;

$$\mathrm{GalNAc}(\alpha 1\rightarrow 3)\mathrm{GalNAc}(\beta 1\rightarrow 3)\mathrm{Gal}(\alpha 1\rightarrow 4)\mathrm{Gal}(\beta 1\rightarrow 4)\mathrm{Glc\text{-}ceramide}.$$

REFERENCES

1 Yamakawa, T. and Suzuki, S., *J. Biochem.*, **38**, 199 (1951).
2 Klenk, E., *Z. Physiol. Chem.*, **273**, 76 (1942).
3 Klenk, E. and Wolter, H., *Z. Physiol. Chem.*, **291**, 259 (1952).
4 Klenk, E. and Lauenstein, K., *Z. Physiol. Chem.*, **288**, 220 (1951); *Ibid.*, **291**, 249 (1952); *Ibid.*, **295**, 164 (1953).
5 Yamakawa, T. and Suzuki, S., *J. Biochem.*, **39**, 175 (1952).
6 Yamakawa, T. and Suzuki, S., *J. Biochem.*, **40**, 7 (1953).
7 Yamakawa, T., Glycolipids of mammalian red blood cells; 16. Mosbach Coll. d. Ges. Physiol. Chem., ' Lipoide ' ed. by Schütte, E. (Springer, 1966), p. 87.
8 Yamakawa, T. and Iida, T., *Japan. J. Exp. Med.*, **23**, 327 (1953).
9 Yamakawa, T., Matsumoto, M., Suzuki, S. and Iida, T., *J. Biochem.*, **43**, 41 (1956).
10 Yamakawa, T., Ota, R., Ichikawa, Y. and Ozaki, J., *Compt. Rend. Soc. Biol.*, **152**, 1288 (1958).
11 Yamakawa, T., Irie, R. and Iwanaga, M., *J. Biochem.*, **48**, 490 (1960).
12 Yamakawa, T., Nishimura, S. and Kamimura, M., *Japan. J. Exp. Med.*, **35**, 201 (1965).
13 Klenk, E. and Padberg, G., *Z. Physiol. Chem.*, **327**, 249 (1962).
14 Handa, S. and Yamakawa, T., *Japan. J. Exp. Med.*, **34**, 293 (1964).
15 Handa, N. and Handa, S., *Japan. J. Exp. Med.*, **35**, 332 (1965).
16 Yamakawa, T., Yokoyama, S. and Handa, N., *J. Biochem.*, **53**, 28 (1963).
17 Jones, J. K. N., *Bull. Soc. Chim. Biol.*, **42**, 1516 (1960).
18 Kuhn, R., Trischmann, H. and Löw, I., *Angew. Chem.*, **67**, 32 (1955).
19 Yamakawa, T., Kiso, N., Handa, S., Makita, A. and Yokoyama, S., *J. Biochem.*, **52**, 226 (1962).
20 Rapport, M. M., Graf, L. and Yariv, J., *Arch. Biochem.*, **92**, 438 (1961).
21 Makita, A., *J. Biochem.*, **55**, 269 (1964).
22 Rapport, M. M., Graf, L. and Schneider, *Arch. Bioch. Biophys.*, **105**,

431 (1964).
23 Makita, A., Iwanaga, M. and Yamakawa, T., *J. Biochem.*, **55**, 202 (1964).
24 Miyatake, T., Handa, S. and Yamakawa, T., *Japan. J. Exp. Med.*, **38**, 135 (1968).
25 Kint, J. A., *Science*, **167**, 1268 (1970).
26 Handa, S., Ariga, T., Miyatake, T. and Yamakawa, T., *J. Biochem.*, **69**, 625 (1971).
27 Hakomori, S., Siddiqui, B., Li, Y.-T., Li, S.-C. and Hellerqvist, C. G., *J. Biol. Chem.*, **246**, 2271 (1971).
28 Clarke, J. T. R., Wolfe, L. S. and Perlin, A. S., *J. Biol. Chem.*, **246**, 5563 (1971).
29 Kawanami, J., *J. Biochem.*, **62**, 105 (1967).
30a Abe, T., Handa, S. and Yamakawa, T., *Seikagaku*, **39**, 555 (1967); *J. Biochem.*, **70**, 1027 (1971).
30b Hakomori, S. and Saito, T., *Biochemistry*, **8**, 5082 (1969).
30c McCluer, R. H. and Evans, J. E., ' Ganglioside inner esters ' in Sphingolipids, Sphingolipidoses and Allied Disorders, ed. by Volk, B. W. and Aronson, S. M. (Prenum, 1972), p. 95.
31 Eto, T., Ichikawa, Y., Nishimura, K., Ando, S. and Yamakawa, T., *J. Biochem.*, **64**, 205 (1968).
32 Vance, D. E. and Sweeley, C. C., *J. Lipid Res.*, **8**, 621 (1967).
33 Sweeley, C. C. and Dawson, G., Lipids of Erythrocyte in " Red Cell Membrane ", ed. by Jamieson, G. A. and Greenwalt, T. J. (Lippincott Publ., 1969), p. 172.
34 Eberlain, K. and Gercken, G., *J. Chromatogr.*, **61**, 285 (1971).
35 Ohashi, M. and Yamakawa, T., *J. Lipid Res.* (in press) (1973).
36 Wiegandt, H. and Baschang, G., *Z. Naturforsch*, **20**, 164 (1965).
37 Evans, J. E. and McCluer, R. H., *Biochim. Biophys. Acta*, **270**, 565 (1972).
38 Hallauer, C., *Z. Immforsch.*, **83**, 114 (1934).
39 Hamasato, Y., *Tohoku J. Exp. Med.*, **52**, 17, 29, 35 (1950).
40 Kabat, E., Blood-Group Substances (New York, Acad. Press, 1956).
41 Yamakawa, T. and Irie, R., *J. Biochem.*, **48**, 919 (1960).
42 Radin, N. S., *Fed. Proc.*, **16**, 825 (1957).
43 Klenk, E., *Angew. Chem.*, **72**, 482 (1960).
44 Nowotny, A. and Backhausz, E., *Acta Physiol Acad. Sci. Hung.*, **12**, 53 (1957).
45 Hakomori, S. and Jeanloz, R. W., *J. Biol. Chem.*, **236**, 2827 (1961).
46 Koscielak, J., *Biochim. Biophys. Acta*, **78**, 313 (1963).
47 Handa, S., *Japan. J. Exp. Med.*, **33**, 347 (1963).
48 Hohorst, H. J., *Z. Hyg.*, **139**, 561 (1954).
49 Yamakawa, T., Mucosubstances of Mammalian Erythrocyte Stroma in ' Biochemistry and Medicine of Mucopolysaccharides ', ed. by Egami, F. and Oshima, Y. (Maruzen, Tokyo, 1962), p. 136.

50 Hakomori, S. and Strycharz, G. D., *Biochemistry*, **7**, 1279 (1968).
51 Ando, S. and Yamakawa, T., *Seikagaku*, **42**, 412 (1970); *J. Biochem.*, **73**, 387 (1973).
52 Marchesi, V. T. and Andrews, E. P., *Science*, **174**, 1247 (1971).
53 Brunius, F. E., Chemical Studies on the True Forssman Hapten, the Corresponding Antibody and their Interaction (Stockholm, 1936).
54 Papirmeister, B. and Mallette, M. F., *Arch. Biochem. Biophys.*, **57**, 94 (1955).
55 Makita, A. and Yamakawa, T., *J. Biochem.*, **51**, 726 (1962).
56 Cheese, I. A. F. L. and Morgan, W. T. J., *Nature*, **191**, 149 (1961).
57 Makita, A., Suzuki, C. and Yosizawa, Z., *J. Biochem.*, **60**, 502 (1966).
58 Ando, S. and Yamakawa, T., *Chem. Phys. Lipid*, **5**, 91 (1970).
59 Siddiqui, B. and Hakomori, S., *J. Biol. Chem.*, **246**, 5766 (1971).
60 Seyama, Y. and Yamakawa, T., *Proc. Japan. Conf. Biochem. Lipids*, **15**, 61 (1973); *J. Biochem.*, in press.

ATP-Requiring Phenomena in Red-Cell Membranes

M. NAKAO

Department of Biochemistry, Tokyo Medical and Dental University, School of Medicine, Tokyo, Japan

Simultaneous addition of adenine and nucleoside to mature erythrocytes not only maintained the ATP concentration in the erythrocytes, but also restored it within a few hours to the normal level in fresh cells from one-twentieth of this concentration. By this means, the relationship between the ATP level in the erythrocytes and various membrane phenomena was clarified. The shape, surface area, post-tranfusional viability and electromobility depended reversibly on the ATP level in the erythrocytes. On the other hand, osmotic resistance became weak once the ATP level went down.

0.6 *M* NaI or KI solubilized an ATPase from erythrocyte membranes. By treating the residue or intact erythrocyte membranes with 2 *M* NaI, Na^+,K^+-sensitive ATPase was obtained. The former ATPase was quite different from the Na^+,K^+-ATPase with regard to sensitivity to Na^+ and/or K^+ requirements, divalent cation requirement, ouabain sensitivity, pH optimum curve, and nucleotide specificity. The latter ATPase showed almost no activity in the absence of Na^+ and K^+ and various properties of the activity showed that it was a typical transport ATPase, as discovered by Skou. Recent progress in purification of the ATPase from pig brain in our laboratory is briefly summarized in relation to the function of the ATPase in erythrocyte membranes. Newly synthesized macromolecular SH inhibitors are described. They inhibited the active transport of rubidium and Na^+,K^+-ATPase, but not ATPase insensitive to ouabain. Based on these data, the behaviour of the Na^+,K^+-ATPase in situ is discussed.

INTRODUCTION

Matured animal erythrocytes consist of a soluble fraction and the cell membrane. The cell membrane is considered to be a typical cell membrane, electron micrographically less than 100Å thick, with many characteristics of the plasma membrane, although the shape of the cell is characteristic. Recently, extensive studies of lipid composition, etc., have been undertaken,[1)] but nothing was known regarding the molecular basis of the dynamic membrane behaviour before in 1960, when Post described an intimate relationship between the active transport of Na^+

and K^+ across the erythrocyte membranes and the part of ATPase activity which was activated by Na^+ and K^+. Afterwards the membrane was used as materials for studies on physichochemical and chemical properties of membrane proteins. In addition to this simple structure, the metabolism is also simple as described in other chapters of this book. The soluble fraction without organella except the cell membranes, contains only a large amount of hemoglobin and glycolytic enzymes with a few associated enzymes. The simple structure and simple metabolism permit us to clarify the relationship between the structure and the metabolism. The main role of glycolysis in the cell is to supply ATP to various energy-requiring systems. Therefore, the cell is certainly one of the most convenient systems for the elucidation of the physiological significance of ATP in the utilization of energy in the cell.

1) Assumed Pathway of ATP Breakdown in the Cells

The importance of energy metabolism and ATP level for the maintenance of cell integrity was pointed out by Professor Rapoport about 25 years ago, when the ACD solution for blood preservation was developed.[1)] During preservation, the ATP level in the cells gradually fell with a decrease in glycolysis or glycolytic activity. The amount of ADP increased at the initial stage and then decreased, followed by the changes in the amounts of AMP and IMP. A hypothesis regarding the pathway of ATP breakdown during storage is shown in Fig. 1.[2)] Compared with other steps, adenosine deaminase activity is relatively

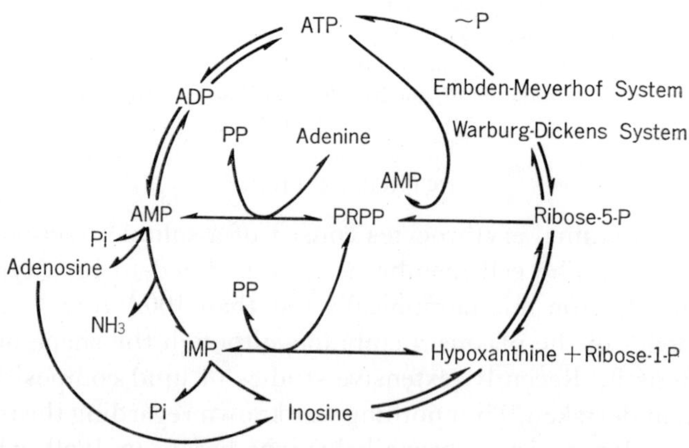

Fig. 1. Assumed pathway of ATP breakdown in preserved erythrocytes.

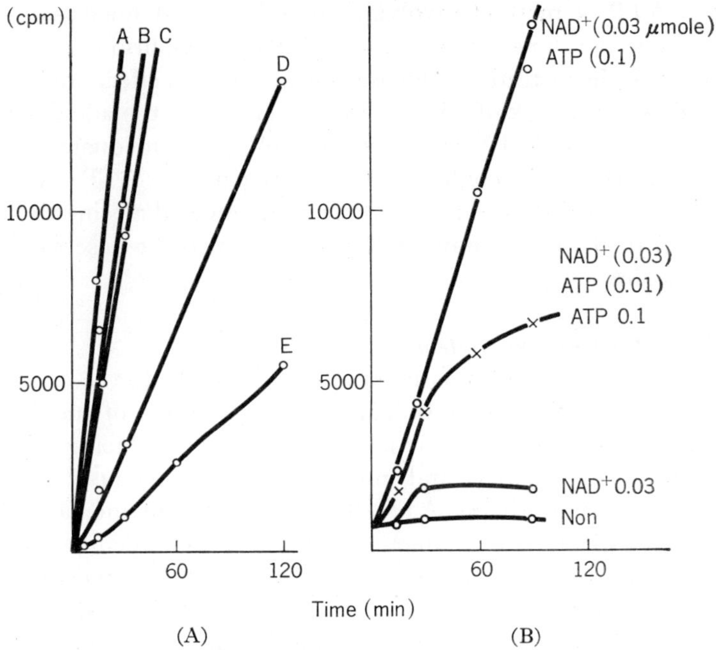

Fig. 2. Existence of a lag period in ATP synthesis in intact red cells (A) and in nucleotide-free hemolysate (B).

Nucleotide-free hemolysate was incubated with C^{14} adenine+inosine in the presence of inorganic phosphate and Mg^{++}. Abscissa shows ^{14}C uptake into ATP.

high in fresh human erythrocytes. The amount of AMP accumulated was relatively small during the whole of the preservation period. Therefore, the deamination step may play a key role in the degradation of ATP. Inosine produced by phosphatase activity was phosphorolyzed to ribose-1-P by a powerful nucleoside phosphorylase and the ribose-1-P was converted to ribose-5-P. With the cooperation of hexose monophosphate and glycolytic systems, the inosine supplied energy to ADP. Thus, ATP is degraded via a cyclic pathway providing some of the energy required to regenerate ATP. The remainder of the inosine is converted to hypoxanthine, which is accumulated in the cell and—may be transferred to other cells *in vivo*, which convert it to uric acid.

It is impossible to introduce preformed nucleotides into the cell directly because the cell membranes are almost impermeable to these phosphate compounds. In order to avoid a kinase step, which requires ATP, a method involving the addition of nucleoside to the medium was developed in a series of papers by Gabrio *et al.*[3–8] They used nucleoside instead of glucose. However, the effect was not sufficient, due to the lack of adenine in the cell. Once the adenine moiety of ATP, ADP and AMP was lost to the cell, the inadequate aminating capacity of the cells could no longer regenerate ATP. Adenosine seemed to be of little use for this purpose, since adenosine deaminase activity in fresh cells is powerful[9] in contrast to the case for inosine and guanosine.

2) *ATP-Regeneration System*

Therefore, adenine plus inosine were added[10] to the cell suspension, with the results shown in Table I. The addition of adenine alone or inosine alone was only partially effective in producing ATP, but the addition of adenine and nucleoside simultaneously was very effective for resynthesizing ATP. The ATP content increased to the normal level within 2 to 3 hours. In this reaction, adenine cannot be replaced by another purine base in nucleic acids, but guanosine, adenosine, deoxyguanosine and deoxyadenosine can be used instead of inosine.[10] The stoichiometry of ATP synthesis in nucleotide-free hemolysate, the action of various inhibitors, and the existence of a lag in the case of erythrocytes stored for a long period, in contrast to fresh cells, led us to propose the following hypothesis for the ATP regeneration mechanism. Nucleoside is rapidly phosphorolyzed by nucleoside phosphorylase, and ribose-1-P is changed into ribose-5-P by ribosephosphate kinase, which is powerful and remains stable

TABLE I. Regeneration of ATP with adenine plus inosine in blood stored for 8 weeks.

	Control	Inosine	Inosine+adenin
AMP	—	—	1.9
IMP	4.7	15	6.8
ADP	—	0.4	7.2
ATP	1.5	2.5	27.4
2, 3-DPG	1.5	74	43.5
HDP fraction	20.5	44	7.0
HMP	8.5	70	35

Incubation: 3 hrs at 37°C. All values are expressed as μmoles/100 ml blood suspension.

during storage. Ribose phosphate reacts with the small amount of ATP remaining in the cell to produce phosphoribose-pyrophosphate (PRPP) which reacts with adenine added externally to produce AMP and inorganic pyrophosphate. AMP, ATP and ADP equilibrate with each other inside the cell, On the other hand, a large amount of ribose-5-P is readily metabolized by way of the hexose monophosphate

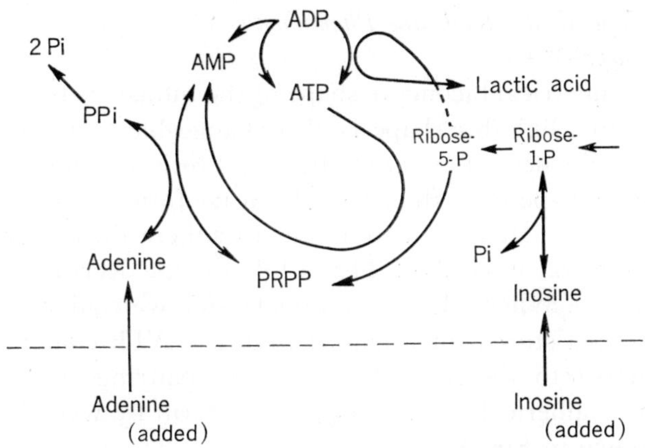

Fig. 3. A positive feedback mechanism for ATP generation in stored blood with the addition of adenine and inosine.

n-Inosine + nPi ⇌ *n* Ribose-1-P + *n* Hypoxanthine
(added) (remaining)

n Ribose-1-P ⇌ *n* Ribose-5-P

Ribose-5-P + ATP ⇌ AMP + PRPP
(remaining)

PRPP + Adenine AMP + PPi
(Added)

PPi ⟶ 2Pi

2ADP + 2ATP ⇌ ADP
(remaining)

4ADP + *m* Ribose-5-P ⟶ 4ATP + X + (Via glycolytic pathway)

Sum: *n*-Inosine + Adenine + 3ATP + qPi
(added) (remaining)(remaining)

⟶ 4ATP + X

pathway and glycolysis to phosphorylate ADP to ATP. Thus the following scheme shows that the more the reaction proceeds, the more the level of substrate increases. This may be a sort of positive-feedback mechanism.[11] The addition of adenine and a nucleoside is a useful method for the investigation of ATP-dependent membrane phenomena, because we can control the ATP level in the cell.

3) ATP-dependent Membrane Phenomena

a) Shape[2,12,13]

The symmetrical biconcave shape of the human red cell is familiar to most people, but this shape is also changeable to almost any form under the influence of external forces. Fresh human erythrocytes changed their shape from the usual biconcave form to a crenated form, and from the crenated form to a smooth sphere during preservation at 4°C for several weeks.[14,2] The ATP content decreased gradually, as shown above. When adenine and nucleoside were added to red cells which had been stored for a long period, the ATP content increased rapidly, almost to the normal level, accompanying their change of shape from a spherical form to a discoidal form by way of a crenated form, as shown in Fig. 4.

When the ATP in fresh cells was depleted by adding deoxyglucose, sodium fluoride or sodium arsenite, the shape of these erythrocytes changed into the crenated form and then the spherical form. If the poison was washed out and adenine and a nucleoside were added to the medium and incubated for 2 hours at 37°C, the shape changed

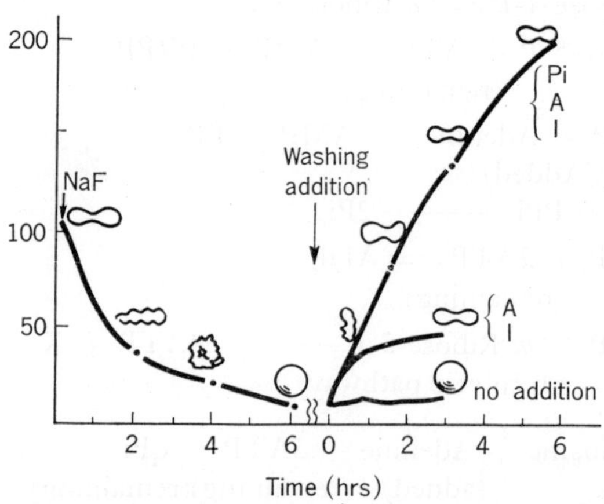

Fig. 4. Reversible shape changes of red cells ATP level depending. . . .

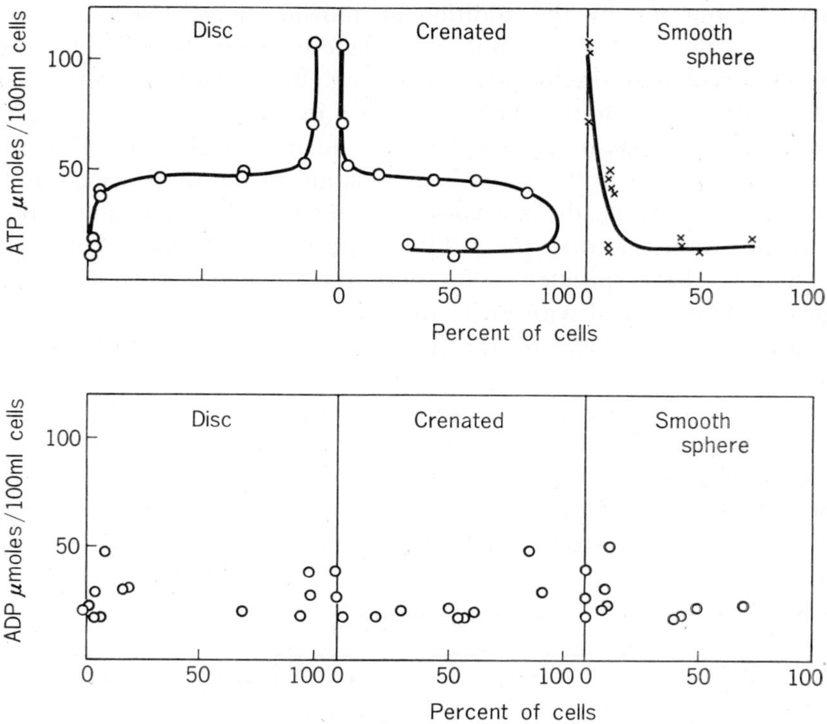

Fig. 5. Relationship between ATP or ADP and the shape of erythrocytes.

back into the disc by way of the crenated form. The disc-sphere transformation is entirely independent of the ionic composition of the medium and the presence or absence of serum proteins. Even in KCl solution, reversible changes occurred.

There seem to be 2 levels of ATP in cells. Above 50% of the normal level, *i.e.*, approximately 50 μmoles/100 ml cells, the shape remained discoid, but below 10% of the normal level, erythrocytes became spherical and between 2 levels they appeared to be crenated.[13]

In Fig. 5, the relationship between the ATP content (abscissa) and the percentage of each of the 3 types (ordinate) is illustrated. This disc-sphere transformation was entirely reversible, depending merely on the ATP level. In regard to the ADP content, no such correlation was observed. Other phosphate compounds did not seem to have any specific relationship to the shape transformation, either. As mentioned above, the sphere-disc transformation of erythrocytes stored for a long period was induced by the addition of adenine and inosine simultaneously, but not by the addition of inosine alone. However, very similar patterns of acid-soluble phosphate compounds were obtained by Dowex-2 anion-exchange resin column chromatography in the case of simultaneous addition of adenine and inosine, and in the case of addition of inosine only, except for the adenine nucleotides. Accordingly, adenine nucleotides have some relation to the transformation.[10] In addition to this, the nucleoside specificity for the transformation was the same as that for ATP generation, and the purine and pyrimidine base specificities for both the transformation and ATP generation coincided with each other. The disc-sphere transformation is reversibly dependent on the ATP content in the cell and may be different from prehemolytic sphering in a hypotonic medium and prehemolytic sphering with some hemolytic reagents. As described below, energy-dependent transformation seems to take place without any volume change. Neither serum albumin and other protein components nor pH have any relation to this phenomenon, because the change occured without any changes in pH or protein components.

TABLE II. Diameter, volume and surface area of red cells.

Red cell	Shape	Diameter μ	Volume μ^3	Surface area μ^2
Fresh	Disc	8.5	87	163 (Ponder)
Stored 8w	Sphere	5.0	65.5	75.5
Stored 8w+(A+1)	Disc	7.8	68.4	138

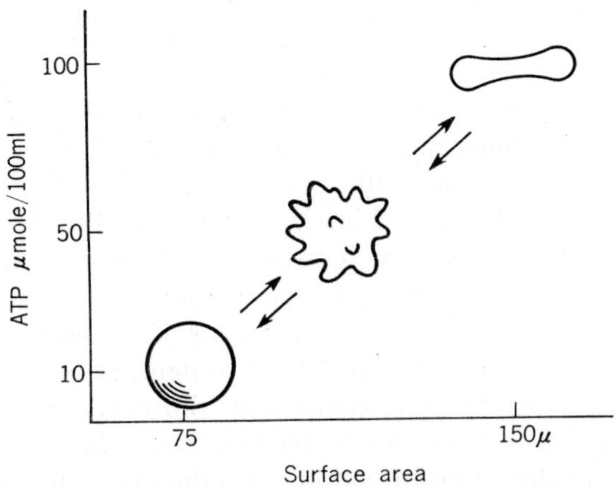

Fig. 6. ATP level and surface area of red cells.

b) *Surface Area*[15)]

Surprisingly enough, the volume of red cells did not change during the ATP-dependent transformation described above. The volume of erythrocytes was measured by 2 methods. One was to determine hematocrit (packed cell volume) and the other was to measure intercellular space with the acid of ^{131}I allumin. The volume of erythrocytes stored for 8 weeks did not change at all after incubation at 37°C for 3 hours with the addition of adenine alone, inosine alone, both adenine and inosine, or with no addition. After incubation of the specimen with adenine and inosine, the erythrocyte changed its shape from spherical to discoid. In contrast, erythrocytes with adenine alone, nucleoside alone, or control solvent only, did not change their shape as described above. This change accompanied the change in the ATP level in the cells. Moreover, the diameter of the erythrocytes was measured directly by microscopic observation and the volume and surface area of the erythrocytes were calculated under appropriate assumptions. Table II and figure 6 indicates that the volume of the cells did not change during the transformation, but the surface area changed remarkably, by about 60–70%. This change in the surface area was also reversible, and depended on the ATP level in the cell. This change might suggest that a part of the surface area which is exposed to the inside or outside of the cell when the membrane spreads, is buried when the surface area becomes smaller with the decrease in the ATP content.

c) *Electrophoretic Mobility and Some Other Properties*

The change in the surface area during the transformation might accompany changes in various properties of the membrane, especially in the outside surface of the membrane. The electrophoretic mobility of the red cells was measured with a Zeiss cell electrophoresis apparatus. Fresh cells showed a mobility of 1 μ/sec/v/cm while the mobility of cells stored for 8 weeks decreased to 0.3 μ/sec/v/cm. After incubation for 1 hour with adenine plus inosine, the mobility increased somewhat in the direction of the original rate. The shape of the red cells changed after incubation as described above. Although the contribution of the shape to the change in cell mobility in an electric field was difficult to estimate, the increase was often too large to be explained only by the transformation of the shape.

Hemolysis time on the addition of various reagents, for example cholic acid, was restored slightly with the increases in ATP in the erythrocytes stored for a long period. The mechanism of action of

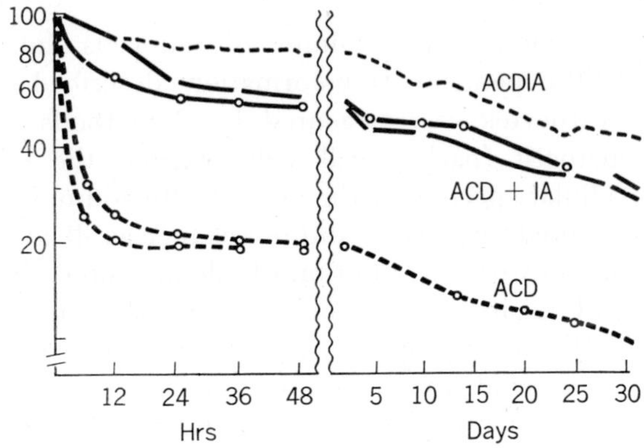

Fig. 7. Post-transfusion viability of erythrocytes stored for 8 weeks. See the legend for Table III.

TABLE III. The same specimen was preserved with ACD (*)(***), ACD +adenine 12.5μmoles per ml+Inosine 25μmoles per ml(**).
After 8 weeks the ACD blood was incubated for three hours with adenine and inosine(***).

Preserved medium	ACD*	ACDIA**	ACD*** (rejuvenated)
ATP μmoles/100 ml cells	5.9	89	77
Osmotic fragility NaCl % at 50% hemolysis	0.61	0.49	0.66
Shape	Sphere	Disc	Disc
Glucose utilization	31	61	51

detergents might not be simple, but this may have some relation to the spreading of the cell surface which accompanied the increase in the ATP content.

d) *Ageing*

The level of ATP and the ATP-generating activity in human red cells decrease gradually during storage. Adenine and inosine were added to erythrocytes stored for 8 weeks, which had an ATP level less than one-twentieth that of fresh cells. After the incubation of the red cells for 3 hours at 37°C, the post-transfusional viability was observed with the cooperation of Prof. Kiku Nakao, using $^{51}CrO_4$.[16] As illustrated in Fig. 7, control ACD red cells which had been stored for 8 weeks were rapidly eliminated from circulation, whereas those which had been previously stored for 8 weeks in ACD medium and then incubated with the addition of adenine and a nucleoside for 3 hours remained in the circulation. The curve, ACD+IA, for these specimens is almost within the normal range for fresh cells.

These data indicated that erythrocytes stored for a long period were rejuvenated when the ATP content was restored to the normal level and glycolytic activity in the intact cells was partially restored. On the other hand, the osmotic fragility of the cells and glycolytic activity in the hemolysate, which was supplied with NAD^+ and ATP, were not restored as shown in Table III. These data lead us to the conclusion that the rejuvenation of red cells aged *in vitro* depended on the ATP level in the cells. Erythrocytes having a low level of ATP were captured by the reticuloendothelial system or by macrophages. The ATP content inside red cells may manifest itself in the membrane ultrastructure, particularly the surface structure, and the signal may be decoded by the surface membrane of the macrophages. The existence of such signals remains to be seen, but the reversible filtrability and electromobility depending on the ATP content in the cells as described above, might suggest that the number of charges, the charge distribution or the ultrastructure of charged groups may be involved in signalling information concerning the age of red cells.

We have dealt with ageing *in vitro* thus far in this paper, but a quite similar process may also be considered for ageing *in vivo*. Some authors suggested that the ATP content decreased also in ageing *in vivo*.[17,18] Therefore, it may be true that the level of ATP is a critical

(a)

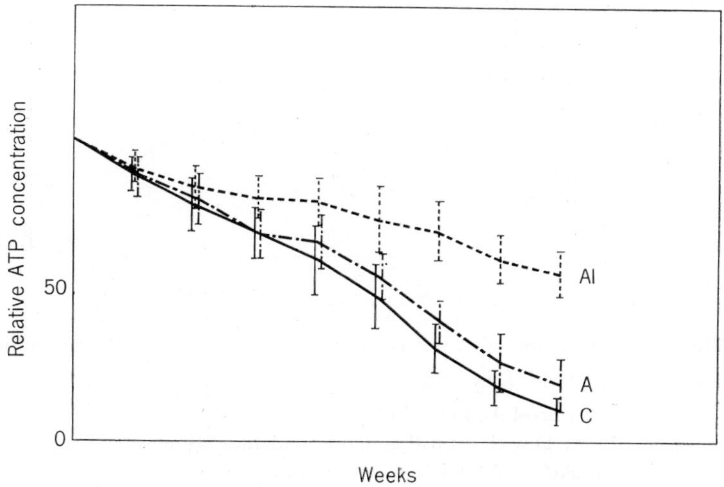

(b)

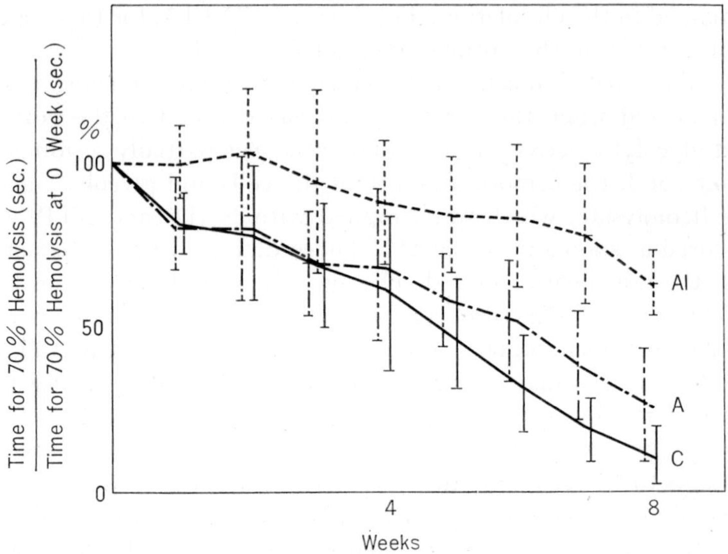

(c)

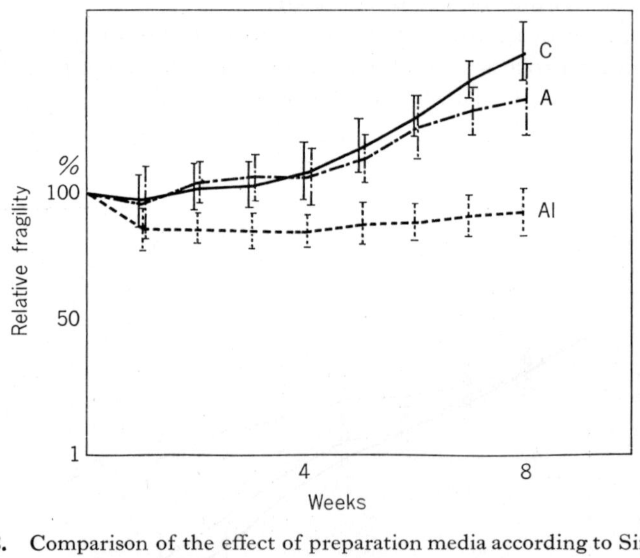

Fig. 8. Comparison of the effect of preparation media according to Simon (A)[19] and Nakao *et al.*[21]

C: Control ACD medium,
A, ACD with a small amount of adenine (Simon[19]),
AI, ACD with adenine and inosine (Nakao[21]).

factor in physiological ageing *in vivo*, even if the mechanism of the decrease of ATP *in vitro* is different from that *in vivo*. The various changes occurring during ageing can be reversed when the ATP level is restored, but there is another kind of ageing process which cannot be reversed by the increase in the ATP level. As mentioned above, the osmotic fragility and the glycolytic activity did not recovered.[16] Specimens of ACD blood were divided into 4 bottles, which contained inosine only, adenine only, inosine plus adenine, or control physiological saline. The amount of adenine and the amounts of adenine and inosine were selected according to Simon *et al.*,[19,20] and Nakao *et al.*,[21-23] respectively. As indicated in Fig. 8, a, b, c, the ATP content was well-maintained even after 8 weeks with adenine plus inosine, and the fragility was also low in contrast to that of the control and the sample with adenine alone. The osmotic fragility increased once the ATP level decreased in the cell and remained constant or became worse after the ATP level was restored by incubation with adenine and inosine at 37°C, as described above. There may be 3 types of ageing processes in the membrane. The first is a process reversibly recovered by restoring the ATP level in the cell. The second is also dependent on the ATP content in the cell, but is irreversible. The third is a process independent of the ATP level in the cells, and including hydrolysis of enzyme proteins and membrane proteins.

e) *Filtrability*

In connection with these ATP-dependent phenomena, the filtrability of erythrocytes was measured. Many years ago, Teitel[24,25] in Rumania described a method for determination of the filtrability, for the first time. According to him, there was no difference filtrability between hereditary spherocytes and normal cells. However, we devised a system which requires only 0.2 ml of red cells in contrast to 2 ml used by Teitel, and found that the filtrability of blood cells preserved for a long period was slow, but accelerated with the increase of ATP following the addition of adenine and a nucleoside. With the addition of adenine alone or inosine alone the rate of filtration did not change. The physiological meaning of this phenomenon is still not clear, but it may mimic the process occurring in the sinus of spleen or elsewhere.

f) *Active Transport of Cations*

The relationship between ATP and the active transport of Na^+ and K^+ is well established.[26] The efflux of 3 moles of Na^+ and the influx of 2 moles of K^+ were coupled with the degradation of 1 mole of ATP.[27] Both movements were inhibited by ouabain. Potassium outside the cell can be replaced by any other monovalent cation. That the rate of potassium uptake depends almost linearly on the ATP content was indicated by results obtained with the ATP-generating system (addition of adenine and inosine) in the range of ATP concentrations from 0.2 to 1.2 μmoles/ml cells.[28] Recently, the low concentration of calcium for example 4×10^{-2} m*M*, inside the cell as compared with the high concentration of blood plasma calcium (5 m*M*) was attributed to active calcium outflux by Schaztmen.[29] Transport is carried out against an electrochemical gradient and with Pi liberation from ATP. The process is highly temperature dependent, with a Q_{10} of 3.5.[30] It is not inhibited by ouabain.[30] As far as human red cells are concerned, there is no concrete evidence for the existence of active transport of substances other than monovalent and divalent cations.

4) ATPases in Red-Cell Membranes

ATP-dependent phenomena in red-cell membranes cover a wide range of subjects, as described above. Generally speaking, the compounds interacting with ATP are proteins. It is evident that some phenomena require not only the existence of ATP in the cells, but also the hydrolysis of ATP. Therefore, ATPases should be investigated first of all. In 1959, Glynn[31] suggested the existence of 2 kinds of ATPase in red-cell membranes from the observation that 10^{-4} *M* calcium suppresses the ouabain-sensitive fraction of ATP hydrolysis, but elevates the ouabain-insensitive fraction. At that time, it was not known whether the Na^+, K^+-ATPase was converted easily into the insensitive ATPase or not. In 1963, T. Nakao *et al.*[32] obtained 2 clearly separated ATPases from human red-cell membranes for the first time. The membranes were treated initially with 0.6 *M* KI. After the supernatant

TABLE IV. ATPases in erythrocyte membranes.

Relative ATPase activity	Cell membranes	0.6*M* KL fraction	2*M* Nal fraction	2*M* Lil fraction
Mg^{2+}				
Ca^{2+}	Activates	Activates		Activates
Mg^{2+}, Na^+, K^+	Activates	Activates	Activates	Activates
Ca^{2+}, (Mg^{2+}, Na^+, K^+)	Inhibits		Inhibits	
Ouabain	Inhibits		Inhibits	
PH optimum		6.8	7.2	
Nucleotide		ATP	ATD	XTP
Specificity		UTP	CTP	XDP

was diluted with 20 times its volume of water, a precipitate was obtained. The precipitate showed ATPase activity. It required Mg^{2+} or Ca^{2+} and in the presence of Mg^{2+}, and the addition of Ca^{2+} activated it further. In addition to this, Na^+ or K^+ slightly accelerated the hydrolysis, at most by 10 to 20% in the presence of Mg^{2+}, but the addition of both Na^+ and K^+ did not stimulate the activity any further. It seems that the stimulating effect of monovalent cations is nonspecific. This enzyme was not inhibited by ouabain, and can split GTP and UTP in addition to ATP. It is evidently distinct from the Na^+, K^+-ATPase.

The residue of the 0.6 *M* KI extract or the original membrane was treated with a very high concentration of NaI, for example 2 *M*. The suspension was diluted to 0.8 *M* NaI and a precipitate was obtained. The precipitate showed very slight ATPase activity in the presence of Mg^{2+} only. The addition of both Na^+ and K^+ increased the activity over 20 times and this fraction was inhibited completely by ouabain. The nucleoside specificity was restricted to ATP and CTP among the nucleoside triphosphates. The purification of the latter enzyme has been attempted in many laboratories, using other tissues, for example brain, kidney, etc., but none of the preparations seem to be pure. Recently we have succeeded in obtaining a highly purified enzyme from pig brain. The specific activity of the best preparation liberated 7,000μmoles Pi/mg protein/hr. Since the specific activity of red-cell membranes is usually 1 or less μmole Pi/mg/hr, the density of Na^+, K^+-ATPase on the surface of red cells may be very low. The number of pumps calculated from ouabain binding on the assumption that 1 ouabain molecule is bound to one molecule of the enzyme is about 250 according to Hoffman.[33] This assumption may be sound on the basis of presently available information.

5) *The Third ATPase*

The red-cell membranes were treated with 2 *M* LiI, as in the case of NaI treatment. The precipitate showed an ATPase activity which required divalent cations, but was inhibited by monovalent cations. The optimum was on the alkaline side. The nucleotide specificity was different from those of the 2 enzymes described above. Whether the enzyme is an artifact obtained from either of the above 2 enzymes or not is not known. To summarize the above description, there are 2 or more ATPases in the red-cell membranes, and the problem of which ATPase corresponds to which function is still obscure, except that Na^+, K^+ATPase is involved in the active transport of Na^+ and K^+, and Ca^{2+} ATPase in Ca^{2+} transport. Since the characteristics of the 0.6 *M* KI-ATPase are not specific, the preparation may still contain several other ATPases. One of them may be calcium-transport ATPase. The shape change accompanying the change in the surface area also seems to occur after change in the external pH or on the addition of chelating agents when ghosts are used instead of intact cells, and it occurs even at low temperatures. Whether the temperature dependence is quantitative or not is still unknown, and whether the other ATP-dependent phenomena require the splitting of ATP or not is also unclear at present. ATPase activities of membranes from cases of hereditary spherocytosis were measured. The Na^+, K^+-ATPase activity increased slightly and the ouabain-insensitive ATPase activity decreased markedly compared with those in normal erythrocytes. This fact might suggest a role for one of the insensitive ATPases in the maintenance of the shape of erythrocytes.

6) The Characteristics of Membrane ATPases in Situ

In order to clarify the mechanism of these ATP-dependent phenomena, the characteristics of membrane ATPases in the intact membrane should be studied. Kinetic data on these phenomena have been extensively complied. However, the physicochemical behavior of the enzyme molecules has not been directly observed yet. We tried to modify the enzyme from one side of the cell membrane, *i.e.*, a sort of polar modificafion. An ideal reagent for this purpose should be a large macromolecular reagent which cannot penetrate the cell membrane.

p-Mercury benzoic acid (PCMB) and p-mercury benzene sulfonate

TABLE V. Distribution of radioisotopes between hemolysate and membranes after incubation of red cells with ^{14}C, ^{203}Hg dextran-acetoxymercurianiline (M. W. 70,000).

	$1.8\times10^{-5}M$ ^{14}C dextran-acetoxymercuri-aniline (dextran : ^{14}C : Hg, 1 : 3.3 : 3)	1.3×10^{-5} ^{203}Hg dextran-acetoxymercuri-aniline (dextran : Hg, 1 : 11.3)
Red cells	15%	19%
Membranes	8.6	6.5
Supernant of hemolysate		
Non hemoglobin	2.4	5.2
Hemoglobin	4.9	7.8

Incubation 37° 54 minutes (J. Matsumoto and M. Nakao).

can cross the membrane rather easily. A large amount of benzimidazolyl-methylmaleiimide, which was kindly donated by Prof. Kanaoka of Hokkaido University, was found in the cell after short-term incubation. Fluorescein mercury was also found in the cell in large amounts when it was added to the medium. It inhibited both Na^+, K^+-ATPase and ouabain-insensitive ATPase activities when the membrane ATPases were tested after hemolysis. A larger mercury derivative of bromophenolphthalein sulfonate, which has 4 bromine atoms and 2 sulfonic acid moieties was newly synthesized, but it was also found in the supernatant of the cell hemolysate, after incubating it with intact red cells. Thus a reagent which has a molecular weight of over 1,000 can penetrate the cell membrane relatively easily. Next, the macromolecule dextran, which has an average molecular weight of 70,000, was newly modified. Acetoxymercurianiline was bound to the dextran by means of bromocyanide treatment. The compound was relatively stable at room temperature. The Na^+, K^+-ATPase and ouabain-insensitive ATPase activities in the ghosts were inhibited 50% at concentrations of roughly 10^{-6} *M*. If it was added to intact cells, both ATPase activities were strongly inhibited at 6.5×10^{-7} *M*. Using ^{203}Hg mercury aniline or ^{14}C mercurianiline, the distribution of radioactivity was measured after incubation of the intact cells for 45 minutes. As shown

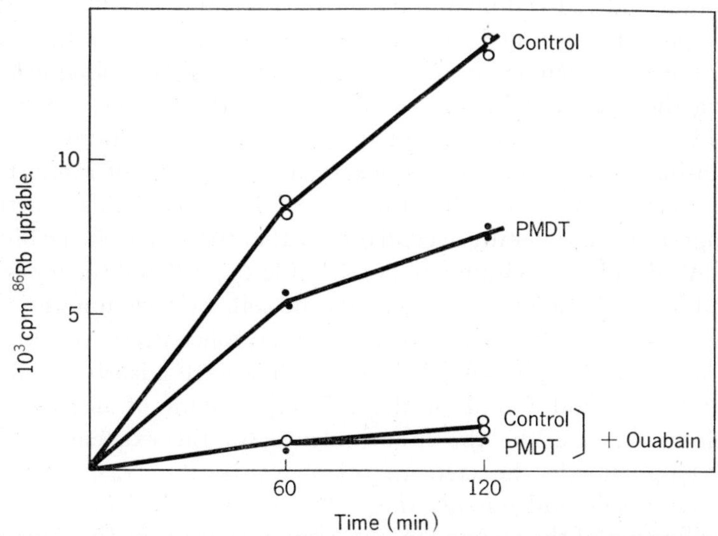

Fig. 9. Inhibition of Rb uptable by a macromolecular Hg compound into erythrocytes.

in Table V, about 10% of the added radioactivity was observed in the red cells.[34]

About one-half or one-third of the radioactivity was recovered in the ghost fraction and the rest was in the supernatant. Though the specific radioactivity per mg protein was far less in the supernatant than in the ghosts, the relatively large amount of radioisotope in the supernatant suggested that the derivative could pass through the cell membranes and was bound to hemoglobin or other soluble proteins. When the compound was added to intact cells, both the Na^+, K^+-ATPase and the ouabain-insensitive ATPase were inhibited, too. The result is easily explicable if the compound penetrates the cell membrane and attacks these ATPases from inside the cell. Finally we synthesized a p-mercuribenzoic acid derivative of a dextran having an average molecular weight of 250,000.[35] The dextran (T 250 Pharmacy) was reacted aminoethylsulfate in strong alkali and the aminoethyldextran obtained was bound to p-amino mercuribenzoate with DCC in DMSO or water soluble DCC.

The stability of the mercury compound was determined using gel chromatography. Usually 10 to 20 mercury atoms were bound per dextran molecule. The compound inhibited the ouabain-sensitive fraction of ^{86}Rb uptake in intact red cells but the ouabain-insensitive fraction was not affected. The compound inhibited Na^+, K^+-ATPase from brain and red-cell membranes with a Ki value of 10^{-7} *M*. When the compound was added to a red-cell suspension and incubated for 30 minutes, the behaviour of the membrane ATPase obtained after washing the cells was different from that mentioned above. The Na^+, K^+-ATPase was strongly inhibited, but almost no inhibition of the ouabain-insensitive fraction was observed. The extent of inhibition of active transport agreed well with that of Na^+, K^+-ATPase activity. Although it is the generally accepted view that the active site or binding site of ATP and the sodium site faces inside the cell and the potassium site and ouabain site may exist outside the cell, we have found no conclusive evidence for this. K^+ is small, and high concentrations of ouabain could affect the Na^+, K^+-ATPase, since they were adsorbed from the small intestine and found in the cell supernatant of heart muscle. Therefore, this may be the first evidence for the existence of Na^+, K^+-ATPase outside the cell. In other words, the Na^+, K^+ATPase faces both inside and outside the cell membrane. Recent progress in the purification of the enzyme in our laboratory leads us to assume that Na^+, K^+-ATPase has only 1 large subunit having a molecular weight of 100,000, although the existence of smaller subunits arround 10,000 or 20,000 has not been ruled out, and it is very interesting that a relatively small peptide might face both inside and outside the cell. The peptide or protein is not an enzyme bound to the cell membrane, but an essential part of the membrane constitution (structure). On the other hand, ouabain-insensitive ATPase has an active site inside the cell, but no reactive group was detected outside the cell in the present experiments. Therefore, we cannot tell whether the ouabain-insensitive ATPase can face both sides or not. Reversible inhibitors might be transferred from a site outside the membrane to other sites during hemolysis. Accordingly, an irreversible inhibitor was also used. An iodacetamide derivative-aminoethyl dextran having an average molecular weight of 250,000 was synthesized in a similar way to the PCMB aminoethyl dextran. The resulting inhibitory effects on the ATPase activities and on active transport were essentially the same as those with the mercury compound.

The technique of polar modification will be a useful tool for observation of the location and behaviour not only of various enzymes in cell membranes, but also of various proteins in cell membranes.

We are continuing studies to clarify the roles of all the enzymes and proteins in the red-cell membranes and the molecular mechanisms of their functions by means of the above lines of investigation.

REFERENCES

1 Rapoport, S., *J. Clin. Inv.*, **591**, 616, 629 (1947).
2 Nakao, M., Tatibana, M. and Yoshikawa, H., *J. Biochem.*, **48**, 672 (1960).
3 Gabrio, B. W. and Finch, C. A., *J. Clin. Inv.*, **33**, 242 (1954).
4 Gabrio, B. W., Stvens, A. R., Jr. and Finch, C. A., *J. Clin. Inv.*, **33**, 247 (1957).
5 Gabrio, B. W., Stvens, A. R., Jr. and Finch, C. A., *J. Clin. Inv.*, **33**, 252 (1957).
6 Gabrio, B. W., Hennesessey, M., Thomasson, J. and Finch, C. A., *J. Biol. Chem.*, **215**, 1509 (1958).
7 Gabrio, B. W., Donohue, D. M., Hunnekens, F. M. and Finch, C. A., *J. Clin. Inv.*, **34**, 1509 (1955).
8 Gabrio, B. W., Donohue, D. M., Hunnekens, F. M. and Finch, C. A., *J. Clin. Inv.*, **25**, 657 (1956).
9 Conway, E. J. and Cooke, R. B., *Biochem. J.*, **33**, 457, 479 (1939).
10 Nakao, M., Nakao, T., Tatibana, M. and Yoshikawa, H., *J. Biochem.*,

47, 661 (1960).
11 Nakao, M., Motegi, T., Nakao, T., Yamazoe, S. and Yoshikawa, H., *Nature*, **191**, 284 (1961).
12 Nakao, M., Nakao, T. and Yamazoe, S., *Nature*, **187**, 954 (1960).
13 Nakao, M., Nakao, T., Yamazoe, S. and Yoshikawa, H., *J. Biochem.*, **49**, 487 (1961).
14 Nakao, M., Nakao, T., Tatibana, M., Yoshikawa, H. and Abe, T., *Biochem. Biophys. Acta*, **32**, 564 (1959).
15 Nakao, M., Nakao, T., Nagano, K., Odaka, T., Adachi, K. and Misugi, K., Proceedings of the 1st International Symposium for Cellular Chemistry, 521 (1965).
16 Nakao, K., Wada, T., Kameyama, T., Nakao, M. and Nagano, K., *Nature*, **194**, 877 (1962).
17 Bernstein, R. E., *J. Clin. Inv.*, **38**, 1576 (1959).
18 Löhr, G. W. and Waller, H. D., *Klin. Wochenens.*, **37**, 833 (1959).
19 Simon, E. R., Chapman, P. G. and Finch, C. A., *J. Clin. Inv.*, **41**, 351 (1962).
20 Simon, E. R., *J. Clin. Inv.*, **41**, 351 (1962).
21 Nakao, M., Ozaki, T., Nagano, K. and Nakao, T., Proc. Intern. Congress of Blood Transfusion (1966).
22 Waka, T., Tanaka, H., Nakao, K., Nako, M. and Yoshikawa, Y., *Proc. Japan Acad.*, **36**, 619 (1960).
23 Nakao, M., Nakao, T., Arimatsu, Y. and Yoshikawa, H., *Proc. Japan Acad.*, **36**, 43 (1960).
24 Teitle, P. P., *Nature*, **206**, 409 (1965).
25 Teitle, P. P., *Neuv. Rev. Franç. d'Hématol.*, **7**, 195 (1967).
26 Post, R. L., Merrit, C. R., Kinsolving, C. R. and Albright, C. D., *J. Biol. Chem.*, **235**, 1796 (1960).
27 Post, R. L., Albright, C. D. and Dayani, K., *J. Gen. Physiol.*, **50**, 1201 (1967).
28 Tatibana, M., Shmamune, A., Nakao, M., Ishii, Y., Hashimoto, T. and Yoshikawa, H., *Folia Haematogyca*, **79**, 470 (1962).
29 Schatzmann, H. J. and Vincenzi, F. F., *J. Physiol.*, **201**, 369 (1969).
30 Lee, K. S. and Shin, B. C., *J. Gen. Physiol.*, **54**, 713 (1969).
31 Glynn, L. M., *J. Physiol.*, **136**, 148 (1957).
32 Nakao, T., Nagano, K., Adachi, K. and Nakao, M., *Biochem. Biophys. Res. Comm.*, **13**, 444 (1963).
33 Hoffman, J. F., *J. Gen. Physiol.*, **54**, 343 (1969).
34 Nakao, M., Nagao, T., Matsumoto, J., Ohta, H. and Nagano, K., VI Internationals Symposium uber Struktur und Funktion uber. Erythrocyten (1970), p. 547, Akademie Verlag. Berlin (1972).
35 Ohta, H., Matsumoto, J., Nagano, K., Fujita, M. and Nakao, M., *Biochem. Biophys. Res. Comm.*, **42**, 1127 (1971).

Glycolysis of the Erythrocyte

G. Jacobasch,* S. Minakami** and S. M. Rapoport*

** Institute of Physiological and Biological Chemistry, Humboldt University, Berlin, GDR, ** Department of Biochemistry, Faculty of Medicine, Kyushu University, Fukuoka, Japan*

Glycolysis of the red cell is regulated by a multistep mechanism, in which HK, PFK, and PK are the control points. The overall flux of glycolysis is determined by HK and PFK, with HK contributing a larger share to the limitation of the flux. They constitute together a common control unit, which reacts to signals such as pH and inorganic P. Most of the signals act on PFK, which represents the chief sensor and master switch of glycolysis. The glycolytic rate increases whenever the HK-PFK system is released from inhibition by positive effectors. The PK reaction, on the other hand, does not limit the glycolytic rate. Rather, it provides a coordinated control of the upper and lower sections of the glycolytic chain. All other steps of the main pathway of glycolysis are equilibrium reactions. Their reversibility provides a type of "buffering" of the glycolytic system. GAPD is not a controlling enzyme either. The ratio $NAD^+/NADH$ is strongly influenced by PFK and PK. Thereby the concentration of the intermediates in the middle section of glycolysis, those above and below GAPD, may vary.

Under steady-state conditions, all of the enzymes of glycolysis work at a low fraction of their capacity. However, the flux may be influenced by external signals. In addition to those mentioned above, pO_2, the lactate/pyruvate ratio of the blood plasma and the body temperature are of importance. Furthermore, the concentration of Mg^{2+} and NH_4^+ may be of significance. The interrelations between the flow of substrates through the upper control unit and the metabolite concentrations set by the degree of control of PK determine the distribution of the flux between the main pathway and the diphosphoglycerate bypass.

INTRODUCTION

Glycolysis is perhaps the best-elucidated metabolic pathway. A large number of the early discoveries relating to its intermediate steps were made on the red cell. In the next period, that of identification and purification of enzymes, studies turned to richer sources such as yeast and muscle. In the present period, the main interest is focused on the clarification of the interplay of the constituent reactions of a metabolic pathway. For this purpose the red cell offers unique advantages, due to the simplicity of its structure and function, whereby the interference of other metabolic interrelations are largely eliminated.[1] Despite its simplicity, the erythrocyte exhibits sufficient variability both in phylogeny and ontogenetic development, to offer deep insights from comparative studies.[2] Further information may be gained from intensive studies of genetic defects. The clarification of the metabolic consequences of mutant enzymes with lowered stability or decreased catalytic efficiency leads to a better understanding of the mechanism of the anemias caused by them, as well as of the glycolytic mechanism. In connection with the elucidation of the mechanism of regulation of glycolysis, it became necessary to isolate the participant enzymes from red cells, since their kinetic parameters differ from those obtained from the sources mentioned previously. Furthermore, there is now a good chance of establishing a mathematical model to describe the over all process of glycolysis.

Even before the elucidation of the mechanism of glycolysis, studies were performed to define the pH optimum and temperature dependence of glycolysis. An optimum pH of 8.2–8.5 and a temperature quotient of two were found.[3–5] Species differences became apparent, with the sequence pig∠beef∠goat∠dog∠horse∠guinea pig∠man∠rabbit∠rat, with a range from less than 0.5, to 2.7 mmoles of glucose consumed per ml cells per hr at pH 7.4 and 37°C.[6] The enzyme activities and the concentrations of various intermediates of glycolysis also vary by more than one order of magnitude.[7] The present review will deal mostly with the red cells of man, with some reference to other species, mostly rat and dog. Within the glycolytic chain the maximal activities of the different enzymes vary by more than 3 orders of magnitude (Fig. 1). The enzymes with the highest activity include PHI, TIM, GAPD and LDH, while aldolase, HK and 2,3-DPGase exhibit the lowest capacities. Although one cannot judge directly from the maximal activity the actual rate of an enzymatic reaction, there exists a fair correlation between the capacities of a number of enzymes, particularly HK, PFK, PK, DPGM and LDH and the glycolytic rates of different species. Most of these enzymes catalyze irreversible reactions of glycolysis.

The actual activity of any enzyme in the glycolytic chain is determined by the concentration of one or more substrates, which means that all of them work under conditions below saturation. It is further influenced by products and various effectors. The controlled reactions,

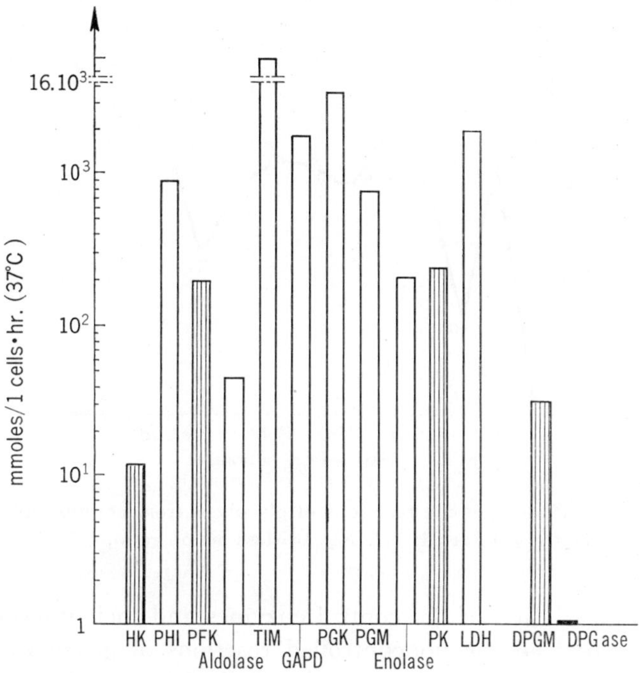

Fig. 1. Capacities of the glycolysis enzymes of the human erythrocyte. The shaded columns indicate enzymes which are not in thermodynamic equilibrium.

catalyzed by the three kinases of glycolysis, namely HK, PFK and PK, are characterized by being far from thermodynamic equilibrium, and being highly sensitive to the influence of effectors.[8] Two of them, PFK and PK strongly exhibit allosteric properties, showing positive cooperativity. Thus both the stability of the glycolytic rate in the flat portion of their substrate activity curves and a steep rise beyond a threshold are provided for, which may be of biological significance. The uncontrolled reactions are near equilibrium. It may be assumed that similar regularities hold for a wide range of biological systems. Reactions which are controlled and those which are not, may be recognized from an analysis of the relationships between the metabolites (Fig. 2). Those which exhibit mass action ratios far from thermodynamic equilibrium under steady-state conditions may be effector-controlled. The presence of three irreversible reactions indicates multistep regulation of the glycolytic flux. It is an interesting problem to define the

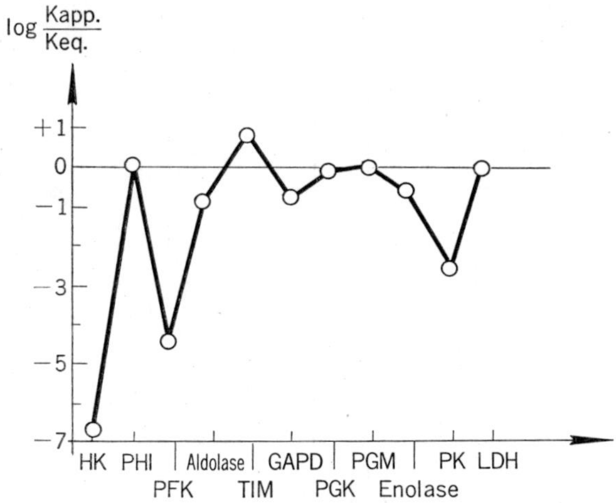

Fig. 2. Deviations of the reactions of glycolysis from equilibrium in the human erythrocyte at pH 7.2. K_{app}=Mass-action ratio.

contribution of each of the control enzymes and their interplay. It is of interest that all the noncontrolled reactions of glycolysis are mediated by enzymes of large capacity and that there exist shuttles between them. This arrangement may provide a type of kinetic "buffering" of glycolysis.

Erythrocyte glycolysis has been considered by a number of symposia, the proceedings of which contain both surveys of various aspects and a wealth of detailed data.[9–14] An overall survey was published in 1968.[15] The present survey is limited to those parts of glycolysis which are of significance for its regulation. Owing to the close connections between GAPD and LDH, mediated by the NAD^+/NADH system, they are discussed together.

1) Hexokinase

Among the enzymes of glycolysis, HK has the lowest capacity. It is characterized by a pH optimum of 8.1–8.3. The activity declines rapidly on the alkaline side of the optimum while the curve slopes gently in the acid range.[16] In the mature red cell of man there may exist three isoenzymes, one of which, type I, accounts for more than 90% of the total activity. Type II occurs only in traces, possibly related to the presence of HbF.[17,18] The enzyme activity declines by about one order of magnitude during maturation of the reticulocytes. The immature cell of rabbits also contains a high-K_M HK, the properties of which are like those of glucokinase of liver and kidney. It is not inhibited by glucose-6-P.[19] In some animal species, particularly the dog, there is a decline of HK activity during the first year of life.[20] This may be connected with the change from high-K_M to low-K_M, cells.

Among the red cells of different species, the HK concentration varies over a 10-fold range. There is a remarkably close correlation between HK content and glycolytic rate, with a ratio of HK/glycolysis of about 4.5 at the pH optimum (or when measured at pH 8.2).[7,15] The dissociation constant of the glucose complex of the enzyme is about 0.05 mM,[147] so that the enzyme in most cells is saturated with glucose. The dissociation constant of the complex with $MgATP^{2-}$, the true substrate of the enzyme, is about 1.6 mM, which is in the range of cellular concentrations. Glucose-6-P[21] and glucose-1,6-P[147] inhibit the enzyme competitive to $MgATP^{2-}$ to an equal degree with a dissociation constant of 0.07 mM. The enzyme is also inhibited by 2,3-DPG again competitive to $MgATP^{2-}$ with a K_i of 2.7 mM.[147] On the other hand, uncomplexed ATP does not appear to inhibit the enzyme. The inhibition by MgADP is under most conditions not important. The activity of HK in the cell is regulated predominantly by the ratio of $MgATP^{2-}$/glucose-6-P. Therefore there is also a close correlation between glycolytic rate and the ATP/glucose-6-P ratio, provided that the Mg^{2+} concentration is constant. Changes of Mg^{2+}, ATP, glucose-6-P or 2,3-DPG will affect the activity of HK in the cell. In some studies it was proposed that high concentrations of P_i activate HK.[22] This effect is not observed in purified preparations and is caused in crude systems probably by release of inhibition of PFK, whereby the glucose-6-P concentration is reduced.[23] Recently, a direct effect of low concentrations of P_i on the type I isoenzyme has been reported in a preliminary communication.[24] Halfmaximal activation is supposed to occur at a P_i concentration of 0.3 mM. At saturating concentrations of P_i the K_i of glucose-6-P is reportedly raised from 2.5 to 25 μM in a noncompetitive manner.

The enzyme has so far not been isolated from red cells. From kinetic studies a random-order mechanism has been established.

2) *Phosphofructokinase*

Dische found in 1935 the first indications for the existence of an enzyme catalyzing the formation of fructose-1, 6-diP from fructose-6-P and ATP.[25] Since it was realized that PFK is a decisive control point of glycolysis, several groups have been engaged in studies to clarify the complicated kinetics of this enzyme. These studies indicate that enzymes from various sources differ to some extent, but always exhibit the properties of allosteric enzymes. So far it has not been possible to establish a satisfactory kinetic model for a mammalian PFK. The maximal activities differ among erythrocytes of different species by more than one order of magnitude.[7] The lowest values are shown by the 2,3-DPG-deficient erythrocytes of deer, sheep and goats with 25–27 μmoles of substrate transformed per ml cells per hour at 37°C. The highest values are found in rat erythrocytes with 500 μmoles per ml cells per hour. In contrast to HK there is no clear-cut correlation between glycolytic rate and PFK activity among different species. The greatest deviations are seen in erythrocytes of the dog, with an unexpectedly high activity of PFK on the one hand and the above 2,3-DPG-deficient erythrocytes on the other.[7,15]

The PFK activity exhibits a distinct decline with maturation, with an additional molecular form in the reticulocyte.[26,34] The enzyme has been purified from the erythrocytes of man, rat and rabbit.[27–29] The highest specific activity determined amounted to 136 IU, comparable to that of pure muscle PFK. The enzyme appears to be a tetramer of molecular weight 420,000, but active aggregates of higher molecular weight are also present.[30] By analogy with the muscle enzyme, it is assumed that the protomer, which is not active, consists of 4 similar but not identical peptide chains.[31] One or two of these may carry the active centers, and others may bind effectors. This assumption corresponds to the results of binding studies[32] on muscle PFK, in which three binding sites for ATP were found, one of which was exchangeable for AMP, 3′,5′-AMP or ADP. In many respects the enzymes of muscle and erythrocytes are similar, but there exist definite differences with regard, to their electrophoretic, immunological and kinetic behaviour.[27,28,33]

There exist a number of kinetic studies of PFK under conditions which are far from those existing in the cell. Mostly the enzyme was studied in systems containing NH_4^+ ions, which significantly affect its allosteric properties.[33] To obtain data which are meaningful for intracellular conditions it is essential to carry out studies in K^+ systems in concentrations of the level obtaining in the cell. Subsequent statements refer exclusively to data in K^+ systems.

The function of the substrates of PFK, which are at the same time effectors which mutually interact in a reciprocal manner, is an

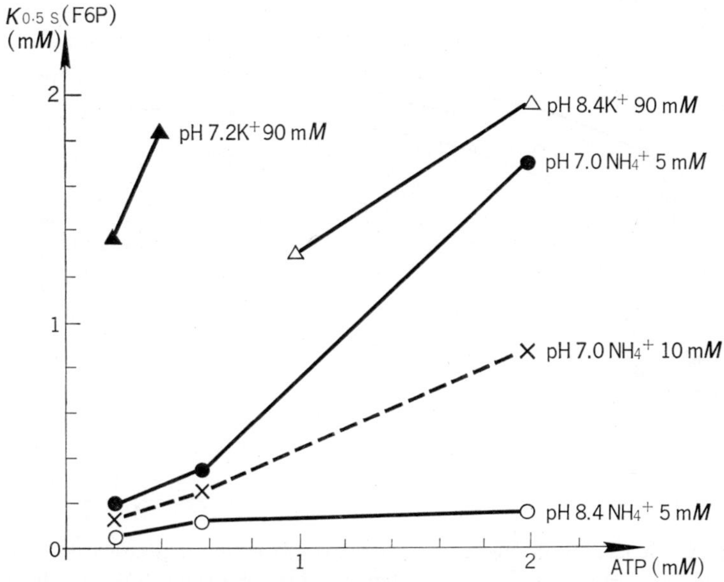

Fig. 3. The influence of ATP, NH_4^+, K^+ and pH on the $K_{0.5\,S}$ values of erythrocyte PFK for fructose-6-P.

essential feature of the regulation of enzyme activity. One of the substrates is $MgATP^{2-}$, the affinity of PFK for which is much greater than that of HK. The affinity is slightly diminished by an increase in the fructose-6-P concentration. From a secondary plot ($1/K_M$ vs. fructose-6-P) one may estimate the $K_{M(ATP)}$ to be 0.1 mM. ATP is at the same time a strong inhibitor, which diminishes the affinity of the enzyme for fructose-6-P. Thus there is a shift to the right of the sigmoidal fructose-6-P substrate activity curve. On the other hand, the other substrate fructose-6-P will release the ATP inhibition, acting as a positive effector. The erythrocyte enzyme appears to be more sensitive to ATP inhibition than the muscle enzyme.[28,33] The ATP inhibition is strongly pH-dependent, the enzyme at pH 7.2 being 10 times more sensitive than at pH 8.4 (Fig. 3). The steepest change of affinity for fructose-6-P is at about pH 7.[27,33] It may been surmised that imidazole groups play a role, an assumption in keeping with the effect of photo-oxidation on the muscle enzyme, following which imidazole groups are destroyed and both the inhibitory effect of ATP and the sigmoidicity of the fructose-6-P substrate curve disappear. The pH optimum of erythrocyte PFK is at 8.4, and the slope towards the acid side depends

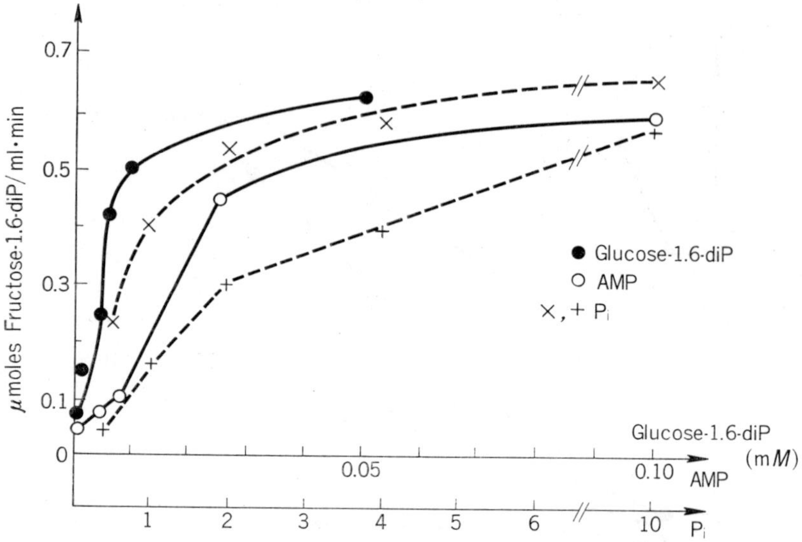

Fig. 4. Release of inhibition of erythrocyte PFK by the positive effectors glucose-1,6-diP, AMP and P_i. The P_i effect is demonstrated both in the KCl (+) and in the NH_4Cl (×) systems. All measurements were carried out at pH 7.2 and 37°C in the presence of 0.5 mM fructose-6-P and 1.25 mM $MgCl_2$. The effects of glucose-1,6-diP and of AMP were tested in the presence of 0.4 mM ATP, that of P_i with 0.2 mM ATP.

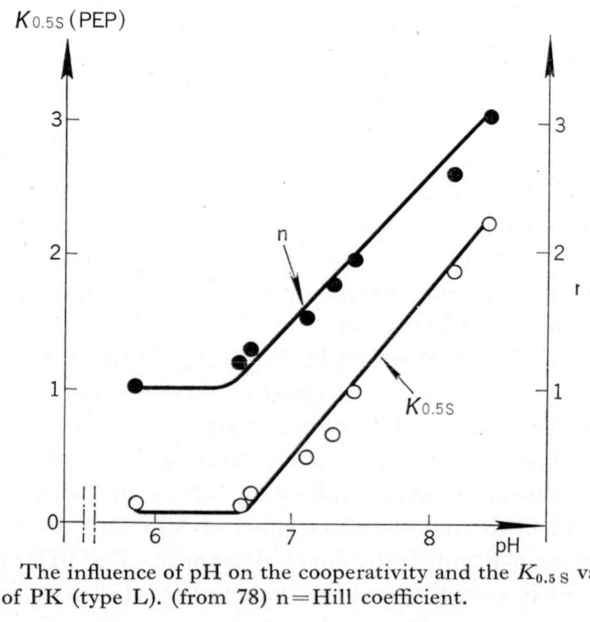

Fig. 5. The influence of pH on the cooperativity and the $K_{0.5\,S}$ values for PEP of PK (type L). (from 78) n=Hill coefficient.

on the ATP concentration.[27] For an understanding of the role of the PFK in the control of glycolysis it is of interest to estimate the extent of the inhibition exerted by ATP at cellular fructose-6-P concentrations. From a secondary plot it may be deduced that in human blood PFK is inhibited 50% at an ATP concentration of 0.015 mM. At the normal ATP concentration of 1.5 mM the enzyme would work only at 0.1% of its capacity, *i.e.*, at one-tenth of the glycolytic rate. This signifies that the physiological activity of the PFK is almost entirely determined by the action of positive effectors which release the ATP inhibition. These are, in the red cell, glucose-1,6-diP, AMP, ADP, fructose-1,6-diP, glucose-6-P and P_i (Fig. 4).[34]

This type of regulation means that the concept of Atkinson on the regulating role of the phosphorylating potential while useful as a heuristic principle, does not apply in detail, since the most effective positive effectors do not take part in the phosphorylation equilibrium.[35]

A particularly powerful positive effector is glucose-1,6-diP the concentration of which in the human cell is about 0.1 mM.[36] In some particularly ATP-sensitive preparations of PFK a 4-fold activation of the enzyme could be achieved by 0.006 mM glucose-1,6-diP. AMP is also a strong effector; levels of 0.02 mM will cause a pronounced activation both at pH 7.2 and at pH 8.4. Maximal activation is observed at concentrations of 0.1–0.2 mM, concentrations which may occur *in vivo*. The activating effect is more pronounced the more the enzyme is inhibited by ATP. ADP is a less effective activator, the action of which can only be demonstrated at alkaline pH values. A more important effect is exerted by inorganic phosphate (Fig. 5). It releases the inhibition by ATP, probably by competing with it at the inhibitory site. The effect of P_i is noticeable at physiological concentrations; its activation constant is 1.6 mM.[148] It was found recently that sulfate ions act identical manner.[149] In a similar manner, but more weakly, glucose-6-P acts by competitively releasing the ATP inhibition. Finally an activation by fructose-1,6-diP which amounts to 40% at concentrations of 0.05–0.1 mM is probably also of physiological significance.[34]

There may also be additional negative effects exerted by multivalent anions, in the first place by 2,3-DPG. For the reticulocyte, citrate has also to be considered.[27,28,37] The PFK of erythrocytes appears to be less sensitive to citrate inhibition than that of muscle. The extent of the citrate effect is strongly dependent on both ATP and fructose-6-P and it increases with rising ATP and decreasing fructose-6-P levels. Similar behaviour but to a less marked extent is exhibited by 2,3-DPG. The low 2,3-DPG level of some species correlates with their low PFK capacity and may explain why the ratio PFK/glycolytic rate is lower in them than in 2,3-DPG-rich erythrocytes. The extent of this effect is, however, limited by the small concentrations of ADP and AMP available.

Cations also play and important role in the activity of PFK, in particular Mg^{2+}, K^+ and NH_4^+. Mg^{2+} exerts primarily an indirect effect by affecting the amount of $MgATP^{2-}$ and of ATP species containing less or no magnesium. This is of significance since free ATP exerts a much stronger inhibition than $MgATP^{2-}$.[38]

Both K^+ and NH_4^+ are cofactors of PFK, with K^+ of course being the physiological factor. The apparent activation constant amounts to about 10 m*M* for K^+ but only 1 m*M* for NH_4^+.[148] The affinity of PFK for NH_4^+ is about 6 times greater than for K^+. The enzyme also exhibits differences in its allosteric behaviour with the two cations. In the K^+ system the Hill coefficient is 3.0 at pH 7.2 and 1.5 at 8.4. NH_4^+ will weaken the cooperativity, so that in the alkaline range, Michaelis kinetics result, with a $K_{0.5S}$ for fructose-6-P which is lower by an order of magnitude (Fig. 3). Correspondingly, the ATP inhibition is 10 times higher in the K^+ as compared with the NH_4^+ system. The specific effect of NH_4^+ consists not only in the weakening of ATP inhibition, since it is still present if ITP, which is not inhibitory, is used as a substrate.[33,34] Addition of NH_4^+ will increase glycolysis by about 40% at pH 7.2–7.4.[39,40] Above pH 8.0, no effect is observed in human erythrocytes, possibly because the breakdown of adenine nucleotides liberates sufficient NH_4^+ to exert a maximal effect. Even at pH 7.4, the steady-state level of NH_4^+, at 0.24 m*M* for human erythrocytes, is in the effective range.[41,137] In reticulocytes it is higher, particularly

TABLE I. Apparent kinetic constants for human GAPD under approximate cellular conditions.[71] The values are expressed in μM. Conditions: pH 7.2, 0.15 *M* KCl, 37°.

Substrate	K'_M	K'_i
NAD^+	50	—
GAP	5	—
P_i	3,900*	—
1,3-DPG	3.5	0.22 (competitive to GAP)
NADH	8.3	0.45 (competitive to NAD^+)

* determined at 10 μM GAP, 50 μM NAD^+.

under anaerobic conditions and may therefore contribute to the Pasteur effect by releasing the inhibition of PFK by ATP. From an analysis of metabolites, it becomes evident that the NH_4^+ effect results in all cases in a reduced inhibition of PFK, resulting in lower fructose-6-P and higher fructose-1,6-diP levels. It is demonstrable even in the presence of high P_i concentrations. The NH_4^+ effect is more pronounced in the K^+-deficient erythrocytes of the dog,[42] in which PFK is working far below the maximally effective K^+ level.[43]

3) Glyceraldehyde-3-phosphate Dehydrogenase

Glyceraldehyde-3-phosphate dehydrogenase catalyzes the following reaction in either direction

$$\text{GAP} + \text{P}_i + \text{NAD}^+ = \text{1,3DPG} + \text{NADH} + \text{H}^+$$

The enzymes from muscle and yeast are among the best understood. However, GAPD has also been purified and crystallized from red cells in several laboratories.[44–46] The enzymes exhibit a fairly steep optimum between pH 8.5 and 8.8. The enzymes from all sources have the same molecular weight (144,000) and four identical subunits.[50,52] Although there have been some indications of differences between the enzymes from red cells, muscle, and liver,[46–51] most evidence indicates that the enzymes are identical. Comparative studies on enzyme preparations from muscle, liver and erythrocytes of man and rabbit carried out with electrophoretic, immunologica and peptide analytic methods failed to show any differences among the organs of any one species. One may conclude therefore that the GAPD is coded by a single gene. Differences among species in the primary structure are also relatively few and so are the variations in the kinetic behaviour. In table I are summarized data on the kinetic constants of the GAPD of man under approximately cellular conditions. There are very similar to those of rabbit enzyme.[150] The constants are strongly interdepended and are furthermore markdly influenced by pH, ionic strength and temperature. It should be mentioned that the values obtained with arsenate instead of phosphate are not applicable for the cell. GAPD is one of the most active enzymes of glycolysis, with a maximal activity of 3,000 μmoles substrate/ml cells hr at pH 7.2 and 37°C in the forward reaction. This is about 150 times the capacity of HK. There are some species differences of about one order of magnitude, apparently related to the 2,3-DPG content. During maturation from the reticulocyte stage, the activity decreases to about one-third.

4) Lactate Dehydrogenase

In all cells with glycolysis, LDH exhibits a high rate of activity. This also holds true for erythrocytes. Its capacity in the human red cell amounts to 2,000 μmoles substrate/per ml cells hr at 37°C. There are some species differences, which again appear related to the amount of organic phosphate compounds. Particularly low values, about one-tenth as high as in the human erythrocyte, are found in species with low 2,3-DPG levels. There is a great variety in the distribution of isoenzymes, without any perceptible correlation to any feature of metabolism. In the human red cell, all isoenzymes have a distribution similar to that in heart muscle, with 44% H_4, 39% H_3M, 14% H_2M_2, 2% HM_3 and less than 1% M_4.[53] In the red cells of rats and rabbits there is, in contrast, only H_4 despite an equal total activity. There is also one isoenzyme in the red cells of sheep, goats, cats and cattle, which have lower LDH capacities. In reticulocytes of rabbits the activity of LDH is about 3 times higher than in erythrocytes, but with the appearance of only a minor amount of an additional isoenzyme.[54]

The pH optimum of the enzyme lies at pH 8.5. The kinetic differences among the various enzyme species are of no regulatory importance and will therfore not be discussed. One should mention that the enzyme reacts not only with NAD^+ but also with $NADP^+$, with about one-sixth the molecular activity and with a pH optimum of 6.0. The biological significance of this reaction is doubtful.[54]

5) The Nicotinamide Adenine Dinucleotide⁺/Reduced Nicotinamide Adenine Dinucleotide Ratio

One of the most important characteristics of glycolysis, but also one of the most contradictory, is the NAD^+/NADH ratio. The value for NAD^+ in human erythrocytes is given by most authors as 0.04–0.09 m*M*/1, and about 4 times as high for rabbit erythrocytes.[55–60] The major discrepancies refer to the values for NADH. They vary for human erythrocytes between 0.055 and 0.002 m*M*. The reasons for the divergences lie in methodical difficulties in determining NADH. Its concentration is very small, while there are sources of large positive errors. The most important ones are the oxidant action of hemoglobin and the incomplete alkaline destruction of NAD^+. A recent study, in which the possible sources of error were eliminated as carefully as possible yielded values of NADH of less than 0.002 m*M* both in human blood as drawn and in cell suspensions at pH 7.2. Thus a ratio of NAD^+/NADH of about 40 results.[61,62] Nevertheless even this value is beset with uncertainties, since the binding of NADH to enzymes and hemoglobin, which certainly would lower the value for free NADH, could not be adequately considered. It would appear that the tenet of Klingenberg, Bücher, Minakami and Krebs, that all pyridine nucleotide-dependent reactions of the cytosol are near equilibrium, is valid for the red cell.[63–65] Therefore one may take the pyruvate/lactate ratio as a basis for the calculated "true" $NAD^+/NADH$ ratio. These values of the $NAD^+/NADH$ ratio differ considerably from those determined experimentally. For human blood the ratio is calculated to be about 1,000, with an NADH concentration of less than 8×10^{-5} mM, which is about 5% of the lowest experimental value.

The lactate/pyruvate ratio of approximately 5 and correspondingly the $NAD^+/NADH$ ratio of flowing blood in the resting state of the body, as established by the activity of the respiring tissues does not correspond to the value found under approximate steady-state conditions *in vitro*. As soon as a blood sample is isolated, the ratios shift in the direction of lower potential due to the production of NADH by the GAPD reaction. With decreasing $NAD^+/NADH$ ratio there is an accumulation of GAP, as may be expected from the equilibrium of the GAPD reaction. Similarly one finds with an increase of the pH, a rather slow further diminution of the $NAD^+/NADH$ ratio with a greater accumulation of GAP. As soon as an oxidant, pyruvate or methylene blue, is added, an increased $NAD^+/NADH$ ratio with a rapid decline of GAP results.

6) *Phosphoglycerate Kinase*

Phosphoglycerate kinase represents the first ATP-generating reaction of the glycolytic chain. The enzyme capacity is very high in the red cells of all mammals, with a maximal value for the forward reaction of 4,700 μmoles per 1 cells per hr at 37°C. The enzyme has been isolated from human red cells.[66–69] There are probably no differences in its kinetic properties compared with the thoroughly studied enzymes from muscle. The enzyme is highly specific for 1,3-PG, for which it has a high affinity, while the adenine nucleotide may be replaced by its inosine analog. A comparison of the metabolite levels with the K_M values indicates that all reactants are in a substrate-sensitive concentration range (Table II). It has been demonstrated that the extent of the reaction is determined by the concentrations of 1,3-DPG and $MgADP^-$. The value of $MgADP^-$ is estimated to be 0.4 times that of ADP. MgADP exerts an activation at a concentration

TABLE II. Kinetic constants for PGK, DPGM and 2,3 DPGase from erythrocytes. (expressed in μM).

Enzyme	Substrate	K_M 37°C	K_i 37°C
PGK	1,3-DPG	2	
pH 7.2	MgADP	100 (12*)	
	Mg2,3-DPG		4,200 (non-comp. to 1,3-DPG)
	$MgATP^{2-}$: mixed inhib.		
	to MgADP		1,870
	to 1,3-DPG		450

* determined at a free Mg^{2+} of 0.85 mM above 100 μM MgADP.

above 100 μM whereby the K_M for it is lowered. Presumably there exist two binding sites. Furthermore Mg^{2+} at high unphysiological concentrations also activate the enzyme. The mass-action ratio of the reactants is near the equlibrium value and a shuttle across this enzyme perhaps up to 15-fold the overall glycolytic rate may be assumed. Even under extreme conditions, such as afterloading with inosine and phosphate, followed by the addition of an oxidant, whereby the flow through GAPD and PGK is increased manyfold there is no noticeable deviation from equlibrium.[70] $MgATP^{2-}$ and MgDPG exert an inhibitory effect in concentrations, which are in the range of the cellular concentration.

7) *Pyruvate Kinase*

This enzyme catalyses the second ATP-generating reaction of glycolysis. It has been studied extensively since it was discovered that mutations of this enzyme are the cause of inherited nonspherocytic hemolytic anemias (see the chapter by Waller), which are frequent in people of middle- and northern-European descent.[72]

In human erythrocytes the capacity of the enzyme amounts to a rate of 235 μmoles of PEP per ml cell per hr at 37°C. There is a paralellism between the glycolytic rate and enzyme activity among different species, except for those with low 2,3-DPG, which have particularly high PK activities. Three types of isoenzymes occur, type I (L) being predominant in liver, type II (LM) in kidney and type III (M) in muscle, but also in brain and leucocytes. The enzyme in erythrocytes is entirely type I.[73] Nevertheless, three molecular forms of the enzyme can be found, which are distinguishible by high-voltage electrophoresis or gelelectrofocusing.[74–76] Two of the three forms may represent conformers, which are interconvertible. They differ in their binding properties with respect to fructose-1,6-diP. In reticulocytes, an additional highly active enzyme species is found, which has not been characterized so far.[77]

PK is similar in some of its kinetic properties to PFK. Both enzymes are inhibited by ATP, in a manner competitive to the non-nucleotide substrate. ATP favors the formation of molecular form one, which has allosteric properties that express themselves in the sigmoidal shape of the activity curve as a function of PEP concentration.[78] The $K_{0.5S}$ for PEP is found to be 0.2 mM. In the presence of low concentrations of fructose-1,6-diP the enzyme is transformed into form two, which does not exhibit cooperative properties, so that the substrate-activity curve for PEP is hyperbolic. The affinity for PEP, but also for MgADP increases severalfold, so that the activity under nonsaturating conditions such as exist in the cell rises to a proportional extent. This form also has a high affinity for potassium. The transition of form one to form two may correspond to that from the R to the T form according to the model of Monod, Wyman and Changeux[79] for allosteric enzymes. Hydrogen ions influence the kinetic behaviour of PK in the same direction as PFK, *i.e.*, both ATP inhibition and the sigmoidicity of the PEP saturation curve decline with increasing pH.[78]

A further metabolite of possible physiological significance is 2,3-DPG, which inhibits PK.[37,80,81] It may be estimated that, in the cell, even minor changes of the concentration of $MgATP^{2-}$, $MgADP^{-}$, PEP, or pH may influence the activity of PK. The most important variable in the cells appears to be MgADP.

THE DIPHOSPHOGLYCERATE BYPASS

There are two bypasses in the glycolytic chain of the erythrocyte: one crossroad is located at glucose-6-P, from which the OPP pathway branches off, and the other is at 1,3-PG. Both bypasses return through their products GAP and fructose-6-P, and 3-PG, respectively, to the main pathway of glycolysis. The diphosphoglycerate bypass includes only two enzymes, DPGM and 2,3-DPGase, both of which catalyze irreversible reactions. It is characterized by the accumulation of the intermediate 2,3-DPG in high amounts in the erythrocytes of some mammalian species.

Despite a multitude of different types of studies there is as yet no complete understanding of the importance of the high concentration of 2,3-DPG in the red cell. Earlier studies demonstrated large changes in concentration of this compound as a function of variations of the pH and of the phosphate concentration of the plasma.[82,83] Decreases were found in various types of acidosis and changes in both directions in parallel with deviations of the plasma phosphate. It was assumed that 2,3-DPG in the red cell reflects the state of the phosphate supply of the body and may serve as a phosphate reserve. Furthermore it plays a role in the Donnan equilibrium between the red cell and plasma and thereby contributes to the stability of the intracellular milieu by keeping both pH and volume changes in the cell at a minimum. Other authors assumed that 2,3-DPG plays a role in potassium transport, possibly by way of 2,3-DPGase or by binding to deoxy-Hb.[84,85] Another suggestion has been that, by means of an increased flow to 2,3-DPG, more NADH may be gained for the reduction of Met-Hb.[86] The conception of 2,3-DPG as a modifier of the function of Hb has gained the widest interest and support.[14,87] So far as the immediate role of 2,3-DPG in glycolysis is concerned, it is recognized as a ubiquitous cofactor for PGM in all animal systems[88] and it is an inhibitor of kinase reactions.[37,80,81] Both of the enzymes of the 2,3-DPG bypass have been isolated from erythrocytes and kinetically characterized.

1) Diphosphoglycerate Mutase

This enzyme catalyzes the transfer of phosphate from its anhydride to an ester form in a bimolecular reaction, with 3-PG as phosphate acceptor.[14,89–92] The maximal activity in human erythrocytes is 240–390 μmoles per 1 cells per hr at 37°C.[24,91] The enzyme has a high affinity both for its substrate, its cosubstrates 3-PG and 2-PG, and its product 2,3-DPG, which exerts competitive inhibition against (Table II) 1,3-DPG. The relations among the metabolites under physiological conditions, with 2,3-DPG levels about 10,000 times as high as 1,3-DPG, indicate that the enzyme works normally at an extremely low percentage of its capacity. Nevertheless one may produce experimental conditions of greatly increased 1,3-DPG concentration under which sizeable rates, exceeding 10 μmoles per 1 cells per hr[14,70,72,92] of 2,3-DPG are formed. A normally functioning mechanism consists of the binding of 2,3-DPG by deoxy-Hb, whereby the product inhibition is decreased. Thus one finds anaerobically up to 40% higher 2,3-DPG concentrations than those occurring in aerobic conditions.[87,93]

2) 2,3-Diphosphoglycerate Phosphatase

This enzymes has the lowest capacity of any connected with glycolysis in the red cell.[17,94–97] It amounts to only 0.06 μmoles per cell per hr at 37°C. It may be activated manyfold by a number of anions. Phosphate and chloride in physiological concentrations increase the rate about 15-fold to 0.84 μmoles per hr. Sixty μM phosphoglycolate, which may occur in the red cell,[98] may stimulate the enzyme 1,500 times (Table II). The activations by bisulfite, sulfite, dithionite and other anions are probably without biological significance.[99] The activators primarily influence the affinity of the enzyme for its substrate. This may be the reason for the more than 1,000-fold variation of the $K_{0.5S}$ values reported. Similarly divergent are the values for the K_i of 3-PG. If one applies the constants of the isolated enzyme to intracellular conditions, the high ratio of 2,3-DPG/3PG would indicate that the enzyme works always at its maximal activity without 3PG inhibition. On the other hand there are indirect indications of possible significance are the inhibitions exerted by PEP and ATP in the phosphoglycolate activated system. 2,3-DPG breakdown by PGM has to be considred as being of possibly equal importance as the reaction catalyzed by the specific 2,3-DPGase.[95]

3) The Adenine Nucleotides

The adenine nucleotides are both substrates and effectors of all three kinase reactions, *i.e.*, of HK, PFK and PK, and serve at the same time as their connecting links. Their ratio also determines the share of the 2,3-DPG bypass. In whole blood about 90% of these nucleotides are in the form of ATP, with 8% and 2% as ADP and AMP respectively. The total amount varies among different species, being 6 times as high in pig erythrocytes as in those of the dog or the goat.[15] The pH is the most important factor influencing adenine nucleotides in the red cell.[7,15,100] With pH values increasing above 7.8 there is a decline in the ATP level, with a corresponding elevation of ADP and AMP.

The reasons for this change are probably two; 1) a greater ATP consumption for cation transport, for which there is some evidence,[134] 2) an unbalance between ATP-consuming and ATP-forming reactions in the glycolytic chain. Due to the release of PFK inhibition there is a relative excess of glucose phosphorylation by both HK and PFK with a resulting accumulation of the products of PFK, as compared with ATP formation by PK. At pH values above 8.0 there is a decrease in the sum of adenine nucleotides, presumably due to their breakdown by phosphatase, which attacks AMP almost exclusively and adenosine deaminase.

The erythrocytes contain high concentrations of adenylate kinase with a maximal activity in excess of 2,000 μmoles per ml cells per hr.[101,139] Surprisingly enough, the mass-action ratio of the adenine nucleotides corresponds only at pH values above 8.0 to thermodynamic equilibrium. The lower the pH the greater the divergence, which may reach 1 order of magnitude.[7,12] The reason has not been clarified yet, but is presumably related to the variation of Mg complexes and the binding of adenine nucleotides.

4) Mg^{2+} and the Mg Complexes

An exact assessment of the role of the adenine nucleotides in the regulation of glycolysis presupposes an exact knowledge of the distribution of their free and Mg-complexed forms. In the kinase reactions the Mg complexes are the true substrates, while the effectors may be either Mg complexes or free adenine nucleotides, which differ in their effects.[38] An indication of the importance of Mg is furnished by the observation that the rate of glycolysis is greatly diminished in Mg-deficient erythrocytes.[102,103]

Recently calculations of the concentrations of free Mg^{2+} and Mg-complexes of the adenine nucleotides and the DPG in the interaction with hemoglobin have been carried out.[104,136] They yielded for the oxygenated cell at pH 7.2 and an ionic strength of 0.15 a value of Mg^{2+} of about 0.5 m*M*,[47] of 1.1 m*M* for free $MgATP^{2-}$ and about 0.1 m*M* for $MgADP^{-}$.[16,77] The free ATP would amount to 0.2 m*M*, *i.e.*, 14%. The binding of ATP and of DPG by oxy-Hb is estimated at about 15%; half of the ATP is bound as MgATP complex. This estimate is in good agreement with an independent assessment based on an $MgATP^{2-}$ value derived from the activity of HK. Matters are different under anaerobic conditions. Here, at least 50% of the ATP is bound, so that an increase of free Mg^{2+}, and a decline of free uncomplexed ATP result.[104] The release of the inhibition of PFK in anaerobiosis is therefore presumably due to both an increase of pH as well as a decline in the stronger inhibition by the free ATP species. These estimates are somewhat higher than those given by Rose on the basis of the Mg dependence of the adenylate kinase reaction.[24,105]

5) The Influence of ATP-consuming Processes in the Membrane

One of the most important functions of energy production is the maintenance of cation transport. One would expect therefore that changes in the activity of cation-transporting ATPase will influence the state of phosphorylation of adenine nucleotides and thereby the glycolytic flux. This prediction is borne out by the fact that agents which specifically affect cation transport, such as oubaine, will also influence the glycolysis rate. The changed ADP/ATP ratios primarily affect the PFK reaction.[106)]

THE CONTROL OF GLYCOLYSIS

The following section will deal with selected problems in the regulation of glycolysis, which are illustrative of its multistep control. The pattern of metabolites which is found under various steady-state conditions exhibits regularities which are the basis of the discussion. They are; 1) Only a few of the metabolites exhibit large changes; they are reactants of the controlled reactions. 2) One finds reciprocal relations between particular pairs of metabolites. Such pairs are listed in the following (Table III).

The interaction of controlled and uncontrolled reactions leads to a division of glycolysis into two main units, which will be discussed together. 1) The HK-PFK system and 2) the PK-GAPDH system. Furthermore, the influence of the external signals such as inorganic phosphate, magnesium and temperature will be dealt with.

1) The Hexokinase Phosphofructokinase System

The hexokinase phosphofructokinase system is a functional unit

TABLE III. Reciprocal relations among metabolites of glycolysis.

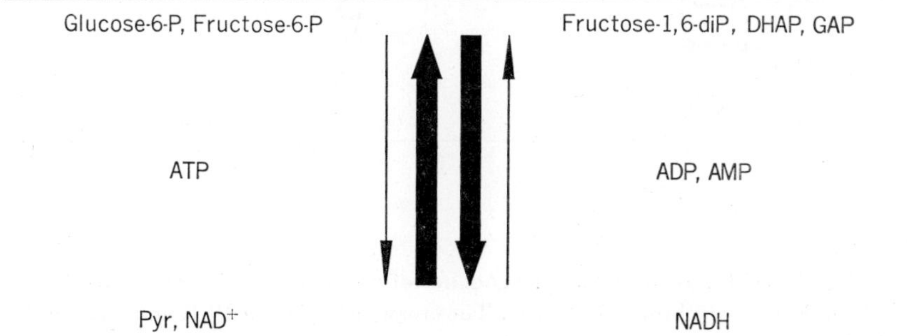

which is linked by glucose-6-P/fructose-6-P on the one hand and ATP on the other. The ratio of glucose-6-P to fructose-6-P is rigidly fixed by the large equilibrium enzyme PHI. Glucose-6-P inhibits HK in a competitive manner to ATP; fructose-6-P on the other hand increases the activity of PFK competitively to ATP. ATP may increase HK activity by providing a higher concentration of the substrate $MgATP^{2-}$, but inhibits PFK. The resulting accumulation of glucose-6-P leads to a product inhibition of HK. The interrelations have been dealt with theoretically in an approximate manner, leading to the prediction that for a given glycolytic rate, two levels of glucose-6-P may be expected and therefore possibly an oscillation.[107)] Furthermore one may expect a consonant increase of both ATP and glucose-6-P, which has actually been observed.[7,108)]

Changes of the pH demonstrate impressively the interrelations of the HK-PFK system. An increase of pH produces an elevation of the glycolytic rate. The changes in the metabolite levels indicate that PFK is a crossover point of the glycolytic chain (Fig. 6). The mass-action

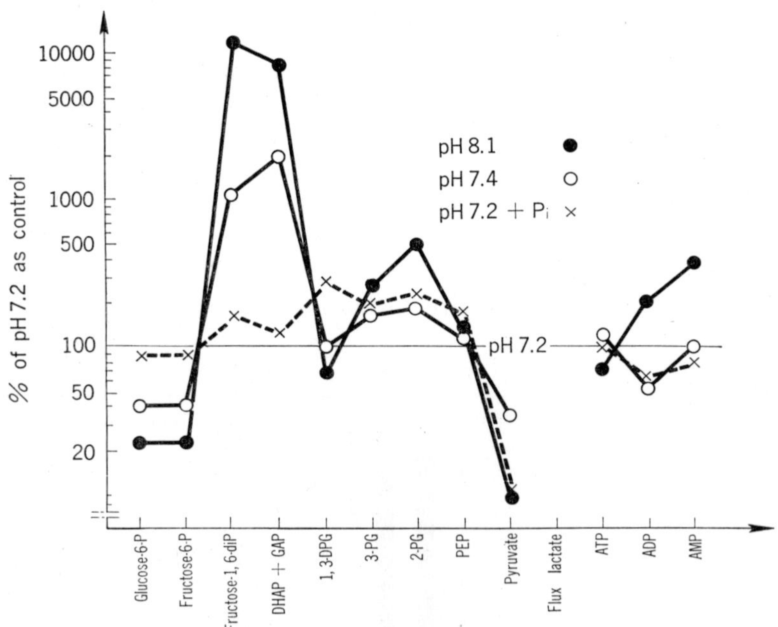

Fig. 6. pH and phosphate dependence of glycolysis and its intermediates in human erythrocytes at 37°C. The crossover points at PFK and PK are shown.

ratio rises by three orders of magnitude and approaches thermodynamic equilibrium within one and a half orders of magnitude (Fig. 2). The reason for this change is complex. Most important are the lessened sensitivity of PFK to ATP inhibition, the decline of ATP and the increase of AMP. Thereby the $K_{0.5S}$ for fructose-6-P is greatly decreased (Fig. 3). The phosphorylation of glucose rises despite a decline of ATP owing to the decrease of glucose-6-P inhibition by one order of magnitude. A further example is provided by differential changes in the enzyme capacities such as occur during blood preservation. With a preferential decline of PFK, the steady-state concentration of glucose-6-P is increased.

2) *The Role of the Pyruvate Kinase-Glyceraldehyde-3-phosphate Dehydrogenase System*

The regulatory properties of PK have been described above. It has been stated that PK, although far from thermodynamic equilibrium does not limit the glycolytic flux. In addition to theoretical consideration, this conclusion rests on the facts that addition of PK to hemolysates of normal cells does not increase the metabolite flux, and its addition to those of PK-deficient cells increases the flux only to normal values.[109] In heterozygotes for PK deficiency, which contain about half the normal enzyme activity, the glycolytic flux in hemolysates is not depressed.[72] Thus the normal complement of PK is at least twice that required for an uninhibited flux limited by the preceding HK-PFK system. The role of PK becomes apparent when pH changes are imposed. This role consists of the regulation of the middle and lower sections of the glycolytic chain and the distribution of the flux between the main pathway and the diphosphoglycerate bypass.

When pH is increased to 8.2, F1, 6P and the triosephosphates accumulate[7,15,27,110,111] (Fig. 6). Previously the erroneus conclusion was drawn that GAPD becomes a limiting step.[112] While at pH 7.2 PFK contributes significantly to the control of the overall flux of glycolysis, its contribution becomes very small at pH values above 7.6. Thus the metabolites beyond PFK but preceding PK increase in concentration. This effect is reinforced by the influence of PK on the levels of the preceding metabolites. Also important is the existence of a restriction on the lower part of the glycolytic chain, namely, the constancy of the sum of all oxidezed metabolites. These factors reduce the $NAD^+/NADH$ ratio by two orders of magnitude, if the pH is shifted from 7.2 to 8.2. This changed ratio is expressed in the GAPD reaction.

Since this step is in equilibrium, the diminished NAD^+ and increased NADH is compensated for by an increase in GAP. This is further reinforced by a lower inorganic P level. As a result, the GAP increases nearly fiftyfold. Since GAP is in equilibrium with both DOAP and F1, 6P by way of TIM and Ald, these metabolites increase correspondingly.

A calculation of the kinetic constants of both the forward and the reverse reaction of the GAPD indicates that at pH 7.2 the enzyme works predominantly in the forward reaction, but at alkaline pH values an extensive shuttle exists.[47] Thus, there is no true limitation of the GAPD at alkaline pH values. The total rate of the enzyme at low pH values is controlled by PFK, while at high pH values the net flux is determined by the PK reaction. Obviously one has to distinguish between a true thermodynamic irreverstibility such as exists in the controlled reactions and a kinetic one-way flux such as may occur by GAPD at pH 7.2. Therefore this enzyme is not a true controlling step. An additional indication that the increase of fructose-1,6-diP and of triose phosphates is determined by the interplay between PFK and PK is given by comparison of the effect of an alkaline pH shift in erythrocytes of different species. While the ratio of PK/PFK capacities in the red cells of man, rat and rabbit is about 1, it amounts to about 10 in the cells of goats (Table IV). Therefore one may expect a reduced accumulation of fructose-1,6-diP and triose phosphates at higher pH values. This was indeed found.[7]

Further support for the thesis that the lowered NAD^+/NADH ratio is the main reason for the large accumulation of the products of PFK above GAPD is given by the effect of oxidizing agents. Addition of methylene blue for instance, leads to an immediate rise of the NAD^+/NADH[113] ratio and a depletion of fructose-1,6-diP and triose phosphates.[7,114,138,115] The opposite effect may be observed on addition of reductants such as sorbitol or xylite, or at high glucose levels, when sorbitol is produced.[116,117] Above a pH of 8.5 both fructose-

TABLE IV. Interrelations between the concentration of 2,3-DPG and the PK/PFK ratio in erythrocytes of various species.

	Man PK deficiency	Rabbit	Rat	Man	Goat	Deer
2,3-DPG	12	7.2	5.5	4.5	≈0.03	∠0.03
PK/PFK	0.3	0.8	0.9	1.1	12.6	16.0

Concentrations are given in mmoles/l cells at 37°C.

1,6-diP and triose phosphates decrease again. At these pH values the ATP concentration declines to levels which decrease the rate of phosphorylation by HK. Thus there is a reduced flux and a smaller accumulation of intermediates. The unbalance between the upper and lower sections of the glycolytic chain at alkaline pH values expresses itself also in the adenine nucleotides. The relative excess of glucose phosphorylation by the HK and PFK reactions and the consequent accumulation of intermediates is no longer balanced by ATP formation, and a lowered ADP/ATP ratio results. The PK reaction also influences the distribution of the metabolic flux from 1,3-DPG in combination with the PFK and ATP consuming processes (Fig. 7).

The rate of 2,3-DPG formation is determined by the ratio 1,3-DPG/2,3-DPG, while that of the PGK forward reaction is determined by the concentration of 1,3-DPG and the ratio $MgADP^-/MgATP^{2-}$. Thus competition results between the two pathways, which is influenced

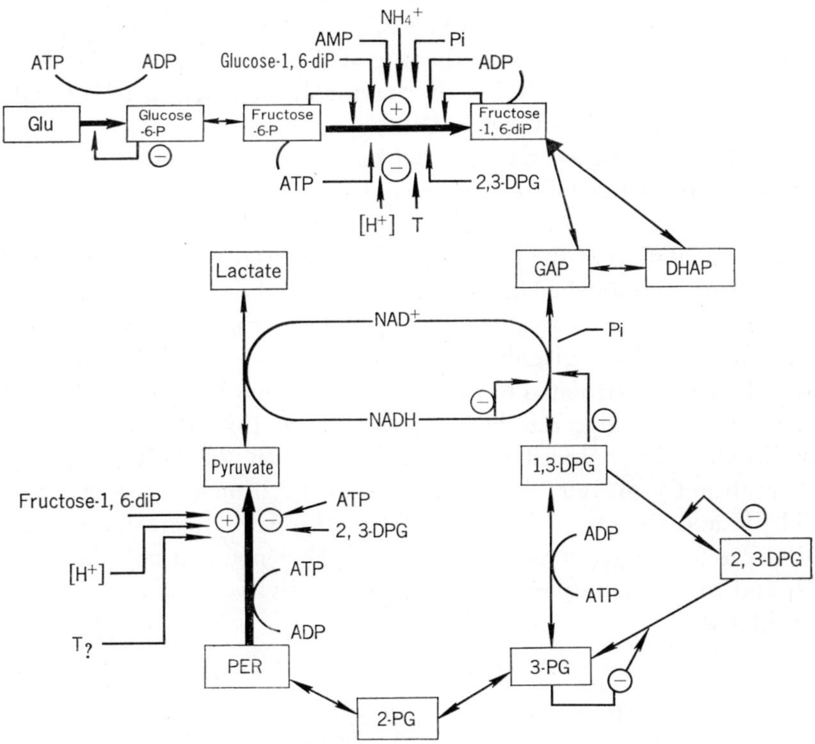

Fig. 7. Overall scheme of control of glycolysis. The influence of activators (+) and inhibitors (—) is shown.

by several factors, each of which in turn depends on other processes. The steady-state level of 2,3-DPG is a resultant of synthesis and breakdown, which is primarily dependent on product inhibition by 3-PG and the degree of activation (perhaps by phosphoglycolate), about which little is known. While a complete kinetic description of this complicated interplay is not available at present, certain regularities are apparent. Whenever there is a relative preponderance of the PFK over the PK reaction, by released inhibition of PFK or reduced activity of PK, the steady-state concentration of 2,3-DPG is found to be increased.[72] This is true, for instance, in PK-deficient erythrocytes. In these cells all relevant intermediates, including PEP, 3-PG and 2-PG as well as 1,3-PG are increased. This results in both higher DPGM and possibly lower 2,3-DPGase activities, which overshadow the tendency to increased ADP concentration. An interspecies comparison shows the same results. The higher the ratio of PFK/PK, the more 2,3-DPG is found (Table IV). The increase of 2,3-DPG with pH, which reaches a maximum at pH 8.2,[118] is also in favor of this interpretation. A preponderance in the rate of 2,3-DPG formation is found under conditions of repletion of previously depleted 2,3-DPG such as exists in stored erythrocytes.[119]

Various estimates, all beset with uncertainties, have been given for the share of the DPGM pathway.[15,120–123] The most conservative ones give values of one-tenth to one-eighth of the total glycolytic flux. A calculation of the actual activity of DPGM at pH 7.2 and 37°C on the basis of published kinetic parameters and determined metabolite concentrations, yields a value of 0.24 μmoles per ml cells per hr, which is about 10% of the glycolytic flux. In presence of high P_i concentrations the rate is calculated to increase two and one-half times; the share of the diphosphoglycerate bypass increases to 13%. Under anaerobic conditions, with reduced product inhibition by 2,3-DPG, the share is significantly greater. A mechanistic explanation for the decline at acid pH and the increase at high pH of the steady-state level of 2,3-DPG cannot be given at present. Both pH-dependent changes in the K_M and the K_i values and in the level or activity of activators may be considered.

THE EFFECTS OF EXTERNAL SIGNALS

1) *The Influence of Phosphate Variations*

High concentrations of inorganic phosphate will increase the glycolytic rate more than twice at pH values above 7.0.[15,106,112,124–128] The cause of the activation of the HK-PFK system below pH 7.6 is a reduced ATP inhibition of PFK with a consequent increase of affinity for F6P. Thus, both F6P and G6P concentrations decline as does the product inhibition of HK. At pH values above 7.6, the main effect is the maintenance of a high ATP level, whereby HK works at higher saturation with its substrate $MgATP^{2-}$.[127] Both the alkaline pH and the inorganic phosphate combine to release PFK nearly completely from its inhibition.[27,33] On the other hand, PK is probably unchanged owing to the compensatory effect of a decreased affinity of the enzyme for PEP on the one hand and the increase of MgADP on the other.[78] Consequently, there is an accumulation of the preceding metabolites (Fig. 6). The NAD^+/NADH ratio declines to values as low as 2–3, due to the greater flux. Under these conditions, the inhibition of the forward reaction of GAPD by NADH and 1,3-DPG becomes significant.

Phosphate deficiency produced by dietary means will produce

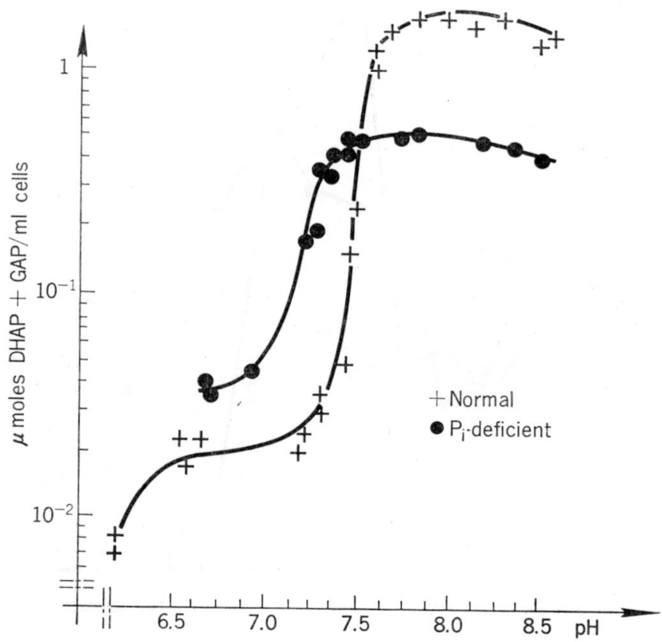

Fig. 8. pH dependence of triose phosphate concentrations in erythrocytes of normal and phosphate-deficient rats.

within weeks a decline of glycolytic rate, with decreased ATP and 2,3-DPG levels.[127,129,130] The time course of the changes of the metabolites indicates that the primary effect is exerted on GAPD by displacement of the equilibrium in favor of the triosephosphates.[47] Below pH 7.6 a compensatory increase of triosephosphates and F1, 6P results, and the levels of the succeeding metabolites decline (Fig. 8).[127,131] The low concentration of 1,3-DPG results both in lower 2,3-DPG and lower ATP synthesis.[132] The decreased ATP concentration means a depressed rate of HK. At pH levels above 7.6 there is less discrepancy between upper and lower sections of the glycolytic chain, a less pronounced decline of the $NAD^+/NADH$ ratio, and a lesser accumulation of metabolites preceding the PK reaction.

2) Mg Deficiency

By dietary means it is possible to reduce the Mg concentration of red cells of rats and dogs to about one-half.[133] Such cells exhibit a

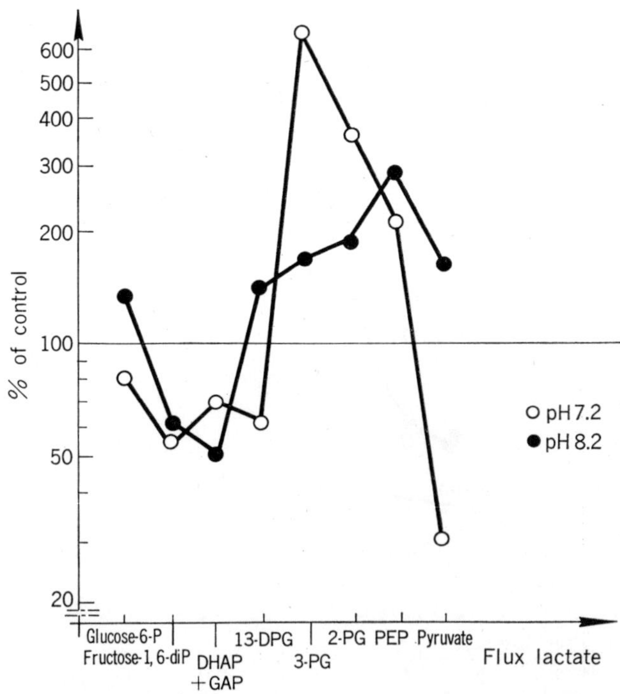

Fig. 9. Glycolysis and its intermediates in erythrocytes of magnesium-deficient rats.

lowered glycolytic rate.[102,103,127] Since Mg in form of adenine nucleotide complexes is a substrate of 4 glycolytic reactions (those catalyzed by HK, PFK, PGK, and PK), the effect of a change in Mg concentration may be expected to be complex and the Mg^{2+} activation. The predominant effect reponsible for the decline of glycolysis appears to be exerted on HK, which is the first controlling step owing to the decrease of the MgATP complex and the Mg^{2+} activation. A second inhibitory effect is probably exercised on PK. The lowering of the MgADP concentration is presumably the cause for a severalfold accumulation of the metabolites preceding the PK reaction (Fig. 9).

3) The Influence of Temperature

Very interesting changes in the overall rate and in the metabolite pattern may be observed with variation of temperature. The temperature optimum of glycolysis is 48°C, independent of pH, with a Q_{10} of 2.1, which is higher than that of any control enzyme.[5,135] Thus lactate formation is decreased to one-thirteenth at 4° as compared to 37°, while the capacity of the HK declines only to about one-fifth.

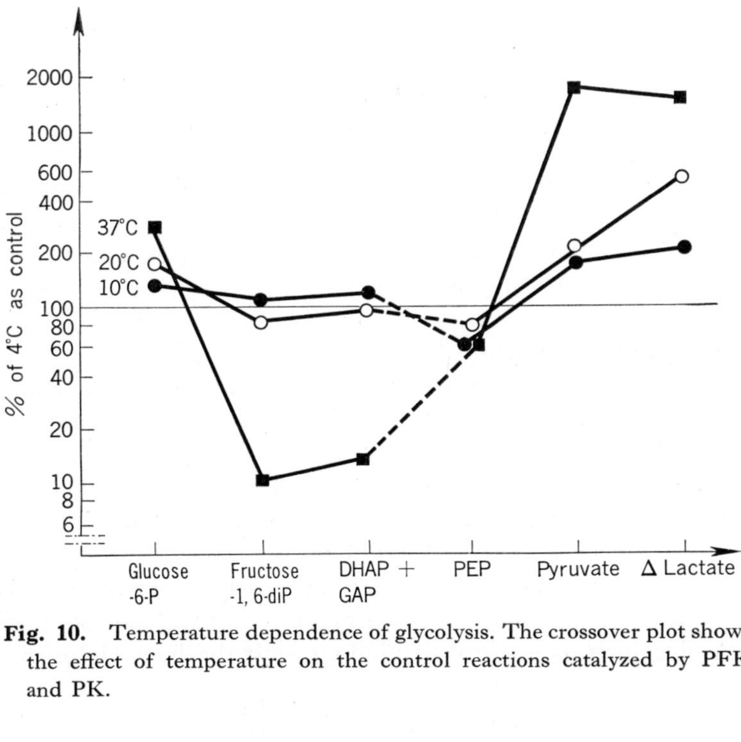

Fig. 10. Temperature dependence of glycolysis. The crossover plot shows the effect of temperature on the control reactions catalyzed by PFK and PK.

TABLE V. Temperature dependence of the $K_{0.5S}$ values for fructose-6-P and of the interaction coefficient of erythrocyte PFK.

Temp. °C	pH 7.2		pH 8.4	
	$K_{0.5S}$ (mM)	Hill Coeff. (n)	$K_{0.5S}$ (mM)	Hill Coeff. (n)
10	0.14	1.88	0.01	1.19
20	0.51	2.60	0.16	1.37
37 } 45 }	1.37	3.00	1.29	1.48
			0.98	2.15

Experimental conditions: 1.25 mM $MgCl_2$, 1 mM P_i and 90 mM KCl. At pH 7.2 the ATP concentration was 0.2 mM and at pH 8.4, 1.0 mM.

The main reason is the increased inhibition of HK by glucose-6-P and glucose-1,6-P, the K_i for both compounds being decreased to less than one-third.[147] Other changes tend to compensate each other which are due to the increased binding of organic phosphate compounds by hemoglobin at low temperatures. There are a decrease of $MgATP^{2-}$, of free 2,3-DPG and Mg 2,3-DPG as well as an increase of Mg^{2+}. At pH 7.2 there and temperatures near O°C there are high F1,6P and triose phosphate levels, which decline steeply with rising temperature to a minimum at 37°C. The reverse change occurs in the G6P, F6P, and pyruvate levels and consequently in the NAD^+/NADH ratio. The crossover plots may be explained by interaction with PFK alone (Fig. 10).[135] The results suggest that at low temperature the cooperative behavior of PFK is weakened. This prediction could be verified on partially purified PFK. It was demonstrated that from 4 to 37°C the sensitivity of the enzyme to ATP inhibition rises, and the $K_{0.5S}$ for F6P increases tenfold (Table V).[33]

4) The Influence of Oxygen Tension

Although mitochondria are absent in the red cell, a phenomenon similar to "Pasteur-effect" was observed; the glycolytic rate of the red cell under nitrogen is higher than that of the cell under aerobic conditions.[93] The level of 2,3-DPG was found to be higher in the anaerobic state than in the aerobic condition. The inhibition of glycolysis and the decrease of the 2,3-DPG are not related to any oxidative reaction as the replacement of oxygen with carbon monoxide leads to the same results. This implies that oxygen or carbon monoxide affect red cell glycolysis as a result of binding with the hemoglobin in the cell.

This alteration of red cell metabolism by oxygen has some practical importance as the increased level of 2,3-DPG has been observed in subjects at high altitudes or in anemic patients.[87] Since 2,3-DPG is known to depress the oxygen affinity of hemoglobin[140,141] and thereby facilitate transport of oxygen to tissues, the increase of the 2,3-DPG under these conditions has teleological significance (see chapter by Tyuma).

The mechanism for the depression of the glycolytic rate and the reduction of the 2,3-DPG level was thought at first to be due to the intracellular acidification caused by the dissociation of proton from hemoglobin bound to oxygen or carbon monoxide.[93] However, the study of the glycolytic intermediates revealed that the pattern of the intermediate changes was not exactly the same as that expected from the acidification. Besides the PFK step, another cross over point appeared between GAP and 3PG: 3PG, 2PG and PEP increased when the red cell was oxygenated or treated with carbon monoxide (Fig. 11).[142] The cross over between GAP and 3PG was explained by the release of 2,3-DPG from hemoglobin and the inhibition of DPGM by free 2,3-DPG released. However, since the level of the 2,3-DPG is determined by several factors,[143] and it may also be explained by an interplay of PFK and PK, further elucidation of the diphosphoglycerate cycle is necessary for quantitative explanation of the oxygen effect.

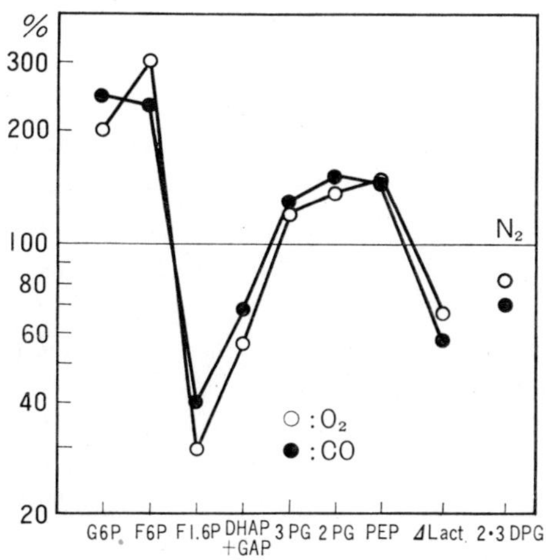

Fig. 11. Effect of oxygen or carbon monoxide on glycolytic intermediates. (from 142).

ENERGETIC CONSIDERATIONS

The red cell is one of the exceptional cell types that can be treated thermodynamically because steady-state concentrations of glycolytic intermediates and coenzymes can be accurately determined and the reaction sequence of glycolysis can be regarded as taking place only in homogeneous cytoplasma so that ambiguous assumptions, such as "compartmentations to particulate fractions," may be unnecessary. Furthermore, number of metabolic systems present in the cells are quite limited.

Free energy changes of the various steps of glycolysis in human red cells under physiological conditions are calculated from the equation, $\Delta F = \Delta F' + 1.42 \log K_{app}$, where $\Delta F'$ is the standard free energy change and K_{app} is the mass action ratio calculated from Table VI.[8,14] The free energy changes thus calculated can be used to illustrate an intuitive model made of two water reservoirs representing substrates and products and a connecting pipe representing the enzymes (Fig. 12).[144] The free energy changes are expressed as the differences in water levels corresponding to the driving forces necessary for the re-

TABLE VI. Concentrations of glycolytic intermediates in human red cell.

Glucose	5.0 mM
G6P	38.5 μM
F6P	15.7 μM
FDP	7.0 μM
DHAH	17.0 μM
GAP	5.7 μM
1,3-DPG	0.4 μM (estim.)
2,3-DPG	5.7 mM
3PG	68.5 μM
2PG	10.0 μM
PEP	17.0 μM
Pyruvate	85.0 μM
Lactate	1.43 mM
ATP	1.83 mM
ADP	180.0 μM
P_i	1.0 mM
[NAD+]/[NADH]	985 (calculated)
Intracellular pH	7.0

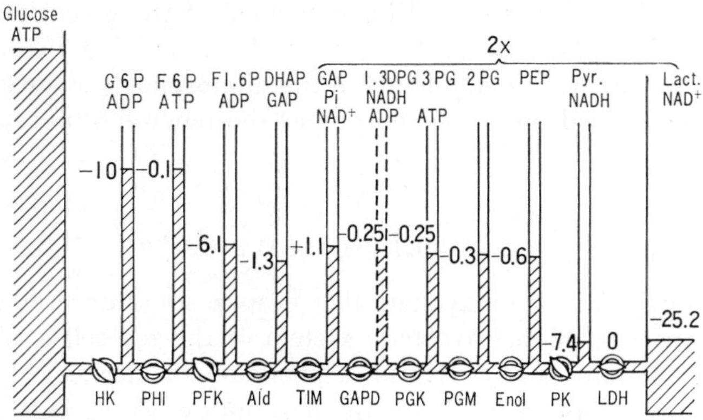

Fig. 12. The free energy changes in erythrocyte glycolysis. The values at the right side of columns are the free energy changes expressed as kcal per mole glucose. (from 144).

actions to proceed. If the activity of any step in the reaction sequence is reduced, the free energy change of the step will increase. This may be visualized in the appearance of a pressure difference seen when water flow is throttled by closing the cock. Three steps corresponding to HK, PFK and PK show big free energy changes indicating that these three steps are important for the regulation of glycolysis.

Similarly the intracellular free energy changes associated with the formation of ATP may be calculated. The free energy change for ATP hydrolysis in the cell is calculated from the concentrations of ATP, ADP and P_i to be −14.3 kcal, assuming the standard free energy for the hydrolysis to be −8.6 kcal. The overall free energy change for the production of lactate from glucose is calculated to be −50.5 kcal per mole glucose using the value of −47.4 kcal as the standard free energy. Thus the efficiency of ATP formation by erythrocyte steady state glycolysis is about 50%, if the contributions of the pentose phosphate cycle and the diphosphoglycerate cycle are not considered.

Finally the free energy changes associated with the active cation transport will be mentioned. According to Sen and Post,[147] one mole ATP is utilized for the transport of 3 meq. Na and 2 meq. K. The free energy required for the transport is 8.5 kcal,[2] which corresponds to about 60% of the energy released by the hydrolysis of ATP. Further, if we assume the active cation fluxes are 3 for Na and 2 for K in meq./1 cell per hour, one mole of ATP will be utilized for the transport by one liter cell per hour which corresponds to about one-third of the

ATP formed, as 3 moles of ATP is formed at the glycolytic rate of 1.5 mmoles/1 cell per hour. The fate of the remaining two-thirds is not clear: a part will be dissipated in the diphosphoglycerate cycle and a part will be used for reactions such as the renewal of phospholipids by acylation.[146]

CONCLUDING REMARKS

In conclusion one may state that despite some uncertainties and gaps, knowledge of the glycolytic system of the red cell is close to a state that should permit at least a phenomenological, even a partly mechanistic, mathematical kinetic description as successful effort in this direction for the steady state conditions has been made.[151–153] This opinion is supported by the extensive correspondence on the conclusions derived from studies on purified enzymes, hemolysates and intact cells. The regularities of the interplay of controlled and uncontrolled reactions, of effector and mass-action influences, and the responses to external and internal signals have general significance and should hold for other types of cells. The knowledge gained from the erythrocyte may be used as a starting point for analysis of the more complex situation of the immature red cell and other respiring cells. In such complex systems the clearcut crossover points found in the erythrocyte are apt to be overbalanced by several other processes. Some of them may be enumerated: 1) the presence of glucokinase, circumventing the HK-PFK control unit, 2) the activity of the glycogenolysis system, including the action of glucose-6-Pase, 3) the activity of the gluconeogenesis system and of fructose-1,6-diPase, 4) the interaction with metabolites of the citrate cycle and of the breakdown of fatty acids, 5) interactions with the metabolism of amino acids, 6) the activity of the respiratory chain and the translocation and compartmentalization of the adenine and pyridine nucleotides, 7) the function of additional bypasses such as formation of glycerol phosphate. The disentanglement of this complexity should not be a hopeless task.

REFERENCES

1 London, I. M., *Harvey Lectures*, **56**, 151a (1961).

2 Whittam, R., Transport and Diffusion in Red blood Cells, ed. by Barcroft, H., Davson, H. and Paton, W. P. M., Monographs of the Physiological Society (The Camelot Press Ltd. London, 1964).

3 Rona, P. and Wilenko, G. G., *Biochem. Z.*, **62**, 1 (1914).
4 Mauriac, P. and Servantie, L., *Comptes rendues de l'Academic des Sciences*, **87**, 200 (1922).
5 Murphy, J. R., *J. Lab. Clin. Med.*, **55**, 286 (1960).
6 Engelhardt, W. A. and Ljubimowa, M., *Biochem. Z.*, **227**, 6 (1930).
7 Jacobasch, G. and Thesis, Dr. Sc., Biowissenschaftliche Fakultät der Humboldt-Universität (Berlin, 1970).
8 Minakami, S. and Yoshikawa, H., *Biochem. Biophys. Res. Comm.*, **18**, 345 (1965).
9 Jacobasch, G., *et al.*, III. Internationales Symposium über Fragen der Struktur und Funktion der roten Blutkörperchen Berlin, 1960. *Folia Haematol.*, **78** (1962).
10 Jacobasch, G., *et al.*, IV. Internationales Symposium über Struktur und Funktion der roten Blutkörperchen, Berlin, 1964. *Folia Haematol.*, **83** (1965).
11 Jacobasch, G., *et al.*, V. Berliner Symposium über Struktur und Funktion der Erythrozyten, 1967. *Folia Haematol.*, **89**, 90 (1968), and 91 (1969).
12 Jacobasch, G., *et al.*, I. Internationales Symposium, Wien, 1968. Stoffwechsel und Membranpermeabilität von Erythrozyten und Thrombozyten, ed. by Deutsch, E., Gerlach, E. and Moser, K. (Georg Thieme Verlag, Stuttgart, 1968).
13 Jacobasch, G., *et al.*, VI. Internationales Symposium über Struktur und Funktion der Erythrozyten, Berlin, 1970. *in*: Abhandlungen der Deutschen Akademie der Wissenschaften (Akademie-Verlag, Berlin, 1971).
14 Brewer, G.J. (ed. by), Red Cell Metabolism and Function, Advances in Experimental Medicine and Biology, **6** (Plenum Press New York-London, 1970).
15 Rapoport, S., *in*: ed. by Campbell, P. N. and Greville, G. D., *Essays in Biochem.*, **4**, 69 (Academic Press London and New York, 1968).
16 Hinterberger, U., Gerischer-Mothes, W., Suckrow, D. and Rapoport, S., *Acta Biol. Med. German.*, **7**, 57 (1961).
17 Eaton, G. M., Brewer, G. J. and Tashian, R. E., *Nature*, **212**, 944 (1966).
18 Holmes, E. W., Jr., Malone, J. I., Winegrad, A. J. and Oski, F. A., *Science*, **156**, 646 (1967).
19 Gerber, G. K. G., Schultze, M. and Rapoport, S. M., *Europ. J. Biochem.*, **17**, 445 (1970).
20 Jacobasch, G., Syllm-Rapoport, I., Wolf, K., Müller, R. and Rymon, J., *Folia Haematol.*, **83**, 310 (1965).
21 Rose, I. A. and O'Connell, E. L., *J. Biol. Chem.*, **239**, 12 (1964).
22 Rose, I. A., Warms, J. V. B. and O'Connell, E. L., *Biochem. Biophys.*

Res. Comm., **15**, 33 (1964).
23 Gerber, G., Kloppick, E. and Rapoport, S., *Acta Biol. Med. German.*, **18**, 305 (1967).
24 Rose, I. A., *Exp. Eye Res.*, **11**, 264 (1971).
25 Dische, Z., *Biochem. Z.*, **280**, 248 (1935).
26 Jacobasch, G., Kühn, B. and Grieger, M., VII. Internat. Symp. über Struktur und Funktion der Erythrozyten 1973. *in*: Abhandlung der Akademie der Wissenschaften der DDR, Berlin, 1974.
27 Kühn, B., Jacobasch, G. and Rapoport, S., *Acta Biol. Med. German.*, **23**, 1 (1969).
28 Layzer, R. B., Rowland, L. P. and Bank, W. J., *J. Biol. Chem.*, **244**, 3823 (1969).
29 Wenzel, K.-W., Gauer, J., Zimmermann, G. and Hofmann, E., *FEBS Letters*, **19**, 281 (1972).
30 Wenzel, K.-W., Zimmermann, G., Gauer, J., Diezel, W., Liebe, St. and Hofmann, E., *FEBS Letters*, **19**, 285 (1972).
31 Paetkau, V. H., Youna Than, E. S. and Lardy, H. A., *J. Mol. Biol.*, **33**, 721 (1968).
32 Kemp, R. G. and Krebs, E. G., *Biochemistry*, **6**, 423 (1967).
33 Jacobasch, G., Kühn, B., Gerth, C. and Rapoport, S., VI. Internationales Symposium über Struktur und Funktion der Erythrozyten, Berlin, 1970, *in*: Abhandlungen der Deutschen Akademie der Wissenschaften (1971), p. 297.
34 Jacobasch, G. and Kühn, B., 1. Joint Symposium Reactions Mechanism and Control Properties of Phosphotransferases, Reinhardtsbrunn-Friedrichsroda, DDR, 1971 (Akademie-Verlag, 1972), in press.
35 Atkinson, E. D., *Annu. Rev. Biochem.*, **35**, 57 (1966)
36 Cartier, P., Leroux, J. P., Balsan, S. and Royer, P., *Clin. Chim. Acta*, **29**, 261 (1970).
37 Jacobasch, G. and Rapoport, S., 2nd Meeting of the Federation of European Biochemical Societies (Wien, 1965).
38 Passonneau, J. V. and Lowry, O. H., *J. Biol. Chem.*, **241**, 2268 (1966).
39 De Loecker, W. C. J., *Clin. Chim. Acta*, **10**, 157 (1964).
40 Kloppick, E., Jacobasch, G. and Rapoport, S., *Acta Biol. Med. German.*, **18**, 37 (1967).
41 Seligson, D. and Hirahara, K., *J. Lab. Clin. Med.*, **49**, 962 (1957).
42 Kerr, S. E., *J. Biol. Chem.*, **117**, 227 (1937).
43 Jacobasch, G. and Rapoport, S., 2. Gemeinschaftstagung der Gesellschaft für experimentelle Medizin (Leipzig, 1970), in press.
44 Oguchi, M., Hashimoto, T., Minakami, S. and Yoshikawa, H., *J. Biochem.*, **60**, 99 (1966).
45 Wolny, M., Wolny, E. and Baranowski, T., *Bull. L'Acad. Pol. Sci.*, **6**, 13 (1968).

46 Maretzki, D. and Rapoport, S., *Acta Biol. Med. German.*, **29**, 207 (1972).
47 Rapoport, S., Maretzki, D., Schewe, C. and Jacobasch, G., Alfred Benzon Symposium IV (1971). (Munksgaard, Copenhagen, 1972), in press.
48 Mills, G. C. and Hill, F. L., *Arch. Biochem. Biophys.*, **146**, 306 (1971).
49 Oguchi, M., *J. Biochem.*, **68**, 427 (1970).
50 Harris, I. J. and Perham, R. N., *J. Mol. Biol.*, **13**, 876 (1965).
51 Heinz, F. and Kulbe, K. D., *Hoppe Seyler Z. Physiol. Chem.*,**351**, 249 (1970).
52 Harrington, W. F. and Karr, G. M., *J. Mol. Biol.*, **13**, 885 (1965).
53 Wieland, Th. and Wachsmuth, E. D., *Biochem. Z.*, **334**, 185 (1961).
54 Priem, F., Diplom-Arbeit Mathematisch-Naturwissenschaftliche Fakultät der Humboldt-Universität (Berlin, 1966).
55 Löhr, G. W. and Waller, H. D., *Nova Acta Leopold. N.F.*, **26**, 143 (1963).
56 Busch, B. and Boie, K., *Klin. Wochenschr.*, **47**, 1172 (1969).
57 Gross, R. T., Schroeder, E. A. and Gabrio, B. W., *J. Clin. Invest.*, **45**, 249 (1966).
58 Cartier, P. M., *Europ. J. Biochem.*, **4** 247 (1968).
59 Omachi, A., Scott, C. B. and Hegarty, H., *Biochim. Biophys. Acta*, **184**, 139 (1969).
60 Glock, C. E. and McLean, P., *Biochem. J.*, **61**, 388 (1955).
61 Hasart, E., Jacobasch, G. and Rapoport, S., *Acta Biol. Med. German.* (1972), in press.
62 Steinbrecht, I. and Kunz, W., *Acta Biol. Med. German.* (1973), in press.
63 Klingenberg, M. and Bücher, T., *Annu. Rev. Biochem.*, **29**, 669 (1960).
64 Minakami, S. and Yoshikawa, H., *J. Biochem.*, **59**, 139 (1966).
65 Krebs, H. A., *Adv. Enzyme Regul.*, **5**, 409 (1967).
66 Hashimoto, T. and Yoshikawa, H., *Biochim. Biophys. Acta*, **65**, 355 (1962).
67 Hashimoto, T. and Yoshikawa, H., *J. Biochem.*, **56**, 279 (1964).
68 Yoshida, A. and Watanabe, S., *J. Biol. Chem.*, **247**, 440 (1972).
69 Reiman, B., Maretzki, D. and Heinrich, R., VII. Internat. Symp. über Struktur und Funktion der Erythrozyten 1973. *in*: Abhandlung der Akademie der Wissenschaften der DDR, Berlin, 1974.
70 Schewe, C., Jacobasch, G. and Rapoport, S., unpublished data.
71 Maretzki, D., Tsamalukas, A. G., Küttner, G., Krüger, S., Groth, J. and Rapoport, S., VII. Internat. Symp. über Struktur und Funktion der Erythrozyten 1973. *in*: Abhandlung der Akademie der Wissenschaften der DDR, Berlin, 1974.
72 Tanaka, K. R. and Valentine, W. N., *in*: Hereditary Disorders of Ery-

throcyte Metabolism, S. 229. ed. by Beutler, E. (Grune & Stratton, New York and London, 1968).
73 Bigley, R. H., Stenzel, P., Jones, R. T., Campos, J. O. and Koler, R. D., *Enzymol. Biol. Clin.*, **9**, 10 (1968).
74 Blume, K. G., Hoffbauer, R. W., Busch, D., Arnold, A. and Löhr, G. W., *Biochim. Biophys. Acta*, **227**, 364 (1971).
75 Ibsen, K. H. and Trippet, P., *Life Sciences*, **10**, 1021 (1971).
76 Hess, B. and Kutzbach, C., *Hoppe Seyler Z. Physiol. Chem.*, **352**, 453 (1971).
77 Grieger, M. and Jacobasch, G., VII. Internat. Symp. über Struktur und Funktion der Erythrozyten 1973. *in*: Abhandlung der Akademie der Wissenschaften der DDR, Berlin, 1974.
78 Rozengurt, E., De Asua, L. J. and Carminatti, H., *J. Biol. Chem.*, **244**, 3142 (1969).
79 Jacobson, K. W. and Black, J. A., *J. Biol. Chem.*, **246**, 5504 (1971).
80 Ponce, J., Roth, S. and Harkness, D. R., *Biochim. Biophy. Acta*, **250**, 63 (1971).
81 Beutler, E., *Nature New Biology*, **232**, 20 (1971)
82 Rapoport, S. and Guest, G. M., *J. Biol. Chem.*, **129**, 781 (1939).
83 Guest, G. M. and Rapoport, S., *Physiol. Rev.*, **21**, 410 (1941).
84 Gardos, G., *Experientia*, **23**, 19 (1967).
85 Parker, J. C., *J. Clin. Invest.*, **48**, 117 (1969).
86 Schröter, W. and Winter, P., *Blut*, **14**, 16 (1966).
87 De Verdier, C.-H., Garby, L., Högman, C. F. and Åkerblom, O. (eds.), Symposium on intracellular Regulation of Hemoglobin Affinity to Oxygen, Försvarsmedicin, **5** (1969), Häfte 4.
88 Sutherland, E., Pasternak, T. and Cori, C., *J. Biol. Chem.*, **181**, 153 (1949).
89 Rapoport, S. and Luebering, J., *J. Biol. Chem.*, **183**, 507 (1950).
90 Rapoport, S. and Luebering, J., *J. Biol. Chem.*, **198**, 583 (1952).
91 Rose, Z. B., *J. Biol. Chem.*, **243**, 4810 (1968).
92 Deuticke, B., Duhm, J. and Dierkesmann, R., *Pflügers Archiv*, **326**, 15 (1971).
93 Asakura, T., Sato, Y., Minakami, S. and Yoshikawa, H., *J. Biochem.*, **5**, 715 (1966).
94 Rapoport, S. and Luebering, J., *J. Biol. Chem.*, **189**, 683 (1951).
95 Harkness, D. R. and Roth, S., *Biochem. Biophys. Res. Comm.*, **34**, 849 (1969).
96 Rose, Z. B. and Liebowitz, J., *J. Biol. Chem.*, **245**, 3232 (1970).
97 Harkness, D. R., Thompson, W., Roth, S. and Grayson, V., *Arch. Biochem. Biophys.*, **138**, 208 (1970).
98 Örström, A., *Arch. Biochem. Biophys.*, **33**, 93 (1951).
99 Duhm, J., Deuticke, B. and Gerlach, E., *Hoppe Seyler Z. Physiol.*

Chem., **350**, 1008 (1969).
100 Mills, G. C., *Fed. Proc.*, **25**, 762 (1966).
101 Cerletti, P. and Bucci, E., *Biochim. Biophys. Acta*, **38**, 45 (1960).
102 Syllm-Rapoport, I., Strassburger, I. and Rapoport, S., *Acta Biol. Med. German.*, **5**, 596 (1960).
103 Jacobasch, G., Syllm-Rapoport, I., Rapoport, S. unter Mitarbeit von Morr, Th., Molzow, F. and Bessenbach, F., *Acta Biol. Med. German.*, **13**, 683 (1964).
104 Berger, H., Gerber, G. and Rapoport, S., *Europ. J. Biochem.* (1973), in press.
105 Rose, I. A., *Proc. Nat. Acad. Sci., U.S.*, **61**, 1079 (1968).
106 Minakami, S. and Yoshikawa, H., *J. Biochem.*, **59**, 145 (1966).
107 Hansen, G., Schott, J., Jacobasch, G. and Rapoport, S., *Acta Biol. Med. German.*, **24**, 253 (1970).
108 Stepanauskas, M., Jacobasch, G. and Boese, C., *Folia Haematol.*, **89**, 490 (1968).
109 Oski, F. A. and Bowman, H., *Brit. J. Haematol.*, **17**, 289 (1969).
110 Minakami, S., Saito, T., Suzuki, C. and Yoshikawa, H., *Biochem. Biophys. Res. Comm.*, **17**, 748 (1964).
111 Reinauer, H. and Bruns, F. H., *Biochem. Z.*, **340**, 503 (1964).
112 Rose, I. A. and Warms, J. V. B., *J. Biol. Chem.*, **245**, 4009 (1970).
113 Wendel, W. B., *J. Biol. Chem.*, **102**, 373 (1933).
114 Saito, T. and Minakami, S., *J. Biochem.*, **61**, 211 (1967).
115 Roigas, H., Zoellner, E., Jacobasch, G., Schultze, M. and Rapoport, S., *Europ. J. Biochem.*, **12**, 24 (1970).
116 Asakura, K., Adachi, K., Minakami, S. and Yoshikawa, H., *J. Biochem.*, **62**, 184 (1967).
117 Travis, S. F., Morrison, A. D., Clements, R. S., Jr., Winegrad, A. J. and Oski, F. A., *J. Clin. Invest.*, **50**, 2104 (1971).
118 Asakura, T., Sato, Y., Minakami, S. and Yoshikawa, H., *Clin. Chim. Acta*, **14**, 840 (1966).
119 Rapoport, S., *J. Clin. Invest.*, **26**, 591 (1957).
120 Dietze, F., Sauer, G. and Rapoport, S., *Acta Biol. Med. German.*, **12**, 312 (1964).
121 Duhm, J., Deuticke, B. and Gerlach, E., *Pflügers Archiv Gesam. Physiol.*, **306**, 329 (1969).
122 Reich, J., Till, G., Günther, J., Zahn, D., Tschisgale, M. and Frunder, H., *Europ. J. Biochem.*, **6**, 384 (1968).
123 Schröter, W., *in*: Metabolism and Membrane Permeability of Erythrocytes and Thrombocytes, ed. by Deutsch, E., Gerlach, G. and Moser, K. (Stuttgart G. Thiemes, 1968), p. 50.
124 Tsuboi, K. K. and Fukunaga, K., *J. Biol. Chem.*, **240**, 2806 (1965).
125 Minakami, S. and Yoshikawa, H., *Biochim. Biophys. Acta*, **99**, 175

(1965).
126 Rose, I. A. and Warms, J. V. B., *J. Biol. Chem.*, **241**, 4848 (1966).
127 Jacobasch, G., *Folia Haematol.*, **89**, 376 (1968).
128 Gercken, G., *Folia Haematol.*, **89**, 401 (1968).
129 Freudenberg, E. and Welcker, A., *Z. Kinderheilk.*, **41**, 466 (1926).
130 Brock, J. and Welcker, A., *Z. Kinderheilk.*, **43**, 193 (1927).
131 Ströder, J. and Garbe, A., *Hoppe Seyler Z. Physiol. Chem.*, **333**, 127 (1963).
132 Rapoport, S. and Guest, G. M., *J. Biol. Chem.*, **126**, 749 (1938).
133 Syllm-Rapoport, I., Habilitationsschrift, Medizinische Fakultät der Humboldt-Universität (Berlin, 1959).
134 Wieth, J. O. and Funder, J., *Scand. J. Clin. Lab. Invest.*, **17**, 399 (1965).
135 Hasart, E., Jacobasch, G. and Rapoport, S., *Acta Biol. Med. German.*, **24**, 725 (1970).
136 Gerber, G., Berger, H., Jänig, G.-R. and Rapoport, S., *Europ. J. Biochem.* (1973), in press.
137 Schweiger, H. G. and Rapoport, S., *Hoppe Seyler Z. Physiol. Chem.*, **313**, 97 (1958).
138 Albrecht, V., Roigas, H., Schultze, M., Jacobasch, G. and Rapoport, S., *Europ. J. Biochem.*, **20**, 44 (1971).
139 Tatibana, M., Nakao, M. and Yoshikawa, H., *J. Biochem.*, **45**, 1037 (1958).
140 Benesch, R. and Benesch, R.E., *Biochem. Biophys. Res. Comm.*, **26**, 162 (1967).
141 Chanutin, A. and Curnish, R.R., *Arch. Biochem. Biophys.*, **121**, 96 (1968).
142 Hamasaki, N., Asakura, T. and Minakami, S., *J. Biochem.*, **68**, 157 (1970).
143 Hamasaki, N. and Minakami, S., *J. Biochem.*, **72**, 981 (1972).
144 Yoshikawa, H. and Minakami, S., *Folia Haematol.*, **89**, 357 (1968).
145 Sen, A.K. and Post, R.L., *J. Biol. Chem.*, **239**, 345 (1964).
146 Feig, S.A., Shohet, S.B. and Nathan, G., *J. Clin. Invest.*, **50**, 1731 (1971).
147 Gerber, G., Preissler, H., Heinrich, R. and Rapoport, S., *Europ. J. Biochem.*, in press.
148 Kühn, B., Jacobasch, G. and Rapoport, S., *Europ. J. Biochem.*, in press.
149 Kühn, B., Jacobasch, G. and Rapoport, S., *FEBS Letters*, in press.
150 Smith, C. M. and Velick, S. F., *J. Biol. Chem.*, **247**, 273 (1972).
151 Heinrich, R. and Rapoport, T., *Europ. J. Biochem.* (1973), in press.
152 Heinrich, R. and Rapoport, T., *Europ. J. Biochem.* (1973), in press.
153 Rapoport, T., Heinrich, R., Jacobasch, G. and Rapoport, S., *Europ. J. Biochem.* (1973), in press.

The Metabolism of the Reticulocyte

S. M. Rapoport, S. Rosenthal, T. Schewe, M. Schultze and M. Miller

Institute of Physiological and Biological Chemistry, Humboldt University, Berlin, GDR

The reticulocyte is defined as an intermediate stage of maturation of the red cell, which is characterized by the inactivation or elimination of the nucleus on the one hand, and on the other by the presence of functional ribosomes and mitochondria. The transition of the erythrocyte occurs by way of the complete degradation of the ribosomes and the mitochondria, the partial breakdown of the cell membrane and the selective decay of key enzymes of the organelles and the cytosol. The degradation is realized by degrading enzymes, primarily ribonucleases, proteases and phospholipases which are inhibited or masked by specific factors. In the selective inhibition of respiration, two inhibitory proteins are instrumental, which are also inactivated during the course of maturation.

The reticulocyte is an excellent model for the study of the energy metabolism of cells. Its physiological metabolic fuels are primarily amino acids, which orginate both from the endogenous breakdown of organelles and from active transport from the plasma. The most important external source of carbon and nitrogen is glutamine. The mechanism of the Pasteur effect and the fate of the amino group of amino acids have been elucidated.

INTRODUCTION

The formation of the erythrocyte is perhaps the best-studied example of a differentiation and maturation process in a multicellular organism. After many years of investigation by morphological methods, it has become lately the subject of extensive experimental research, in particular by biochemical methods. The most detailed knowledge exists on the reticulocyte, which represents a comparatively long-lived intermediate stage of the maturation process. This cell, originally defined empirically by its characteristic network, when stained with basic dyes[1)] can now be characterized on the basis of an understanding of the nature of the maturational changes of the red cell. This maturation process is characterised by two basic features: 1) the synthesis of a specialised protein, hemoglobin, in large amounts 2) the complete or nearly complete elimination or inactivation of the cellular organelles. In the process, their specific functions are also lost. The initial step is a differentiation of the stem cell, most often localised in the bone marrow, which is induced by erythropoetin (see the chapter by Takaku *et al.*). Hormonal induction appears to be a general phenomenon in all types of differentiation. A morphologically distinct cell type, the proerythroblast is produced. All subsequent processes can be defined as maturational. They are characterized by progressive dissociation of the synthesis of RNA from both DNA duplication and protein formation.[1–8] During the next stage, that of the basophilic erythroblast, synthesis of RNA declines and the nucleolus disappears, whereupon the transfer of RNA from the nucleus to the cytoplasm ceases. From the next stage on, that of the polychromatic erythroblast, the complement of cells with ribosomes, mitochondria, mRNA and tRNA can no longer be replenished by synthetic processes. Their lifetime limits the amount and duration of the terminal protein synthesis. Processes of degradation become prominent. The nucleus becomes increasingly pycnotic, but division continues. The cessation of DNA synthesis, whenever it occurs during the maturational sequence, signifies the transition of the reticulocyte stage. Thus, this type of cell may be defined as any nucleated or anucleate cell without DNA synthesis, but still containing functional ribosomes and mitochondria in its cytoplasm. In sauropsids the inactive nucleus remains as a relict, while it is expelled, presumably after an atypical division, in mammalia.[9–10]

The reticulocytes may differ in size, RNA and hemoglobin content, depending as to whether inactivation or expulsion of the nucleus occurs in the stage of the normoblast or the polychromatic erythroblast.[11–13] There are indications that the transition to the reticulocyte may even occur at the level of the basophilic erythroblast. The reticulocyte differs from the most immature cells in two other respects. 1) There is no longer any endoplasmic reticulum, which is still present even though not prominently, in the proerythroblast, and 2) it has only relicts of lysosomes, the cytoplasmic vacuoles.[14–16] The enzymes usually found in lysosomes, *i.e.*, hydrolases with acid pH optima, are to be found mostly in the cytosol or attached to the cell membrane. The last stage of maturation is the transformation of the reticulocyte to the erythrocyte. It is characterized by the disappearance of ribosomes, mitochondria and the cytoplasmic vacuoles, whereby protein synthesis and respiration functions vanish, by the selective partial or complete loss of synthetic faculties, of membrane carriers and individual

TABLE I. A comparison of main constituents and metabolic pathways in reticulocytes and erythrocytes.

Constituent		Reticulocyte	Erythrocyte	Remarks
RNA	mg/ml	25– 4	0.3	
Hemoglobin	,,	300–200	330	
Non-Hb Prot.	,,	45	15	
Lipid	,,	9	5	
Pathway				
RNA synthesis		—	—	
Protein synthesis		+	—	
Heme synthesis		+	—	
Purine synthesis		+	—	some enzymes remain
Pyrimidine synthesis		+	—	
Glycogen synthesis		—	—	
Glycogenolysis		—	—	
Lipid synthesis		(+)	—	Weak in reticulocytes; only phosphatidic acid synthesized in erythrocytes
Respiration		+	—	
Citrate cycle		+	—	some enzymes remain
Glycolysis		+	+	decreased
Gluconeogenesis		—	—	
OPP pathway		+	+	decreased
Fatty acid breakdown		+	—	
Amino acid catabolism		+	—	GPT remains
Active transport amino acids		+	(+)	some carriers remain
Active transport cations		+	+	

enzymes of the cytosol. A comparison between the reticulocyte and the erythrocyte regarding the main constituents and the metabolic pathway, is given in Table I.

Since differentiation and maturation occur in practically every cell type of a multinucleate organism, be it during embryogenesis or in later life in germinal centers, the conclusions from studies on the maturation of the red cell are likely to have general significance.

THE ORGANELLES

1) *Ribosomes and RNA*

SRF and RNA: It took nearly 70 years to establish a definite connection between the characteristically staining material. SRF (Substantia reticulofilamentosa), on the one hand and RNA on the other. In 1936 the occurrence of RNA in the reticulocyte was demonstrated cytophotometrically,[17] but only 20 years later was chemical proof furnished[18] when ribosomes were isolated,[19,20] and the SRF was demonstrated to be an artifact[21,22] and proved to be precipitated ribosomes.[23,14] The amount and appearance of the SRF has been the basis of classification of reticulocytes.[24] There is, under well-defined conditions, a proportionality between the amount of brilliant cresyl blue taken up by reticulocytes and their content of RNA.[21,22] Staining with acridine orange[25] and electron microscopic procedures[26] are more sensitive than brilliant cresyl blue.

Reticulocyte-rich blood or cell suspensions contain 0.1–1.0 gm of RNA/100 ml cells.[18,20,27,28] With increasing maturity, the concentration of RNA declines to values of 10–35 mg/100 ml cells in erythrocytes.[18,20,29,30] The distribution of the RNA also varies during maturation. In immature cells as much as 35% is stroma-bound.[31] Of the RNA in the stroma-free supernatant fluid, 80% is located in ribosomes, 7% in a post-ribosomal fraction, which may represent breakdown products, and 12% is located in the cytosol[29]; this is mostly tRNA.[32] In erythrocytes, nearly 50% is accounted for by the RNA of the cytosol.[29]

The Ribosomes: Among eucaryotes, the ribosomes of reticulocytes and of liver have been standard objects of study.[33,34] They represent nearly spherical bodies (dimensions are 200×185 Å in negative, 180×150 Å in positive contrast) which consist of a larger and a smaller subunit. *In situ*, most ribosomes are arranged in clusters, known as polysomes, of 4–6 with a predominance of pentamers.[35–38] *In situ*, these are frequently arranged in a ring form. In more mature reticulocytes the number of polysome clusters diminishes and eventually only monosomes are found. The number of ribosomes may be calculated from the RNA content to be 3,000/μm^3 in immature reticulocytes and one-hundredth of this number in the old reticulocytes of normal blood.

The sedimentation constant of the monosomes and their subunits is the same as that of others of eucaryotic origin, 78–82 S.[39,40]; older monosomes are supposed to show a lower sedimentation constant of 62 S. Their density ranges from 1.560–1.680.[40] The protein content is from 48–51%, depending on the washing procedure.[41] So far, about 50 different protein species have been identified, which differ from those of *E. coli* in showing a preponderance of acid proteins and of those of molecular weight larger than 40,000.[42] There does not appear to be any change in the protein/RNA ratio during maturation or in different stages of anemia, except under the influence of actinomycin.[43a,b] The protein content of ribosomes prepared from reticulocytes 48 hours after the administration of actinomycin *in vivo* is nearly doubled. The ribosomes contain 3 rRNA species, the 28 S of the larger (58 S) subunit, the 18 S of the smaller (40 S), and the 5 S RNA.[44,45] Their molecular weights are 1.5×10^6, 0.5×10^6 and about 5×10^4, respectively.[46,47] Their RNA's exhibit a pronounced secondary structure, with about 70% double-stranded sections.[48,51] The prevalence of G-C pairs is greatest in the 28 S and smallest in the 5 S RNA.[43,44] In the single-stranded sections of both 18 and 28 S there is a predominance of purine bases, while the number of pyrimidines corresponds to that of the total RNA. In the 5 S RNA there is a prevalence of C. There is an extreme polarization of the bases in the double-stranded sections of the 28 S RNA, with clusters of 5–8 U and A nucleotides, respectively; a corresponding clustering of the G-C bases is postulated.[8,49] The proteins interact extensively with both the single-stranded and double-stranded sections of the RNA. Presumably the peripheral proteins of the ribosomes are attached to the single-stranded regions, while the inner (core) proteins interact with the double-stranded sections. Corresponding to the model derived from sectrophotometric studies and studies on the enzymatic breakdown of RNA,[48–51] the electron microscopically determined length of the rRNA is reduced by 50 to 60% of that calculated from the number of bases.[52]

Stroma-bound Ribosomes: Burka and co-workers reported originally[31] that, independed of the type, on hemolysis about 30% of the cellular RNA is to be found in the stroma in the form of membrane-bound ribosomes, which differ from those of the cytosol with respect to their physicochemical and functional characteristics. In later communications, variable amounts of stroma-bound RNA were reported (11–27%).[53,54] A decline from 30 to 10% during maturation was found others.[55] The membrane-bound ribosomes are reported to be richer in protein, and to contain a higher percentage of heavy polysomes, which are more resistant to ribonuclease action and to lowering of Mg^{2+} concentration.[53] They exhibit a lower rate of incorporation of ^{32}P and of labeled amino acids and are supposed to synthesise an undefined, nonhemoglobin protein having a molecular weight larger than hemoglobin.[56] These claims are open to some criticism. The protein/RNA ratios reported for the cytosolic ribosomes are higher than those found by other groups. The possibility of secondary adsorption of proteins and membranes appears not to have been excluded. The lower rates of synthesis would only be convincing if they were compared on the basis of RNA. Membrane binding *in situ* has not been demonstrated. It is conceivable that ribosomes are attached to filaments arising from the inner membrane.[57)]

a) The Relation between Magnesium and RNA Content

It is known from various studies that a minimal ratio of Mg^{2+}/RNA-P of 0.2 is necessary for the stability of the monosomes and the formation of polysomes with natural mRNA.[33)] Magnesium binding by ribosomes depends on the relationship between monovalent ions, *i.e.*, the intracellular K^+, and the Mg^{2+} concentration, which is also influenced by low and high molecular complexing agents, in particular ATP.[58)] Considering these facts the changes in magnesium concentration during maturation are most interesting. Total magnesium in reticulocytes may exceed 14 m*M*, but it is only 2–3 m*M* in erythrocytes.[59a~c,60)] Based on a content of 30 m*M* of RNA-P in reticulocytes, about 9 m*M* magnesium are ribosome bound with a Mg^{2+}/RNA-P ratio of 0.3. If the 2.5-fold concentration of ATP is also considered, it appears likely that the level of free Mg^{2+} does not differ greatly between reticulocytes and erythrocytes.

The nonribosomal RNA: A minor fraction, about 2% is mRNA, which occurs attached to the polysomes as an mRNA-protein complex[61,62)] and is up to 90% globin messenger. About 20% is found in post-ribosomal fractions.[29,32)] The amount increases relatively and absolutely with maturation of the reticulocytes.[27)] The increase may result from the breakdown of ribosomes, both by liberation of rRNA-split products 55RNA[43)] and ribosome-bound tRNA. In erythrocytes the postribosomal fractions predominate. The occurrence of tRNA is indicated by the base ratios, etc.[63,32)] The pattern of the tRNA's corresponds to the amino acid composition of globin.[64)] It would appear that tRNA and 55RNA are more slowly degraded than other RNA species.

Formation and degradation of RNA: There is little specific information about the formation of RNA during maturation of the red cells except for the time course. Formation of rRNA and tRNA are early events while the mRNA for globin is synthesized at least 24 hours later.[65)] The formation of other types of mRNA preceding that for globin is indicated.[38] In the reticulocytes there is only a renewal of the -pC_3pC_2pA end of tRNA, with a turnover rate of 4–8 hours for A and 30 hours for the C_2.[63]

During incubation of reticulocytes *in vitro* there is a decline of RNA (*in vitro* maturation).[66,67] With preference to the liberation of pyrimidine bases as would be expected from the properties of the ribosomal pyrimidine-specific ribonuclease. In hemolysates, on the other hand, there is less total breakdown with increasing share of the purines.[66] It is possible that this is due both to inhibition of the ribonuclease by its inhibitor in the cytosol and the unmasking of the membrane-bound diesterase. The beakdown leads to the formation of uracil and hypoxanthine[68] as a result of the action of phosphatases and nucleoside phosphorylases, while the degradation of cytosinenucleotides appears to stop with cytidine.[69]

b) The Protein Synthesis of the Reticulocyte

It is not intended to discuss here the mechanism and regulation of hemoglobin synthesis (see the chapter by London). Comment will be limited to some remarks on the question of which factors contribute to the decline of protein synthesis during maturation. The faculty for protein synthesis is larger in immature as compared with the most mature reticulocytes and vanishes completely in the erythrocytes.[70–43a~c] It would appear that neither the amount of ribosomes, nor of mRNA or tRNA are by themselves limiting.[73,74] This is indicated by the fact that addition of protein-containing wash solution from immature reticulocytes may stimulate amino acid incorporation by ribosomes from old reticulocytes up to 3-fold.[75] It would appear that the limitation resides in the factors participating in the initiation reactions of peptide synthesis. In addition, inhibitory factors may be instrumental.[76,78,72] For the synthesis of non-hemoglobin protein, on the other hand, the amount of mRNA's coding for them may be limiting.

2) The Mitochondria

In recent years, increasing information on the mitochondria of reticulocytes with regard to their morphological, chemical and functional properties has become available.[79] These studies appear of general interest since these objects are the best available for the investigation of the ageing and degradation process of mitochondria. In general, they do not differ significantly in their appearance from those of other mitochondria of animal origin. The average area in electron microscopic cuts is 0.07–0.015 μ^2, similar to that of liver mitochondria.[80] Their number, if related to the volume, is probably also equal and so is the amount of mitochondrial protein (30 mg/ml cells) if the immature reticulocyte is considered. Both numbers and levels of mitochondrial protein are less in more mature cells.

The mitochondria of immature reticulocytes exhibit *in situ* mostly orthodox structures with a loose matrix. But there occur also both condensed and vacuolized forms in the same cell.[81a,b,26] In the more mature cells, degraded forms predominate. The degradation involves particularly the cristae and the matrix. Some of the mitochondria contain ferritin granula, perhaps as an expression of an inhibition of heme synthesis.

Isolated mitochondria are likewise multiform. There appears to exist a correlation between the specific activity of succinate dehydrogenase (SDH) and the form of the mitochondria. Those with the highest enzyme activity are predominantly of the condensed type and those with intermediate activity of the orthodox type, while the cells with the lowest SDH activity exhibit mostly degraded forms.[82] The chemical composition of isolated mitochondria shows interesting characteristics if compared with that in the liver (see Table II).[80] It can be seen that their content of cytochromes b, c and c_1 is about double that of rat liver mitochondria.[83] Correspondingly the cytochrome oxidase activity is 2–4 times as high, even though the cyt. a peak is hard to visualise. The content of phospholipids is more than twice as high; it is even higher than that of heart mitochondria. Even in preparations with pre-

TABLE II. Comparision of mitochondria of rabbit reticulocytes with these of rat liver.

Component	Amount/μ moles/mg Protein	Quotient Reti/liver
Cytochrome oxidase	0.3–0.6[1)]	2.4
Cytochrome b	0.58	1.8
Cytochrome c_1	0.42	2.2
Cytochrome c	0.65	1.8
CoQ	1.45	1.0
Phospholipid	0.37[2)]	2.6
NAD^+	0.16	0.04
NADP	0.47	0.09

1) μ moles cyt c/min per mg Protein oxidized.

2) mg/mg Protein.

ponderantly degraded forms there are only traces of lysophosphatides to be found, indicating that phospholipase A_2 activity may be limiting as compared with lysophospholipase. On the other hand, there is a comparatively high percentage of free fatty acids. Their amount appears to be correlated with the proportion of degraded forms.

The mitochondria show only slight incorporation of linoleate.[84] This may well be due to the preceding degradation of the endoplasmic reticulum, which is where, in other cells, the synthesis of mitochondrial lipids takes place. The isolated mitochondria are extremely depleted of both NAD^+ and $NADP^+$ and require the addition of the pyridine nucleotides for function.[85a~c] Their respiratory characteristics correspond to those of other animal mitochondria. They contain the enzymes of the citrate cycle and are capable of oxidizing fatty acids and glutamate. Oxaloacetate is a particularly good substrate. Even earlier, direct and indirect evidence for the occurrence of both enzymes and substrates of the citrate cycle and of other components usually found in mitochondria had been obtained.[86–90b] A peculiarity appears to be the mitochondrial (*i.e.*, stroma-bound) localization of the $NADP^+$-dependent isocitrate dehydrogenase,[89,90b] while no NAD^+-dependent ICDH is found. The activity of the ICDH is high compared with liver mitochondria, similar to that of heart mitochondria. Glutamate dehydrogenase on the other hand behaves in a reverse manner. It is low in the mitochondria of reticulocytes and of heart as compared with those of liver.[85b] Functional intact mitochondria from rabbit reticulocytes contain considerable amounts of hexokinase. Hexokinase activity of mitochondria is in average about 0.13 I.U./mg mitochondrial protein. Freshly isolated mitochondria contain about 70% of the total hexokinase activity of the whole cells.[85a~c]

3) *The Cell Membrane*

No analysis of the isolated cell membrane of reticulocytes has been published so far. The stroma as usually obtained is predominantly a mixture of cell membrane and mitochondria with a complement of stroma-bound ribosomes. The cell membrane contains as a characteristic component an acid phosphatase which is sensitive to fluoride inhibition.[91,92] It exhibits an active incorporation of linoleate in phospholipids, mostly lecithin, which is 4 times as large as that of the erythrocyte.[84] Functionally it is characterized by the presence of carriers for amino acids,[93–96] and glucose,[97] which are either greatly reduced or absent in the erythrocyte.

4) The Cytosol

The cytosol of the reticulocyte, when compared with the erythrocyte, is characterized by a much greater activity of some of the enzymes of glycolysis and of the OPP pathway.[87,98–109] Consequently the reticulocyte possesses a much higher capacity for glucose utilization than the erythrocyte. Particularly striking are the differences with respect to the enzymes controlling the initial steps of the pathways, HK and GPD. A number of enzymes exhibit additional molecular forms in the reticulocyte. These include HK, PFK, PK and also LDH.[99,109–111] Furthermore a high-K_M HK has been found.[112] Among others, a particularly high activity of inorganic PPase should be noted.[113]

The overall content of ATP, is about 3 times higher than in the erythrocyte.[114] A separate analysis for the cytosol has not been carried out, but it is likely that most of the ATP is in the cytosol. Higher concentration of glutathione have also been observed.[115]

THE DEGRADING AND INACTIVATING FACTORS

From the above account, one can conclude that the main processes of maturation of the reticulocyte are the complete degradation of ribosomes and mitochondria, the partial breakdown of the cell membranes and the selective decline of enzymes of the cytosol. The major factor responsible for this degradation is the action of nucleases, proteinases and phospholipases. Their characteristics will be described in this section. The specificity of the onset and time course of the degradation and the selectivity of the changes led to the assumption of the existence of specific factors which might be instrumental in bringing about the selective decay of the characteristic properties of the reticulocyte. This became apparent when reticulocytes and erythrocytes were compared with respect to their enzyme equipment. It was found that the loss of metabolic pathways was caused by the loss of some but not all of the participant enzymes. The search for such factors led to the discovery of two inhibitory proteins of the respiratory chain. One of them, inhibitor F, inhibits both SDH and NADH oxidase systems of mitochondria, the other, inhibitor C, acts on the cytochrome oxidase. Their properties and a mechanism by which enzymes with sensitive and essential SH groups might be inactivated will also be discussed.

7) *The Nucleases*

Enzymes degrading either RNA or DNA have been observed in various types of red cells. Studies relating the enzyme activity to the maturation process were mostly carried out on the rabbit. The results are difficult to assess in a quantitative manner owing to several complicating factors. The enzymes appear to be located in various cell fractions, with most of their activity masked. This is partly caused by a well-defined inhibitor of ribonuclease in the cytosol. Furthermore, the enzymes are highly sensitive to variations of ionic strength. In addition there is the problem of the existence of an endogenous substrate for the enzymatic attack, the accessibility of which depends on the experimental conditions, and lastly the difficulties of comparing various methods for the determination of the enzymatic activity. In this section the enzymes and their inhibitors are reviewed briefly only to the extent that appears germane to the maturational process.

A. The Ribonucleases and Their Inhibitors

So far, two ribonucleases have been clearly defined in the reticulocytes of rabbits.

1. The Pyrimidine-specific Endonuclease with a pH Optimum of 7.5

This enzyme corresponds in some properties to the type I pancreatic ribonuclease.[41,48,58,116,117a,b] The pyrimidine-specific RNases of rabbit reticulocytes and pancreas differ considerably from each other in the molecular structure and in the mechanism of cleavage. The reticulocyte enzyme has a molecular weight of 25,000 daltons, but is not a dimer of pancreatic RNase. Its mobility in the electrophoresis is lower owing to a smaller charge compared with the enzyme of pancreas. The reticulocyte RNase is also more sensitive against temperatures above 65°C and reduction of its disulfide bridges. Clusters of pyrimidine bases are split by this enzyme preferentially. The primary products of cleavage of uracil oligonucleotides are a trinucleotide and the corresponding residue. It is found in ribosomes and cannot be washed away by 0.5 *M* NH_4Cl. This enzyme is responsible for the self-degradation of ribosomes which may be observed *in vitro*. It attacks only singlestranded sections of the RNA. It is practically inactive at low ionic strength; maximal activity is found at 0.15 *M* KCl. For this reason apparently, it has escaped detection by some observers.[118] Mg^{2+} ions (0.01 *M*) do not affect the breakdown of free RNA, but will inhibit the self-degradation of ribosomes. It is likely from all other properties that an enzyme activity with a pH optimum of 8.2 refers to the same protein.[119] This ribonuclease has a pronounced dependency on maturation, and only traces of any activity are left in erythrocytes.

2. *The Acid Phosphodiesterase of the Stroma*

The occurrence of a stroma-bound enzyme activity with a pH optimum of 6.5[120] was reported in rabbit reticulocytes. It was later characterized[121] and partly purified.[10] It is a base-nonspecific diesterase which produces 3′-nucleotides. This enzyme also shows a pronounced decline on maturation to one-thirtieth of its previous level. An enzyme from rat reticulocytes with a pH optimum of 6.5–7.5 may also belong to the same class.[122] Both the enzymes from rabbit and rat reticulocytes are largely masked by RNase inhibitors, which may be inactivated by various means.[123,124]

3. *Other Enzyme Activities*

A further enzyme activity corresponding to a pyrimidine-specific endonuclease has been described in the cytosol, which is similar in its properties to ribosomal RNase.[125] It is uncertain whether it represents a third type of enzyme, or differs only in location from the ribosomal ribonuclease. This enzyme activity also declines with maturation. Lastly, enzyme activities with a pH optimum of 5.4 were described in the bone marrow of rabbits[120] and in chicken reticulocytes. The latter was purified 560-fold.[126]

The RNase inhibitors: The presence of inhibitory proteins for RNase in various tissues is well-known. An inhibitory activity in the cytosol was also described in reticulocytes of rabbits and in small amounts in erythrocytes of various species.[127–129] The inhibitory protein was partially purified.[129] It will inhibit type I RNases of animal origin but not T_1 RNase or type I of *E coli*. A similar inhibitory protein has been demonstrated in rat reticulocytes.[122,123] The inhibitory activity also declines with maturation. The inhibitor appears to contain essential and accessible SH groups.

The inhibitory effect of hemin in low concentration on RNase, which may be of biological significance, should be mentioned.[125,130]

The DNases: In bone marrow and in reticulocytes of anemic rabbits stroma-bound DNase activity has been found.[120,131,132] The pH optimum is at pH 5.0, but there may be additional enzymes with higher pH optima. The enzyme is independent of Mg^{2+}. The enzyme activity is nearly completely masked in hemolysates owing to an inhibitory effect of hemoglobin which apparently forms complexes with the DNA which are protected from enzymatic attack. Similar enzymes have been described in the red cells of amphibia and snakes, where their activity is also completely masked.[133–135] The biological significance of the enzyme may be connected with the expulsion in mammals of the nucleus, which may be disintegrated after its extraction, and in the breakdown of mitochondrial DNA.

2) *The Proteinases*

In early reports a much greater proteinase activity was found in reticulocytes of rabbit and man than in erythrocytes.[136,137] Only the proteinase activity with a pH optimum of about pH 3.5 appears to reside in the red cell, while enzyme activities with pH optima of 7.5 and 10.5[138,139] appear to be due to contamination with leucocytes.[143a] In later studies the characteristics of some of the multitude of enzymes and their changes on maturation were further detailled. The most important *endopeptidase* appears to be a cathepsin which exhibits a pH optimum of 3.5.[140,143a] It is a specific enzyme resembling cathepsin A in its specificity, and has been purified extensively.[143a~c] It is strongly maturity-dependent and is no longer found in the mature erythrocyte. It is localised in the stroma. It is subject to inhibition by GSSG and phenylhydrazine,[141,142] and in a purified state by dithioerythritol.

A multitude of exopeptidases have been described in red cells.[143b] They include gly-gly, gly-leu, imino and imido dipeptidases, amino tripeptidase and leucine aminopeptidase. Their activities are 1 to 3 orders of magnitude higher than those of the endopeptidases. Their pH optima are extremely broad, so that they will exert nearly maximal activity at physiological pH values. They are localised in the cytosol. Since most of these enzymes are localised in the lysosomes of other cells, a primary lysosomal location in earlier stages of maturation of the red cell may be surmised.

The maturation dependence of exopeptidases varies greatly. It is as great as that of the marker enzyme GOT in the case of gly-gly, gly-leu, and imino dipeptidases, wherease imido dipeptidase and amino tripeptidase do not change. Leucine aminopeptidases decrease steeply with maturation in the human red cell, but only slightly in that of the rabbit. The connection of the various enzymes with energy-dependent proteolysis, which furnishes amino acids both for energy metabolism and hemoglobin synthesis, is by no means clear.[144,145] There are some indications that the activity of the proteinases may be masked and unmasked in a manner which is still not clear.

3) The Phospholipases

These enzymes may be presumed to play an important role in maturation processes both in the degradation of mitochondria and of the cellular membranes. Unfortunately, however, there is a complete lack of information on their occurrence and activity in the reticulocyte. Indirect evidence for their activity may be seen in the occurrence of free fatty acids both in mitochondria and in the cytosol, in the decline of the phospholipid content of the red cell during maturation and in the appearance of degraded forms of the mitochondria. These are very similar to forms which may be observed if rat-liver mitochondria are exposed to the action of phospholipase A_2.[146] The occurrence of this enzyme in the outer membrane of mitochondria has been described.[147] In mature rat erythrocytes a phospholipase A_2 has also been described,[148] which may have become located in the cytosol by a secondary process. A membrane-bound lysophospholipase has been observed in human erythrocytes.[149]

4) The Protein Inhibitors of Respiration

Inhibitor F: The presence of this inhibitor has been demonstrated in stroma-free hemolysates of reticulocytes from rabbits,[150,151] and in much smaller amounts in blood cells from anemic chicken[152] and man.[153] No inhibitory activity is demonstrable in red cells from nonanemic blood. However, the detection of traces may be vitiated by the presence of stimulatory respiration factors which are present in mature cells. If experimental anemia is produced by repeated bleeding, the inhibitory activity will appear only after the first peak of reticulocytosis with the outpouring of small (normocytic) reticulocytes,[154] which exhibit extremely high rates of respiration.[155,156] With prolongation of bleeding the inhibitory activity may persist at a high level or decline slowly. There is generally less inhibitory activity if anemia is produced by administration of phenylhydrazine, possibly because of the oxidative destruction of inhibitor F. So far the inhibitor has been purified about 1,000-fold, without as yet achieving homogeneity.[153]

In Table III, some of the properties of inhibitor F are listed.[153,156–158] The estimates of its molecular weight are based on gel filtration, which also indicated a rather uniform size for the molecules. The content of divalent nonheme iron was deduced from the inactiva-

TABLE III. Properties of inhibitor F.

Molecular weight	100,000
Functional groups	Fe (II); SH
Inactivators	SH reagents; oxidants, phospholipids, serum albumins
Action site in the respiratory chain	Fe (III) of the flavin enzyme-associated "iron-sulfur proteins"

ting effect of carbon monoxide, EDTA, o-phenanthroline and other more-or-less selective metal chelators. It has now been confirmed by direct iron analysis.[153] Recently we discovered that serum albumins from man, rabbit and beef suppress the action of inhibitor F in a proportional manner over the range 0.1–1.0%; the biological significance of this effect is obscure.[153] The inhibitor contains essential SH groups and is highly autoxidizable, the more so the purer the preparation.[157]

The finding that the inhibitor F preparations show heterogeneity, *i.e.*, several well-defined activity peaks on ion-exchange resins despite a uniform molecular weight is most intriguing. This is actually what one would expect with any cellular protein which is subject to a decay process, such as inhibitor F itself. We may assume that the various fractions arise from a stepwise terminal proteolytic degradation during the maturation process within the red cell. Thereby a family of "isoproteins" are formed which exhibit biological activity and possess about the same molecular weight but differ in the number of charged groups. The fraction with the largest cationic charge, may well be the last proteolytic product which still exhibits biological activity. It is characterized by great lability and was only discovered after rigorous exclusion of heavy metals and oxygen in all phases of fractionation. We assume it to have a loosened secondary structure, which may make it susceptible to further extensive degradation.

Inhibitor F will suppress nearly completely both the NADH and the succinate systems of intact swollen mitochondria of various origins and electron-transporting particles (ETP).[150,151,159] It will partially inhibit crude soluble SDH[160] and the artificial NADH-cyt c reductase (Mahler enzyme).[161] From a comparison of various systems, its point of action has been determined to be trivalent iron (Fe^{3+}) in the iron-sulfur proteins of the SDH and the NADH-CoQ reductase, respectively (Fig. 1). Its effect is additive in the succinate system with that of

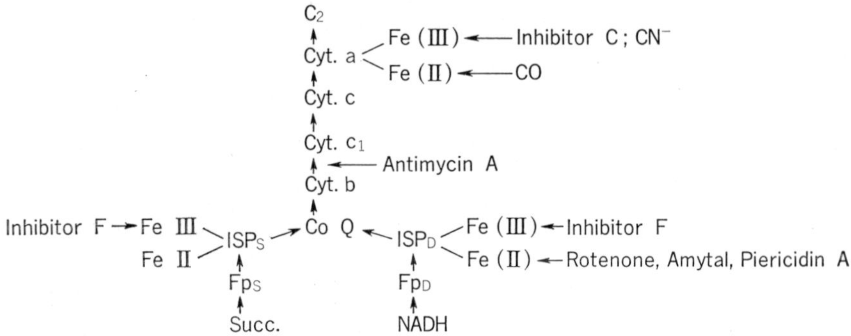

Fig. 1. Scheme of the action sites of inhibitors F and C.

TTFA, and with those of rotenone and amytal in the NADH systems.[159] The reaction rate is slow as compared with low-molecular inhibitors. It takes 15–45 minutes for completion, depending on the type of mitochondrial preparation. The effect is approximately proportional to the amount of inhibitor used and is irreversible. One may conclude, therefore, that there occurs a stochiometric reaction to form a complex with the iron-sulfur proteins, perhaps in the form of an Fe^{2+}-Fe^{3+} charge-transfer complex, as it exists in prussian blue. One may assume that the inhibition is produced by the suppression of valency change in the iron-sulfur proteins. The molar activity of inhibitor F may be estimated to be as high as that of rotenone with a K_i of 5 nM. In addition to the specific binding, there is also nonspecific binding to the ETP proteins, as indicated by the action of chaotropic agents.

As mentioned before, in mature erythrocytes inhibitor F is no longer present. It was shown that inhibitor F is inactivated by various phospholipids in a stoichiometric reaction, preferentially by phosphatidyl ethanolamine and phosphatidylserine containing highly unsaturated fatty acids.[157,158] It would appear that the phospholipids liberated from the mitochondria and the cell membrane during maturation cause inactivation of inhibitor F. Proteases and phospholipases also breakdown inhibitor F and its inactive complex with phospholipids.

It may be assumed that such phospholipids are liberated by the action of proteases during the maturation process, since native stroma of reticulocytes do not affect inhibitor F. It may be mentioned that similar inhibitors have been discovered in various tissues including testicles, mammary glands and the placenta, organs which also exhibit maturation and involution processes.[162]

B. Inhibitor C

The second inhibitory protein, inhibitor C has been studied much less extensively.[163,164] It resembles inhibitor F with respect to its molecular weight, and the inactivating effect of phospholipids and of EDTA. It is therefore presumed to be also an iron protein. It differs from inhibitor F by being activated rather than inhibited by serum albumin and in its dose-effect curve, which is not stoichiometric. Partial separation of the two inhibitors has been achieved. It will act only on the oxidized form of cytochrome oxidase; the presence of oxygen however, is not necessary. Both particle-bound and solubilized cytochrome oxidase will be inhibited. This inhibitor also disappears completely during maturation. The mechanism of its inactivation has not been studied.

5) Inactivation of Proteins with Sensitive SH Groups

Another possible mechanism of enzyme decay may be related to the fact that SH groups are essential for the structure or function of many proteins, whether or not these groups are parts of an active center. It is of interest that enzymes with highly sensitive SH groups, such as HK, PK, GPD, PPase, cathepsin A, glutaminase, δ-ALA synthetase, and GK are among those which show the steepest decline during maturation.[165,166,168] This behaviour appears to be independent of their primary location in the cell. This correlation is, however, not without exceptions. Thus GAPD, which is one of the enzymes with the most sensitive SH groups, declines much less in its activity than the above group of enzymes.[167] In this case, and perhaps in others, the stability may be due to protection of the SH group by a coenzyme or substrate.[6,7,168] As far as the possible oxidants of the SH groups are concerned, at this time only speculation and model experiments are available. The oxidant effects of H_2O_2, superoxide radicals, and of GSSG have been described.[6,7,168] Partial protection is given by GSH and catalase. The actual conditions during maturation have not been defined, but it is likely that the presence of molecular oxygen is essential for the decay of enzymes.

There is also a reduction in the number of isoenzymes in several cases so far investigated. This may be connected with their original location in different cell compartments, *e.g.*, in the case of malate dehydrogenase.[169] It would also appear possible that the disappearance of particular isoenzymes is related to differences in the sensitivity of their SH groups.

THE DYNAMICS AND INTERPLAY OF MATURATIONAL CHANGES

1) Dimensional and Biochemical Differences among Reticulocytes and the Dynamics of Maturation

Indications of morphological and dimensional differences among reticulocytes have been noted by many observers. In this section they will be related to biochemical characteristics and the maturational process.

The normal total differentiation and maturation time of normoblastic erythropoesis is estimated to be 7.5 days.[170] Assuming 20 hours for each cell division there remain about 4 days for the reticulocyte stage. Normally the reticulocytes spend most of the time of their maturation in the bone marrow. Those in the peripheral blood, representing the last stage, differ little in their dimensions from normocytes. They are characterized by a low RNA concentration of 2–4 mg/ml cells,[23,171] and a low respiration.[23] A number of diverse stimuli may induce an outpouring of reticulocytes from the bone marrow, thereby abbreviating their stay there, while prolonging their maturation time in the peripheral blood. These cells are only little larger and more immature than the normal reticulocyte population. More intensive stimuli such as drastic bleeding or hemolysis will induce the outpouring in the peripheral blood of more immature reticulocytes and of those which arise from skipped cell divisions.[12,172–175] Such "stress-reticulocytes" are much larger than normal and may have a poor hemoglobin content.[23,114] The erythrocytes arising from megalo reticulocytes are also large; their survival time in the peripheral blood is much reduced.[43,176] Intensive blood loss and other stimuli may also lead to the activation of previously dormant fatty bone marrow, which will then produce a relatively immature red-cell population even during the recovery from anemia.[177–179]

A complex study was carried out to characterize the different types of reticulocytes which arise during the course of experimental anemia in the rabbit.[180a~h] The cells were fractionated in a density gradient, and their dimensional and biochemical characteristics were determined. The biochemical criteria were chosen so as to represent the ribosomes, the mitochondria and the cytosol. In this way for populations of reticulocytes which appear in sequence could be differentiated (see Fig. 2).[180a~h,181] 1) On the first day normal-sized reticulocytes with about

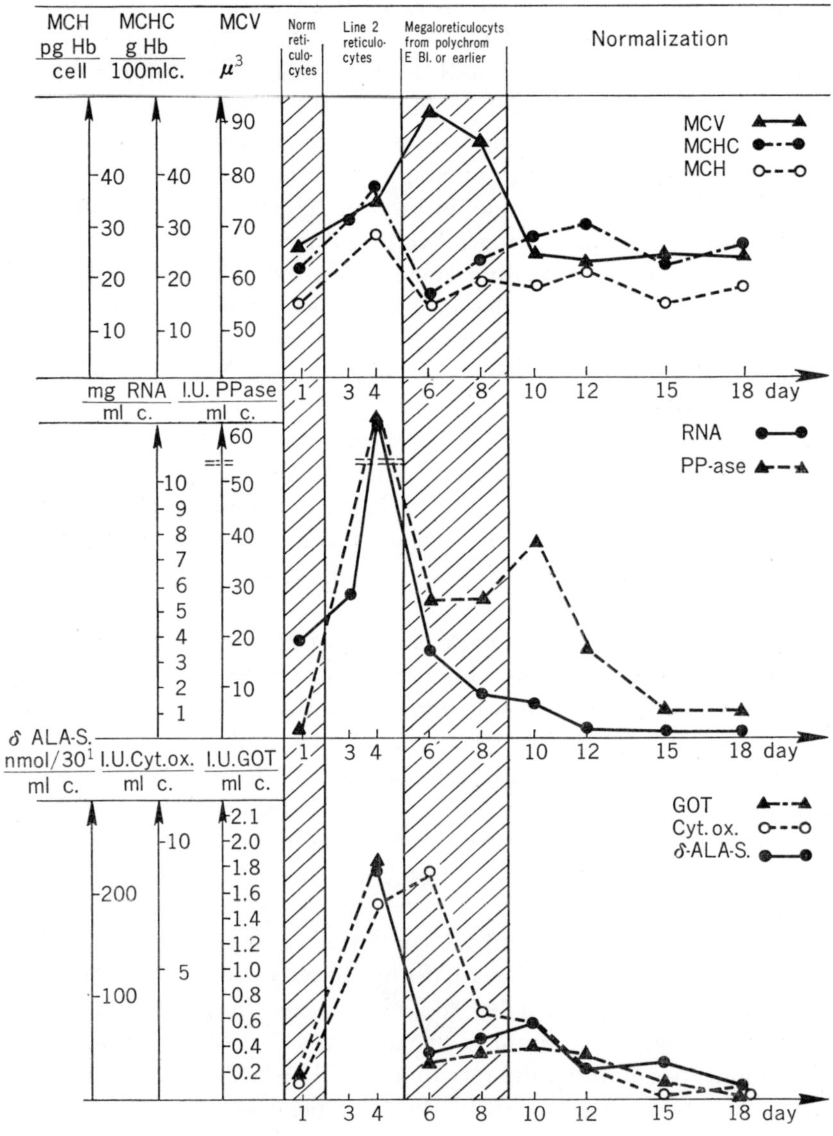

Fig. 2. Changes of cellular parameters and enzymes during, the course of an anemia of rabbits.

4 mgRNA/ml, which have low respiration and low levels of all enzymes investigated, 2) on the fourth day or even on the third, a nearly pure population of cells, which is little larger and fairly rich in hemoglobin.

It is characterized by an extremely large RNA content of 25 mgRNA/ml cells, high respiration and activity of mitochondrial enzymes as well as of the PPase of the cytosol, and by the absence of inhibitor F. They correspond to the "line 2" cells of Borsook.[12,182] 3) From the sixth day on there appear megaloreticulocytes with sizes 2 or 4 times as large as the normocytes, as a result of skipped divisions. These cells are characterized by a low hemoglobin level of 200 mg or less per ml cells, an RNA content of about 5 mg/ml cells and a respiration about half as large as those of the preceding stage. They exhibit high inhibitor F activity. 4) On the twelfth day or thereabouts, a population of large hemoglobin-rich cells with high cytochrome oxidase activity, not yet characterised fully, are produced. They originate presumably from newly activated bone marrow.

The variations in hemoglobin concentration explain the shifts in the distribution of the reticulocytes in a density gradient during the course of anemia. Due to the fact that the sequence of maturational changes is not identical for the various types of reticulocytes, a complex pattern results.

2) *The Pattern of Maturational Changes of Cellular Constituents*

While there is a general concurrence of changes in many constituents during maturation, it was noted early that there exist differences between various criteria.[13,61,183] In the complex study mentioned above, a more comprehensive picture was obtained.[180] It indicates that there exist differences among the criteria which characterize the ribosomes, the mitochondria and the cytosol. Among the constituents of one cellular compartment, in particular, mitochondria and cytosol differences also exist (see Fig. 3).

A number of mitochondrial constituents, represented by cytochrome oxidase, exhibit a plateau of high activity at all RNA concentrations in excess of 2 mg/ml cells.[180c] This indicates that there is no direct correlation between the number of ribosomes and of mitochondria in the various types of immature reticulocytes. The levels of these enzymes decline steeply to nearly zero in the last stages of maturation in the range of RNA concentrations below 1 mg/ml cells. In this class of constituents are included all participants of the respiratory chain which are located in the inner membrane of the mitochondria, which includes SDH, and also some components of the matrix of the mitochondria, such as GOT, δ-ALA synthetase and ICDH.[89a,b,99,184] The same behaviour is also shown by glutaminase[185,186] and DNase which may be part

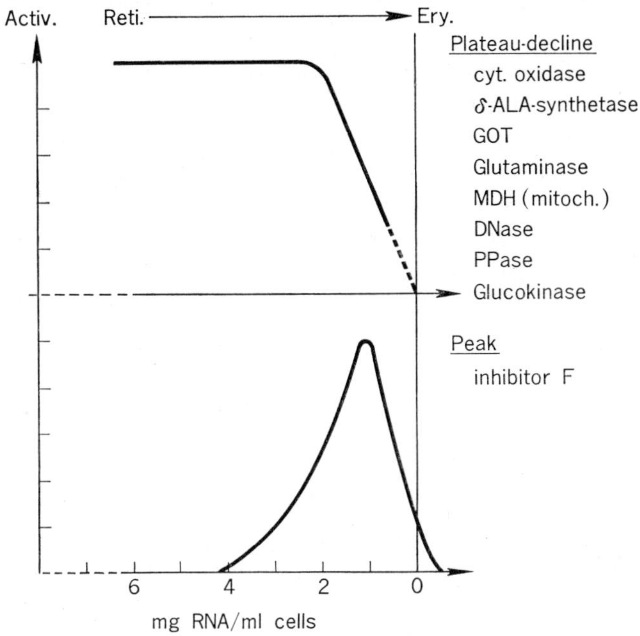

Fig. 3. Scheme of the changes of some enzymes and inhibitor F during maturation.

of the outer membrane. Levels of other mitochondrial enzymes of the matrix, such as fumarase,[86] decline very little. These enzymes may survive the degradation of the mitochondrium and so become constituents of the cytosol. The case of malate dehydrogenase is particularly interesting.[86,169,187] Apparently the mitochondrial enzyme, which accounts for half the activity in the reticulocyte, disappears, while the cytoplasmatic enzyme remains unchanged. The enzyme of the cytosol also show a great divergence. The steepest decline is found for GK and PPase.[180d] This pattern is similar to that of the mitochondrial enzymes. There is some indication that the megaloreticulocytes are particularly rich in PPase.[180e] HK and PK also decline by an order of magnitude while many others change only by a factor of three or less.

Characteristic behaviour is exhibited by inhibitor F. It is very low in its activity in the reticulocyte type 2 population, and it reaches a maximum at the time of the steepest decline of mitochondrial constituents.

3) *Life Span of Organelles and the Maturation Process*

Very interesting parallels may be drawn between the turnover times of organelles in the liver, which has been studied most thoroughly, and their changes during maturation of the red cell. In the liver ribosomes[188,189] and mitochondria[190,191] have biological half-lives of about 7 and 9 days, respectively. The biological half-life of the endoplasmic reticulum is about 3–5 days.[192] If similar life spans hold for the erythropoietic cells, and if the life time of the mRNA species for the synthesis of the organelles is short, one comes to the conclusion that with cessation of RNA synthesis at the stage of the basophilic erythroblast, new-formation of organelles is no longer possible. In that case both the ribosomes and the mitochondria of the reticulocyte may be considered to be near the end of their normal life span. The mechanism of their degradation in the reticulocytes may be representative for other cells. From these considerations, it would also follow that one cannot expect the presence of an endoplasmic reticulum in the reticulocytes derived from the normal maturation process of erythropoietic bone-marrow cells, owing to the short life span of this organelle. Differences in the life spans of the constituents of the mitochondrium[193,194] may be reflected in a varying pattern of decline of their amounts or activities during maturation.

4) *The Interplay of Factors during Maturation*

The time course and selectivity of the changes during maturation require a subtle regulation. One would postulate therefore the existence of reaction chains, which are triggered by key events and the interplay of activating and inhibiting factors. The degrading enzymes as well as the inhibiting and inactivating factors must exist in latent or masked states to come into action when required and to cease after a critical stage. The breakdown processes must be correlated with the synthesis of hemoglobin, as has in fact been found, thus providing an efficient amino acid economy in the cell.

At this time, only one chain of events, discernable in its outlines, is thought to be instrumental in bringing about the degradation of mitochondria and the cessation of respiration. It is summarized in the following scheme (Fig. 4). While the scale of the ordinates is arbitrary, the relative position of the curves corresponds to the actual course of events. It may be seen that respiration declines most steeply at the time of maximal activity of inhibitor F, which strongly supports the idea that the action of the inhibitor is the key event. It is also of interest

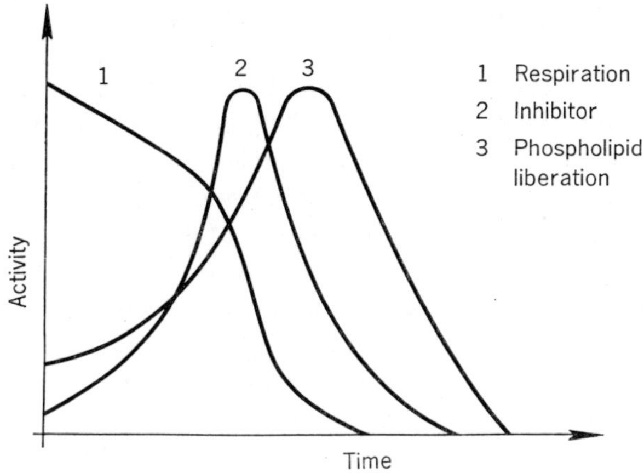

Fig. 4. Scheme of the decline of respiration, activity of inhibitor F, and the liberation of phospholipids.

that the second curve may be considered as a first derivative of the first curve. The third curve is somewhat hypothetical. It indicates the liberation of phospholipids, mainly from the breakdown of mitochondria. These are responsible for the inactivation of inhibitor F, which is absent in erythrocytes. Lately an additional factor has been discovered, which mediates the penetration of inhibitor F across the mitochondrial membranes. It was found that crude, but not purified, inhibitor F inhibits the respiratory chain of intact liver mitochondria, A protein, called the mitochondrial lysis factor, could be separated from both inhibitors F and C. This factor causes the disruption of the outer membranes and a complete disappearance of the inner structure.[195)]

THE REGULATION OF ENERGY METABOLISM OF THE RETICULOCYTE

From the preceding sections it will have become apparent that the reticulocyte contains the complete systems of both aerobic and anaerobic energy-yielding processes. In this section the following aspects will be dealt with: 1) The control of respiration, 2) the metabolic substrates and 3) their interrelations.

1) *Control of Respiration*

The oxygen uptake of the reticulocyte represents about 80% of mitochondrial respiration, the rest involving extramitochondrial pathways which have not been defined precisely.[196b,197] This conclusion is based on the extent of cyanide inhibition of respiration of about 80% on the one hand, and that of 20% produced by 3-amino-1,2,4-triazole, which may be selective for catalase, on the other. One would assume therefore that there may be as much as 20% of oxygen consumption connected with the formation of H_2O_2, presumably by the action of various extramitochondrial flavoproteins, such as NADPH oxidases.[198] Newer data (see chapter on catalase) indicate the existence of an antimycin A-resistent respiration, the organic substrates of which glucose, ribose, serine and glycine, yield $NADPH_2$.[196b]

The oxygen consumption of the reticulocyte varies according to its state of maturation, as judged by other criteria such as RNA content, and according to the stage of anemia. Furthermore there are differences between species. The oxygen consumption of human reticulocytes from cases of erythroblastosis fetalis is about one-third as large as that of those from anemic rabbits.[199] In other cases of reticulocytosis in patients (*e.g.*, pyruvate kinase deficiency) even lower values have been observed.

The values of oxygen consumption of chicken reticulocytes are in the same range of those from mammalian species.[200] The highest rates of oxygen uptake observed range from 25–70 μmoles of O_2 per ml of reticulocytes per hr in various species, which corresponds to values observed in active tissues.[104,200–202] Even the first observers were impressed by the stability of the oxygen consumption of the reticulocyte. It is much the same whether various substrates are present or not.[203] It will continue for many hours, declining slowly with a half-life of about 10 hours.[204] Addition of glucose causes a decrease by about 10–20%[197,204]; some additions, in particular oxaloacetate, cause an increase of about 10%.[197] The oxygen consumption of the rabbit reticulocyte however does not correspond to the maximal capacity of the respiratory chain. Uncoupling by addition of 2,4-DNP produces an initial increase of oxygen consumption of more than 2-fold.[204] Therefore it would appear that the oxygen consumption of intact reticulocytes is strictly controlled, presumably by the concentration of ADP, since variously produced elevations of inorganic phosphate do not increase the oxygen uptake.[205] The limitation of the effect of 2,4-DNP appears to lie in the supply of metabolic substrates, since addition of intermediates of the citrate cycle, in particular of oxaloacetate, will increase the effect of 2,4-DNP severalfold.[203]

The oxygen consumption of isolated mitochondria from reticulocytes under respiratory control with 2-oxoglutarate as substrate corresponds entirely to that observed in intact cells.[85a~c] Estimates of the activities of the cyt a and of the NADH-cyt c system[206] would also indicate that their capacities exceed the oxygen consumption under physiological conditions by severalfold. In keeping with this conclusion, the respiratory control quotient of isolated mitochondria is about 4.[85a~c] Matters may be different in the human reticulocyte. The activity of the cytochrome oxidase, and of the succinate-cyt c system were only one-tenth and one-seventh, respectively, of that of rabbit reticulocytes, while that of the NADH-cyt c system was equal.[199] Therefore it is likely that, for this type of reticulocyte, respiration is limited by the amount of an enzyme, perhaps succinate dehydrogenase.

2) *ATP Formation from Respiration and Glycolysis*

Since there is neither a significant amount of glycogen nor gluconeogenesis in the reticulocyte, glycolysis is dependent on the external supply of glucose. In its absence, only small amounts of lactate (2–5 μmoles per ml cells per hr) are formed.[207] Immature reticulocytes, particularly those obtained on the fifth day of bleeding may not exhibit any aerobic glycolysis at pH 7.4, while those found late in an anemia may produce as much as 30 μmoles lactate aerobically, equal to the anaerobic glycolytic rate of the same blood samples. For the anaerobic rate of glycolysis, peak values of 100 μmoles lactate per ml of reticulocytes per hr have been observed, corresponding to a 30-fold increase in rate as compared with the mature erythrocyte. The same high values are observed in the presence of 2,4-DNP.[207]

ATP formation proceeds practically exclusively by way of oxidative phosphorylation. It amounts to 120–200 μmoles of ATP per ml of reticulocyter per hr, while the contribution of aerobic glycolysis ranges from 0–30 μmoles of ATP. On the other hand, the peak values of ATP formation from anaerobic glycolysis approach those from respiration. It is remarkable that an ATP level of about 3 mM in reticulocytes cannot be maintained without addition of glucose. Apparently cytosolic phosphorylation is essential. The reason may lie in the limitation of the translocase system for adenine nucleotides in the mitochondria or in the necessity of reducing equivalents in the cytosol which are furnished by glucose. It is, of course, not surprising that there is a rapid breakdown of ATP and total nucleotides under anaerobic conditions or in the presence of 2,4-DNP, which is accelerated in the absence of glucose. There have been many speculations on the mechanisms of the Pasteur and Crabtree effects. Following early suggestions, it has been proposed that the suppression of the utilization of glucose by respiration is caused by an increased inhibition of PFK.[208,209] It was further assumed that the level of citrate, which is increased under aerobic conditions, is an important negative effector limiting glucose utilization.[210,211]

In reticulocytes it has been possible to elucidate the mechanism of the Pasteur effect further and to modify it. Undoubtedly, in this cell also, the HK-PFK system is under tighter control under aerobic conditions, as indicated by high levels of the inhibitor ATP, and low ones of the positive effectors, AMP, P_i, ammonia and ADP. Under anaerobic conditions there is a rise of all positive effectors combined with a fall of ATP. Similar changes as in anaerobiosis are observed at high pH values. Aerobic lactate formation greatly increases with rising pH values and reaches 90% of the anaerobic rate at pH 8.5. At this pH, the ATP inhibition of PFK is largely released. Simultaneously there is a decrease in the concentration of ATP while those of ADP, AMP and ammonia increase.[212,232] Nevertheless these changes do not suffice to explain the inhibition of the HK under aerobic conditions at pH 7.2. It was postulated and found that there is considerable compartmentation of the ATP in the mitochondria which exists only under aerobic conditions. It is not certain as yet whether its extent suffices to explain fully the inhibition of glucose consumption an aerobiosis. The Crabtree effect may be explained in a similar manner. Mitochondrial oxygen uptake of reticulocytes is controlled by the cytosolic ADP concentration. It has been demonstrated[205] that addition of glucose will lower the total ADP level and therefore presumably the cytosolic ADP concentration, thereby diminishing the rate of mitochondrial oxygen uptake.

3) *The Metabolic Substrates*

The prolonged oxygen consumption of reticulocytes without substrate raises the question of the endogenous substrate of oxidation. The second aspect to be considered is the interaction between endogenous and external substrates. Warburg surmised from the respiratory quotient of about one, that proteins constitute the metabolic fuel under endogenous conditions.[213] Later studies showed that amino acids which arise from the breakdown of the stroma, *i.e.*, the organelles, mostly mitochondria and ribosomes, constitute a large part of the endogenous substrate.[144,145,214,215] The breakdown of the stroma also furnishes a sizeable proportion, perhaps as much as one-third, of the substrate for hemoglobin synthesis. It includes, besides amino acids, fatty acids and glycerol from phospholipids as well as ribose which originates from ribonucleic acids and low molecular nucleotides, mostly ATP. In the following sections these substrates will be considered.

The amino acids: Complete oxidation of a protein yields a RQ of about 0.8. The higher value found by Warburg[213] would lead one to expect that lower aliphatic amino acids would be metabolised preferentially. A survey of $^{14}CO_2$ formation from tracer amounts ($5 \times 10^{-6} M$) of various ^{14}C-labeled amino acids indicated a pronounced preference for glutamine, glutamate, aspartate, proline, serine and glycine. On the other hand, histidine, phenylalanine and tyrosine yielded only a little $^{14}CO_2$ under such conditions. In these studies possible differences in the uptake of the amino acids and in their intracellular concentrations were not taken into account.[215,216] A complete analysis of the intracellular concentrations of amino acids in the reticulocyte is not available as yet. The concentrations are strongly dependent on the respiratory rate (maturity)[217] presumably as a function of the activity of the specific carriers of the cell membrane[93–96] the intracellular processes liberating amino acids, and their rate of utilization for protein synthesis (see Fig. 5). The concentration of the amino acids is also strongly dependent on the time of incubation. Most of the amino acids diminish by one-half within 10 mins of substrate-free incubation, as result of the cessation of the external influx.[217] Thereafter they increase to levels well in excess of the initial level. This secondary rise may be suppressed by the addition of glucose. It is probably due to the cessation of hemoglobin synthesis in the absence of glucose while the breakdown of the stroma continues.[144] From these observations, one may conclude that the composition of the metabolic mixture undergoes variations both with maturation and during experimental periods under various conditions. Taking the intracellular concentrations and the data on $^{14}CO_2$ formation together, it would appear that for the immature erythrocyte glutamate, aspartate, and alanine furnish the bulk of the metabolic substrate of respiration. With increasing maturity the contribution of glycine is of increasing importance.[218]

Further insights concerning the utilization of amino acids were obtained by the study of the $^{14}CO_2$ formation as a function of their

TABLE IV. The concentration of some amino acids in rabbit reticulocytes.

Amino Acid	(Approximate values) Concentration (m*M*)
Glycine	1.1–1.8
Glutamate	0.6–0.9
Alanine	0.4–0.8
Aspartate	0.4–0.7
Threonine	0.4
Serine	0.2–0.5
Others	<0.05

Initial values of reticulocyte-rich suspensions. The lower values correspond to oxygen uptakes of less than 8 μmoles of O_2, the higher ones to more than 11 μmoles of O_2 per ml cells per hour.

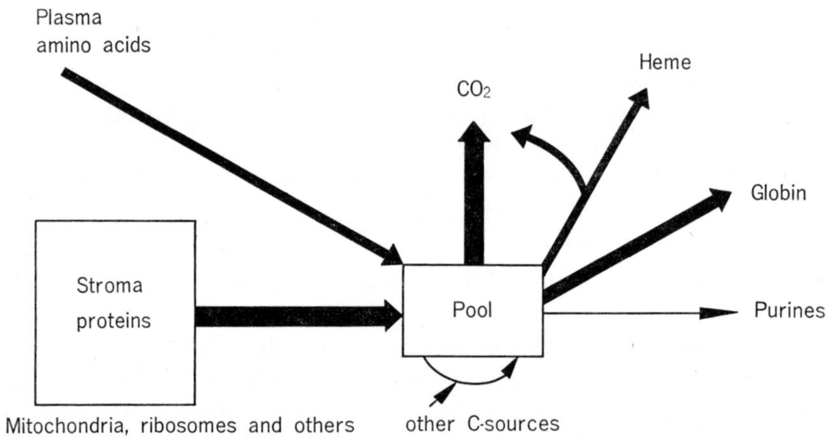

Fig. 5. Influx and efflux of the amino acid pool of the reticulocyte.

external concentrations. Under such circumstances it is possible to calculate the share of the external substrate in the total CO_2 formed. A useful approximate indication of the share is the percentage ratio of the $^{14}CO_2$ formed from a given substrate to the total O_2 consumption, *i.e.*, the "relative CO_2 formation". For precise calculations, the RQ of various substrates has to be taken into account. Since the oxygen consumption does not vary, regardless of which substrate is utilized, an increase in the relative CO_2 formation from 1 amino acid signifies a suppression of the contribution from other substrates. In Fig. 6 are presented some representative examples of the dependence of the relative CO_2 formation on substrate concentration.[216,219] It may be seen that the amino acids exhibit different patterns. Glutamine, glutamate, and aspartate converge to a limit of 80% relative CO_2 formation. Curves similar to those with glutamate were also obtained for proline, lysine, threonine and leucine with values of relative CO_2 formation in excess of 30% at high substrate concentrations. On the other hand glycine, serine, phenylalanine and tyrosine remain below 10% relative CO_2 formation. The curves for individual amino acids show a strong maturity dependence.[218,220] It is particularly pronounced for alanine and leucine which exhibit a decline of relative CO_2 formation to less than onefifth. This means that the capacity for their oxidation declines 5 times more in relation to the total respiration. On the other hand the relative CO_2 formation from glycine increases 2 to 3-fold, *i.e.*, it declines less than the cellular respiration (see Fig. 7). The differences between the amino acids in presence and in absence of external substrate and the changes during maturation appear to be due to the interplay of 3 processes, *i.e.*, 1) their transport across the cell membrane, 2) the endogenous supply of amino acids from intracellular breakdown and

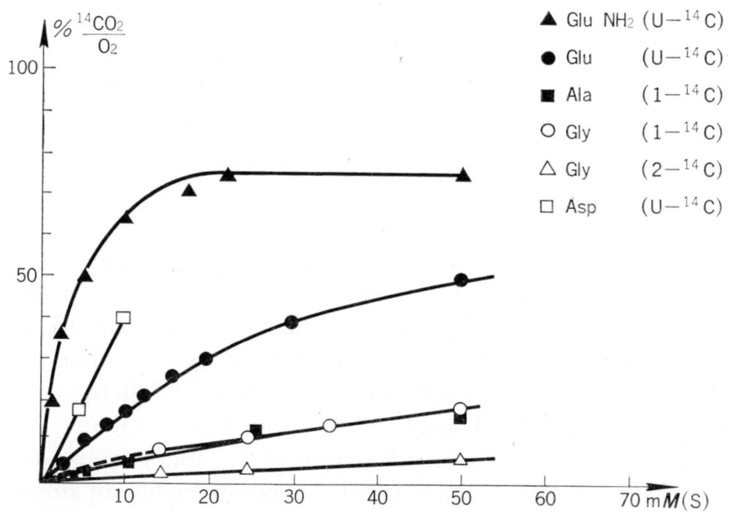

Fig. 6. $^{14}CO_2$ formation as a function of substrate concentrations from some amino acids.

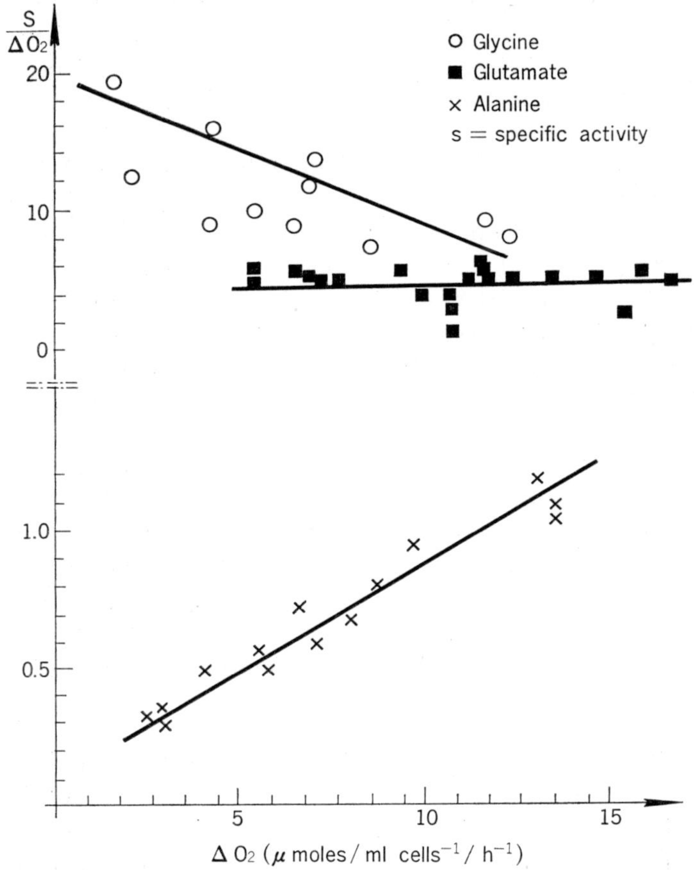

Fig. 7. Maturity dependence of $^{14}CO_2$ formation from tracer amounts of some amino acids.

3) the amount of key enzymes in the metabolic pathways of the individual amino acids. Each of these processes exhibits a different dependence on maturation. The fact that it is possible to increase greatly the relative CO_2 formation from most of the amino acids by elevation of their external concentration indicates that the decline of oxidation is primarily determined by the first 2 factors, *i.e.*, the disappearance of carriers and exhaustion of the endogenous sources.

At this point, a closer analysis of the metabolic fate of amino acids in the reticulocyte is appropriate. So far the metabolism of only 2 groups of amino acids has been studied in any detail: 1) those which are metabolized via the citrate cycle, *i.e.*, glutamine, glutamate, aspartate and alanine and 2) glycine and serine.

a) The Metabolism of Glutamine, Glutamate, Aspartate and Alanine

All these amino acids have in common the fact that they tend to reach 80% relative CO_2 formation. This permits two conclusions: 1) that the enzymatic capacities of their pathways are very large and unsaturated under endogenous conditions and *in vivo*, and 2) that each of them may monopolize the basic CO_2-forming system, *i.e.*, the citrate cycle, suppressing the utilization of other substrates draining into it. It has been demonstrated that there exist close interrelation among the amino acids and their deamination products. Glutamate is utilized almost exclusively via aspartate by means of transamination with oxaloacetate (Borst pathway), which may yield acetyl-CoA via pyruvate (see Fig. 8).[221] In this manner, either from glutamate or aspartate, the complete citrate cycle, *i.e.*, both acetyl-CoA and oxaloacetate, may be derived. Thus the high relative CO_2 formation from each single amino acid is accounted for. A consideration of the equilibrium constant and the steady state concentrations of ammonium ions, 2-oxoglutarate, and glutamate as well as direct proof of the low yield

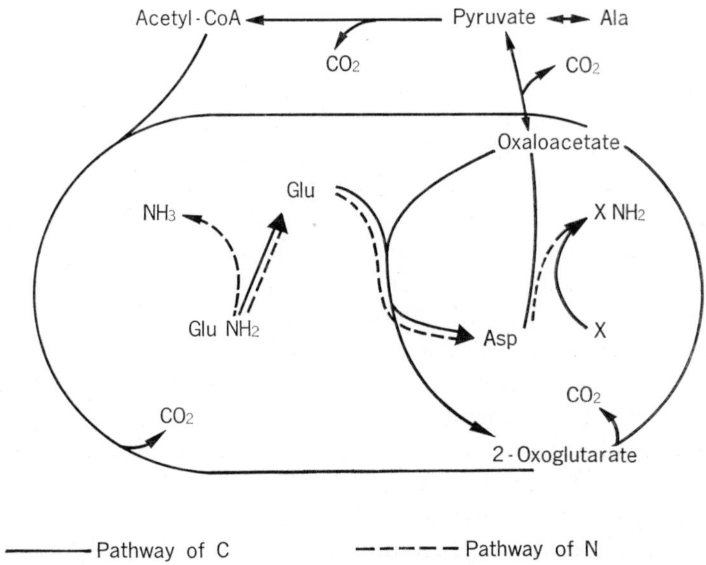

Fig. 8. Scheme of the pathway of glutamate (and alanine) oxidation in the reticulocyte.

of $^{15}NH_3$ from ^{15}N-labeled glutamate indicate the insignificance of the glutamate dehydrogenase reaction for the catabolism of glutamate. The enzyme may rather serve for ammonia fixation.[221] CO_2 formation from substrate amounts of alanine is surprisingly low and does not exceed 15% of relative CO_2 formation. The limitation in its utilization may lie in the low activity of the GPT.

The reticulocyte is probably the first cell for which a clarification of the pathways and interactions of the amino acids connected with the citrate cycle has been achieved. The differences between the amino acids with respect to the substrate dependence of CO_2 formation (Fig. 6) are mainly caused by their transport properties. The exceptionally steep rise from glutamine, with an apparent K_M of 2 mM, is caused both by its concentrative transport and ease of passive permeation. On the other hand, glutamate, which exhibits an apparent K_M of 40 mM[216] is known to permeate slowly.[222] Since glutamine is utilized via glutamate, by means of the action of a powerful glutaminase within[185,186] the cell, permeation is the only factor responsible for the difference between them. Aspartate which is next highest in relative CO_2 formation presumably permeates better than glutamate while alanine permeation may vary according to the state of maturity of the reticulocyte.[95]

b) The Metabolism of Glycine and Serine

The metabolism of glycine and serine will be discussed on the basis of the accompanying scheme (Fig. 9) which summarises the available evidence. Apparently the only pathway of serine degradation is by way of the pyridoxal phosphate-dependent serine hydroxymethylase, with the formation of glycine and of N(5), N(10)-methylene-FH_4.[223,224] This reaction is probably localized in the cytosol. The conversion of serine to pyruvate could be excluded.[225] Thus the subsequent fate of serine coincides with that of glycine.

Glycine is utilised under physiological conditions mainly in the synthesis of porphyrins and globin and, to a minor extent, of purines.[226,227] In a representative experiment it was estimated that about 0.6 μmoles per ml of reticulocytes per hr were incorporated into porphyrins and 0.8 μmoles into globin. The total of 1.4 μmoles per ml of reticulocytes per hr represents nearly one-fifth of the total turnover of amino acids under such circumstances. The only pathway of CO_2 formation from glycine is by way of the reactions of the Shemin cycle.[228] The proposed pathway via glyoxalate[229] plays only a suboradinate role,

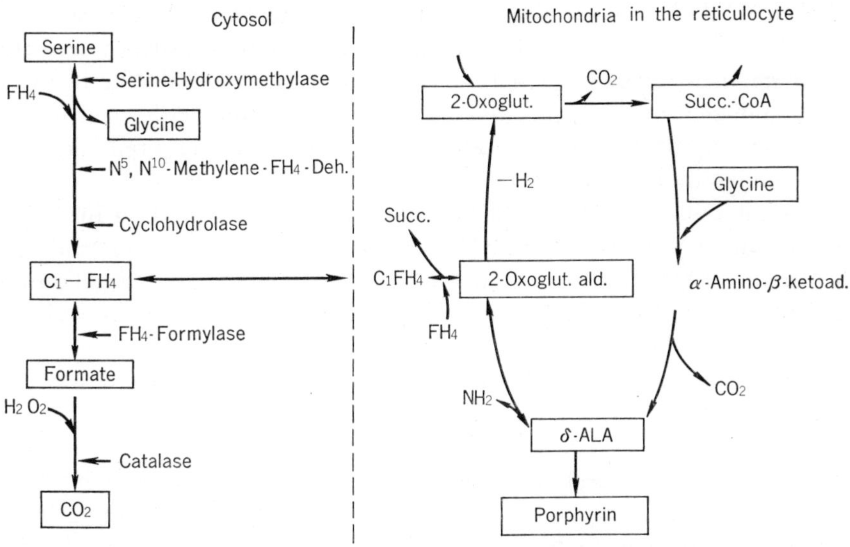

Fig. 9. Scheme of serine and glycine metabolism in the reticulocyte.

if any.[230] The first reaction by means of δ-ALA synthetase liberates CO_2 from the carboxyl group of glycine. Under physiological or substrate-free conditions, the δ-ALA formed is utilized practically completely for porphyrin synthesis, with CO_2 formation from the α-carbon of glycine amounting to only 3% of that from the carboxyl carbon. If the substrate concentration of glycine is increased, the subsequent reactions of the Shemin cycle acquire greater prominence, presumably due to an increased concentration of δ-ALA. By transamination, 2-oxoglutaraldehyde is formed, from which two possible pathways have been demonstrated: 1) dehydrogenation to 2-oxoglutarate and 2) C_1-transfer to FH_4 and formation of succinate, or rather succinyl-CoA. The reactions from δ-ALA via 2-oxoglutaraldehyde to succinate appear to be freely reversible, while the dehydrogenation of 2-oxoglytaraldehyde to 2-oxoglutarate is not. At high glycine concentrations the pathway via 2-oxoglutarate, which yields CO_2 by way of the citrate cycle, predominates over that via succinate.

The fate of the α-carbon of glycine, *i.e.*, of δ-ALA has not been accounted for completely. At high concentrations of glycine (50 m*M*) one-fourth is converted into CO_2, an equal amount into porphyrins and 3% as C_1 unit into purines.[226] The metabolism of both serine and glycine is closely connected with that of the C_1 group. Both the C-3 and the C-2 of serine or glycine, respectively, yield C_1-FH_4 compounds, which are either utilized for synthesis, primarily of purines or yield formate in a reversible reaction (FH_4-formylase).[223,224] The formate is catabolized to CO_2 by means of catalase, depending on the availability of H_2O_2. Utilization of one-carbon units for syntheses predominates, of course, in the immature reticulocyte. The share of one-carbon units catabolised to CO_2 via formate by means of catalase increases with maturity, being practically zero in the most immature and approaching 100% in the most mature reticulocyte, which is the situation in the erythrocyte. The reverse is true for the CO_2 formation via 2-oxoglutarate and the citrate cycle.[225]

The limitation of CO_2 formation from the C-2 of glycine via the catalase pathway appears to be in the reaction leading from 2-oxoglutaraldehyde to the C_1-FH_4 compound, since increase of H_2O_2 supply (by addition of methylene blue) will not augument the yield of $^{14}CO_2$ from [2-^{14}C]-glycine. Under such conditions, CO_2 formation from serine and formate increases 6 to 7-fold.[227] All the enzymes of the Shemin cycle are localized in the mitochondria, while those of the one-carbon metabolism, including catalase, are to be found in the cytosol. They decline, except for catalase, to about one-tenth during maturation, but do not disappear.[224]

c) *Glucose, Ribose and Glycerine*

Glucose appears to be a minor substrate of the immature reticulocyte of rabbits and rats, accounting for 20% or less of the total CO_2 formation. Its share increases with maturation and may reach 50% in the most mature reticulocyte. Four-fifths of the glucose is catabolized by the OPP pathway, the rest via pyruvate through the Embden-Meyerhof (EM) pathway.[231] The formation of $^{14}CO_2$ from labeled glucose is dependent on the concentration of glucose over a wide range, increasing 2.5-fold from 5 to 100 m*M* glucose. This effect is due to the action of a high-K_M HK, which is similar in its properties to the GK in liver and kidney. This enzyme is no longer present in mature erythrocytes. Its functional significance for the reticulocyte is questionable. It provides an alternative route of formation of glucose-6-P, which is not subject to product inhibition, while the persistent HK of red cells is extremely sensitive to it. It is conceiveable that the action of GK safeguards a supply of glucose-6-P for the function of the OPP pathway.[112] The utilization of glucose is not limited by permeation since the same results are obtained with rat reticulocytes, which are easibly permeable to glucose, as in rabbit reticulocytes, which are not.

No definite answer can be given at present as to how the utilization of glucose by the two pathways is regulated. 2,4-DNP increases the share of glucose in the total CO_2 formation more than threefold.[234] The flux through both the OPP and the EM pathways is greater more so through the latter pathway. There are obviously several possible reasons for such an effect.

The relative decline of CO_2 formation from alanine during maturation, while that of glucose increases, may be connected with damage to the inner mitochondrial membrane, which loses its properties as a barrier, as can be demonstrated electron microscopically.[81] Thus intramitochondrial GPT may be liberated from the matrix into the cytosol.

The oxidation of glucose via the OPP pathway is limited by the concentration of $NADP^+$, both in erythrocytes and in reticulocytes.[235,236] This is well-illustrated by the effect of methylene blue, which affects only the state of oxidation of cytosolic pyridine nucleotides without causing uncoupling of the oxidative phosphorylation.[236,237] Under its influence, $^{14}CO_2$ formation from glucose by way of the OPP pathway may increase 30-fold, while that via the EM pathway is unchanged. The large proportion of the OPP pathway in reticulocytes would indicate a high state of oxidation of $NADP^+$ in the cytosol. This may be connected with the production of H_2O_2 from the extramitochondrial pathway of oxygen consumption. It is also possible that under certain conditions (see chapter on catalase) there may be mitochondrial H_2O_2 formation. This perhaps is how 2,4-DNP increases $^{14}CO_2$ formation from glucose both via the EM and the OPP pathways.

Another carbohydrate which may contribute to the metabolic mixture is ribose, or rather ribose phosphate, which originates both from the breakdown of ribonucleic acids and to smaller extent from low-molecular nucleotides. The ratio of $^{14}CO_2$ formation from [2-^{14}C]-glucose as compared with that from [6-^{14}C]-glucose indicates that the rate of recombination from pentose phosphates to hexose phosphates amounts to about 10% of the glucose turnover.[231] Thus ribose may be metabolized, like glucose, both by the EM and the OPP pathways.

Glycerol is a substrate closely related to the carbohydrates. The formation of $^{14}CO_2$ from labeled glycerol proceeds in a linear manner as a function of substrate concentration. It may reach 10% relative CO_2 formation at a concentration of 50 m*M* glycerol.[238] The details of its metabolism have not yet been elucidated. Under physiological condition its contribution as a respiratory substrate is negligable.

d) The Fatty Acids

The fatty acids, particularly octanoate are good substrates of both reticulocytes and their isolated mitochondria.[239] They originate both from intracellular breakdown and form external sources. They permeate the cellular membrane freely. Activation for the subsequent degradation occurs both by the carnitin-dependent systems of the outer mitochondrial membrane and by the carnitin-independent systems of the inner membrane. The first mechanism predominates for palmitate, the second for octanoate. The contribution of palmitate reaches a ceiling of about 10%, due to limitation of the capacity of the activating system for long-chain fatty acids or their translocation through the mitochondrial membrane. On the other hand, octanoate may contribute as much as 65% of the respiratory substrate. It is thus evident that the steps of fatty acid degradation subsequent to their activation, which are identical for palmitate and octanoate, have a large capacity. Under physiological conditions fatty acids may furnish about 10% of the respiratory substrate of reticulocytes.

e) The Interrelations among the Metabolic Substrates

There exist a multitude of competitive and cooperative interactions among the metabolites which have not been analysed throughly so far. Some of them may be mentioned. Most of the metabolic effects are related to the citrate cycle and to the compartmentalization of the metabolic pathways. Addition of glucose, despite its minor contribution to CO_2 formation, produces multiple effects: 1) It will decrease oxygen consumption (Crabtree effect) by the mechanism previously discussed. There is some indication of a correlation of the magnitude of this effect with the rate of aerobic glycolysis. 2) It will decrease the concentration of amino acids within the cells, presumably due to the increase and maintainance of hemoglobin synthesis in the presence of glucose.[213] 3) It will decrease $^{14}CO_2$ formation from alanine, glutamate, aspartate, proline, valine and serine. The metabolism of all these substrates includes reactions of the citrate cycle; on the other hand $^{14}CO_2$ formation from leucine, threonine and lysine are unaffected. 4) It will decrease the extent of liberation of ammonia, both by preserving the nucleotides in their phosphorylated forms, which are thus protected from deamination, and by its nitrogen-sparing effect on the metabolism of amino acids.[145]

Oxaloacetate in low concentrations will increase the formation of fatty acids, presumably by providing an acceptor for the acetyl-CoA from fatty acids in the citrate synthetase reaction. At higher concentrations, mutual competition between oxaloacetate and fatty acids is observed, since both yield acetyl-CoA.[239] In high concentrations, oxaloacetate will decrease the extent of the OPP pathway of glucose, probably by decreasing the state of oxidation of $NADP^+$ in the cytosol. This may be an expression of functional competition between $NADP^+$-consuming reactions. The interactions between pyruvate and amino acids are essentially the same as those described for glucose.

f) The Metabolic Mixture under Substrate-free Conditions and In Vivo

In Fig. 10 the composition of the metabolic substrate of the rabbit reticulocyte in the presence of blood plasma and under substrate-free conditions is compared in a schematic manner. The situation for the erythrocyte is also shown. The main influence of the plasma as source of metabolites appears to be the influx of glutamine, the concentration of which ranges from 0.4–0.7 m*M* in the plasma.[240,241] It may contribute from 20–50% of the CO_2 formation.[216] Of the other

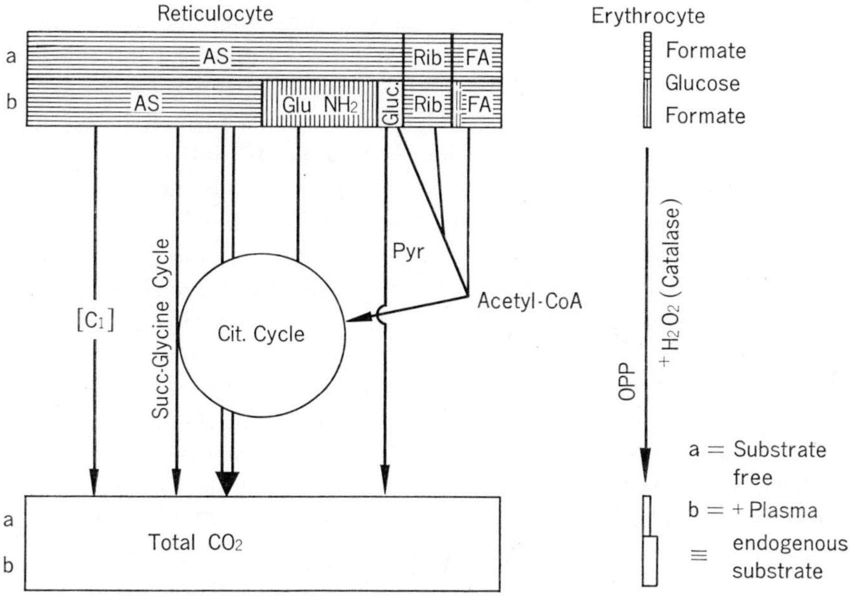

Fig. 10. The metabolic fuel of the reticulocyte.

amino acids, alanine with a plasma concentration of 0.2–0.3 mM[242] may participate significantly in CO_2 formation of the most immature reticulocyte. The reverse is true for glucose, the share of which in energy production increases with maturation. The contribution of fatty acids from the plasma, which are mostly protein-bound is unknown[243]; it certainly represents less than 10% of the total CO_2 formed.[239]

g) *The Fate of Nitrogen from the Amino Acids*

Reticulocytes form ammonia in varying amounts, depending on their degree of maturity and experimental conditions. The formation of ammonia is greatest in immature reticulocytes.[145,216] It is diminished in the presence of glucose and is increased greatly in anaerobiosis or in the presence of 2,4-DNP.[23] A large part of the ammonia may be accounted for by the deamination of nucleotides, particularly those of adenine.[145] This pathway was elucidated some time ago. The lack of rephosphorylation of ADP to ATP leads to the formation of AMP by means of adenylate kinase. AMP is hydrolysed by the ubiquitous acid phosphate monoesterase (pH optimum, 5.5).[244] The resultant adenosine is deaminated by a powerful specific deaminase.[245,246] There is, of course, ammonia formation from glutamine by mean of glutaminase.[135,186] Glutamate dehydrogenase apparently has only a minor role, if any, in ammonia formation, since there is only a small liberation of ammonia of 3% from ^{15}N-glutamate under conditions in which glutamate furnishes 30% of the respiratory substrate.[221] From a consideration of the ratio of CO_2 and ammonia formed it was apparent that the liberation of ammonia falls far behind that expected from the share of amino acids in the respiratory substrate. This discrepancy becomes even greater if the deamination of nucleotides is taken into account. Therefore an acceptor for the amino group has to be postulated. Glycine appeared to be the candidate for such an amination product, since it exhibits a high intracellular concentration, which even rises under substrate-free conditions despite its utilization for the synthesis of porphyrins, globin and purines. Indeed, incorporation of ^{15}N into glycine from ^{15}N-glutamate could be demonstrated.[227] Its extent lies in the predicted range. The source of the carbon atoms for glycine formation, has been found to be glucose. Glycine arises presumedly via serine and hydroxypyruvate from 3-PG or 2-PG by way of transamination and formyl-transfer.[233]

REFERENCES

1 Ehrlich, P., *Berl. Klin. Wochenschr.*, **18**, 43 (1881).
2 Thorell, B., *Folia Haematol.*, **78**, 7 (1961).
3 Seno, S., *Acta Pathol. Jap.*, **16**, 457 (1966).
4 Marks, P. A., Fantoni, A. and De la Chapelle, A., *Vitam. Horm.*, **26**, 331 (1968).
5 Cameron, I. L. and Prescott, D. M., *Exp. Cell Res.*, **30**, 609 (1963).
6 Grasso, J. A., Woodard, J. W. and Swift, M., *Proc. Nat. Acad. Sci.*, **50**, 134 (1963).
7 Grasso, J. A. and Woodard, J. W., *J. Cell Biol.*, **31**, 279 (1966).
8 Fantoni, A., De la Chapelle, A., Rifkind, R. A. and Marks, P. A., *J. Mol. Biol.*, **33**, 79 (1968).
9 Skutelsky, E. and Danon, D., *J. Cell Biol.*, **33**, 625 (1967).
10 Skutelsky, E. and Danon, D., *Exp. Cell Res.*, **60**, 427 (1970).
11 Brecher, G. and Stohlman, F., Jr., *Proc. Soc. Exp. Biol. Med.*, **107**, 887 (1961).
12 Borsook, H., Lingrel, J. B., Sacro, J. L. and Milette, R. L., *Nature*, **196**, 347 (1962).
13 Stohlman, F., Jr., Ebbe, S., Morse, B., Howard, D. and Donovan, J., *Ann. N. Y. Acad. Sci.*, **149**, 156 (1968).
14 Bessis, P. M. and Breton-Gorius, J., *Nouv. Rev. Franc. Hematol.*, **4**, 72 (1964).
15 Orlic, D., Gordon, A. S. and Rhodin, J. A. G., *Ann. N. Y. Acad. Sci.*, **149**, 198 (1968).
16 Kent, G., Minick, O. T., Volini, F. I., Orfei, E. and Madera-Orsini, F., *J. Cell Biol.*, **27**, 51A (1965).
17 Caspersson, T., *Scand. Arch. Physiol.*, **73**, Suppl. 8, 98 (1936).
18 Holloway, B. W. and Ripley, S. H., *J. Biol. Chem.*, **196**, 695 (1952).
19 Rabinovitz, M. and Olson, M. F., *Exp. Cell Res.*, **10**, 747 (1956).
20 Dintzis, H. M., Borsook, H. and Vinograd, J., *in*: Microsomal Particles and Protein Synthesis, Washington, Academy of Sciences, Washington DC, ed. by Roberts, R. B. (Pergamon Press London-New York-Paris-Los Angeles, 1958), p. 95.
21 Coutelle, R., Rapoport, S. and Lindigkeit, R., *Naturwissenschaften*, **42**, 127 (1955).
22 Coutelle, R. and Rapoport, S., *Folia Haematol.*, **73**, 326 (1955).
23 Rosenthal, S., Künzel, W. and Wagenknecht, C., *Folia Haematol.*, **78**, 135 (1962).
24 Heilmeyer, L., Lehrbuch der Inneren Medizin, Band II (Blut und Blutkrankheiten) 4. Auflage (Springer-Verlag, Berlin-Göttingen-Heidelberg, 1951).
25 Kosenow, W., *Acta Haematol.*, **7**, 360 (1952).

26 Rosenthal, S., David, H., Uerlings, I. and Gross, J., *in*: VI. Internationales Symposium über Struktur und Funktion der Erythrozyten; Abhandlungen der Deutschen Akademie der Wissenschaften zu Berlin (Akademie-Verlag, Berlin, 1971) p. 525.
27 Coutelle, Ch., Rosenthal, S., Gross, J., David, H. and Uerlings, I., *Acta Biol. Med. German.* (in the press).
28 Goetze, E., Lindigkeit, R. and Rapoport, S., *Biochem. Z.*, **326**, 48 (1954).
29 Rosenthal, S., Künzel, W. and Wagenknecht, C., *Acta Biol. Med. German.*, **13**, 281 (1964).
30 Burka, E. R., *J. Lab. Clin. Med.*, **68**, 833 (1966).
31 Burka, E. R., Schreml, W. and Kick, C. J., *Biochemistry*, **6**, 2840 (1967).
32 Burka, E. R., *Bioch. Biophys. Acta*, **166**, 672 (1968).
33 Petermann, M. L., The physical and chemical properties of ribosomes (Elsevier, Amsterdam, London, New York, 1964).
34 Cox, R. A., *in*: Biochemistry of ribosomes and messenger RNA, International Symposium, Castle Reinhardsbrunn 1967; Abhandlungen der Deutschen Akademie der Wissenschaften zu. Berlin, ed. by Lindigkeit, R., Langen, P. and Richter, J. (Berlin, Akademie-Verlag, Berlin, 1968), p. 23.
35 Warner, J. R., Rich, A. and Hall, C. E., *Science*, **138**, 1399 (1962).
36 Slayter, H. S., Warner, J. R., Rich, A. and Hall, C. E., *J. Mol. Biol.*, **7**, 652 (1963).
37 Mathias, A. P., Williamson, R., Huxley, H. E. and Page, S., *J. Mol. Biol.*, **9**, 154 (1964).
38 Rifkind, R. A., Luzatto, L. and Marks, P. A., *Proc. Nat. Acad. Sci.*, **52**, 1227 (1964).
39 TS'O, P.O.P. and Vinograd, J., *Biochim. Biophys. Acta*, **49**, 113 (1961).
40 Dejimenez, E. S., Webb, F. H. and Bock, R. M., *Arch. Biochem. Biophys.*, **125**, 452 (1968).
41 Prehn, S. and Rosenthal, S., *Acta Biol. Med. German.*, **24**, K 51 (1970).
42 King, H. W. S., Gould, H. J. and Shearman, J. J., *J. Mol. Biol.*, **60**, 143 (1971).
43a Wilner-Zehavi, T., Izak, G. and Mager, J., *Blood*, **27**, 319 (1966).
43b Zehavi-Willner, T. and Danon, D., *FEBS Letters*, **26**, 151 (1972).
44 Kruh, J., *Biochim. Biophys. Acta*, **129**, 631 (1966).
45 Zehavi-Wilner, T., *Biochem. Biophys. Res. Comm.*, **39**, 161 (1970).
46 Cox, R. A., Gould, H. and Kanagalingham, K., *Biochem. J.*, **106**, 733 (1968).
47 Cox, R. A., *Biochem. J.*, **117**, 101 (1970).
48 Prehn, S., Rosenthal, S. and Rapoport, S. M., *Europ. J. Biochem.*, **24**, 456 (1972).
49 Prehn, S., Rosenthal, S. and Rapoport, S. M. (in preparation).
50 Cox, R. A., *Biochem. J.*, **114**, 743 (1969). *Ibid.*, **114**, 753 (1969).

51 Cox, R. A. and Bonanou, S. A., *Biochem. J.*, **114**, 769 (1969).
52 Ladhoff, A. M. and Rosenthal, S., David, H., Grupe, M. and Metzler, E., *Acta Biol. Med. German.*, **29**, 621 (1972).
53 Schreml, W. and Burka, E. R., *J. Biol. Chem.*, **243**, 3573 (1968).
54 Burka, E. R. and Schickling, L. F., *Biochemistry*, **9**, 459 (1970).
55 Rosenthal, S., Habilitationsschrift der Medizinischen Fakultät der Humboldt-Universität zu Berlin, 124 (1968).
56 Bulova, S. I. and Burka, E. R., *J. Biol. Chem.*, **245**, 4907 (1970).
57 Baker, R. F., *Fed. Proc.*, **26**, 1785 (1967).
58 Rosenthal, S., Jagemann, K., Prehn, S. and Heinemann, G., *Acta Biol. Med. German.*, **18**, 329 (1967).
59a Ginzburg, S., Smith, J. G., Ginzburg, G. M., Reardon, J. Z. and Aikawa, J. K., *Blood*, **20**, 722 (1962).
59b Benbassat, J. and Karpas, S., *Isr. J. Med. Sci.*, **8**, 1840 (1972).
59c Valberg, L. S., Card, R. T., Paulson, E. J. and Szivek, J., *Brit. J. Haematol.*, **13**, 115 (1967).
60 Guest, G. M. and Rapoport, S., *Physiol. Rev.*, **21**, 410 (1941).
61 Marbaix, G. and Burny, A., *Biochem. Biophy. Res. Comm.*, **16**, 522 (1964).
62 Burny, A., Huez, G., Marbaix, G. and Chantrenne, H., *Biochim. Biophys. Acta*, **190**, 228 (1969).
63 Holt, C. E., Joel, P. B. and Herbert, E., *J. Biol. Chem.*, **241**, 1819 (1966).
64 Smith, D. W. E. and McNamara, A. L., *Science*, **171**, 577 (1971).
65 Gaskill, P. and Kabat, D., *Proc. Nat. Acad. Sci. U.S.*, **68**, 72 (1971).
66 Rost, G. and Rapoport, S., *Acta Biol. Med. German.*, **7**, 226 (1961).
67 Schweiger, H. G., Schweiger, E. and Vollertsen, I., *Z. Naturforsch.*, **19 B**, 248 (1964).
68 Bertles, J. F. and Beck, W. S., *J. Biol. Chem.*, **237**, 3770 (1962).
69 Sandberg, A. A., Lee, G. R., Cartwright, G. E. and Wintrobe, M. M., *J. Clin. Invest.*, **34**, 1823 (1955).
70 Glowacki, E. R. and Milette, R. L., *J. Mol. Biol.*, **11**, 116 (1965).
71 Rowley, P. T., *Nature*, **208**, 244 (1965).
72 Lodish, H. F. and Desalu, O., *J. Biol. Chem.*, **248**, 3520 (1973).
73 Schulman, H. M., *Biochim. Biophys. Acta*, **155**, 253 (1968).
74 Rowley, P. T. and Morris, J. A., *J. Biol. Chem.*, **242**, 1533 (1967).
75 Herzberg, M., Revel, M. and Danon, D., *Europ. J. Biochem.*, **11**, 148 (1969).
76 Levy, E., Tichonicky, L. and Kruh, J., *Biochemie*, **53**, 671 (1971).
77 Howard, G. A., Adamson, S. D. and Herbert, E., *Biochim. Biophys. Acta*, **213**, 237 (1970).
78 Maxwell, C. R., Kamper, C. S. and Rabinovitz, M., *J. Mol. Biol.*, **58**, 317 (1971).
79 Guggenheim, S. J., Bonkowsky, N. L. and Harris, J. W., *J. Lab. Clin.*

Med., **69**, 357 (1067).
80 David, H., Uerlings, I., Rosenthal, S. and Schulz, W., *Acta Biol. Med. German.*, **27**, 533 (1971).
81a Krause, W., David, H., Uerlings, I. and Rosenthal, S., *Acta Biol. Med. German.*, **28**, 779 (1972).
81b Gasko, O. and Danon, D., *Exptl. Cell Res.*, **75**, 159 (1972).
82 Schulz, W., Neymeyer, H. G. and Rosenthal, S., *Acta Biol. Med. German.*, **26**, 439 (1971).
83 Schewe, T., Wiesner, R. and Schulz, W., *Acta Biol. Med. German.*, **28**, 1 (1972).
84 Warrendorf, E. M. and Rubinstein, D., *Canad. J. Biochem.*, **49**, 919 (1971).
85a Augustin, H. W. and Kunzendorf, H.-J., VI. Internationales Symposium über Struktur und Funktion der Erythrozyten; Abhandlungen der Deutschen Akademie der Wissenschaften zu Berlin (Akademie-Verlag, Berlin, 1971), p. 455, 459.
85b Grecksch, G., Wiswedel, I. and Augustin, W., VII. Internationales Berliner Symposium über Struktur und Funktion der Erythrozyten, *in*: Abhandlungen der Akademie der Wissenschaften der DDR (Akademie Verlag, Berlin, 1974).
85c Gellerich, F. N. and Augustin, W., VII. Internationales Berliner Symposium über Struktur und Funktion der Erythrozyten, *in*: Abhandlungen der Akademie der Wissenschaften der DDR (Akademie Verlag, Berling, 1974).
86 Rubinstein, D. and Denstedt, F., *J. Biol. Chem.*, **204**, 623 (1953).
87 Rubinstein, D., Ottolenghi, P. and Denstedt, O. F., *Canad. J. Biochem., Physiol.*, **34**, 222 (1956).
88 Dajani, R. M. and Orten, J. M., *J. Biol. Chem.*, **231**, 913 (1958).
89a Sarkar, S. R. and Rapoport, S., *Acta Biol. Med. German.*, **11**, 323 (1963).
89b Rapoport, S. and Sarkar, S. R., *Acta Biol. Med. German.*, **11**, 335 (1963).
90a Gasko, O. and Danon, D., *Brit. J. Haematol.*, **23**, 525 (1972).
90b Gasko, O. and Danon, D., *Brit. J. Haematol.*, **23**, 535 (1972).
91 Rost, G. and Rapoport, S., *Acta Biol. Med. German.*, **3**, 142 (1959).
92 Berry, D. H. and Hochstein, P., *Arch. Biochem. Biophys.*, **131**, 170 (1969).
93 Riggs, R., Christensen, H. N. and Palatine, I. M., *J. Biol. Chem.*, **194**, 53 (1952).
94 Winter, Ch. G. and Christensen, H. N., *J. Biol. Chem.*, **240**, 3594 (1965).
95 Anatonioli, J. A. and Christensen, H. N., *J. Biol. Chem.*, **244**, 1505 (1969).
96 Yunis, A. A. and Arimura, G. K., *J. Lab. Clin. Med.*, **66**, 177 (1965).

97 Augustin, H. W., Häcker, M. R. and Hofmann, E., *Hoppe Seyler Z. Physiol. Chem.*, **339**, 42 (1964).
98 Rapoport, S., *Folia Haematol.*, **78**, 96 (1962).
99 Grieger, M., Jacobasch, G. and Gerth, Ch., VII. Internationales Berliner Symposium über Struktur und Funktion der Erythrozyten, *in*: Abhandlungen der Akademie der Wissenschaften der DDR (Akademie Verlag, Berlin, 1974).
100 Marks, P. A., *Science*, **127**, 1338 (1958).
101 Schapira, F., *Rev. Franc. Etud. Clin. Biol.*, **4**, 151 (1959).
102 Hinterberger, U., Ockel, E., Gerischer-Mothes, W. and Rapoport, S., *Acta Biol. Med. German.*, **7**, 50 (1961).
103 Coltorti, M., DiSimone, A. and Budillon, G., *Boll. Soc. Ital. Biol. Sper.*, **35**, 1630 (1959).
104 Kahrig, C. and Rapoport, S., *Acta Biol. Med. German.*, **6**, 238 (1961).
105 Oski, F. A., Brigandi, E. and Noble, L., *Pediatrics*, **44**, 84 (1969).
106 Maretzki, D. and Rapoport, S., *Acta Biol. Med. German.*, **29**, 207 (1972).
107 Arnold, H., Blume, K. G., Busch, D., Lenkeit, U., Löhr, G. W. and Lübs, E., *Klin. Wochenschr.*, **48**, 1299 (1970).
108 Kühn, B., Jacobasch, G., Gerth, Ch. and Rapoport, S., I. Intern. Symposium of the Biochem. Soc. GDR and the All-Union Biochem. Soc. Acad. Sci. USSR, Reinhardsbrunn 1971, Reaction Mechanism and Control Properties of Phosphotransferases (Akademie Verlag, Berlin, 1973), p. 421.
109 Jacobasch, G., Grieger, M. and Kühn, Bl, VII. Internationales Berliner Symposium über Struktur und Funktion der Erythrozyten, *in*: Abhandlungen der Akademie der Wissenschaften der DDR (Akademie Verlag, Berlin, 1974).
110 Eaton, G. M., Brewer, G. J. and Tashian, R. E., *Nature*, **212**, 944 (1966).
111 Starkeweather, W. H., Cousineau, L., Schock, H. K. and Zarafonetis, C. J., *Blood*, **26**, 63 (1965).
112 Gerber, G. K. G., Schultze, M. and Rapoport, S. M., *Europ. J. Biochem.*, **17**, 445 (1970).
113 Malkin, A. and Denstedt, O. F., *Canad. J. Biochem. Physiol.*, **34**, 121 (1956).
114a Bartlett, G. R., VI. Internationales Symposium über Struktur und Funktion der Erythrozyten, Berlin; *in*: Abhandlungen der Deutschen Akademie der Wissenschaften zu Berlin (Akademie-Verlag, Berlin, 1972), p. 495.
114b Rapoport, S., Guest, G. M. and Wing, M., *Proc. Soci. Exp. Biol. Med.*, **57**, 344 (1944).
115 Wagenknecht, C., *Folia Haematol.*, **78**, 77 (1962).

116 Rosenthal, S., Repoport, S. M. and Heinemann, G., *Acta Biol. Med. German.*, **13**, 946 (1964).

117a Rosenthal, S., Prehn, S. and Rapoport, S., *Acta Biol. Med. German.*, **17**, 667 (1966).

117b Prehn, S., Manuscript submid

118 Stavy, L., Feldman, M. and Elson, D., *Biochim. Biophys. Acta*, **91**, 606 (1964).

119 Rowley, P. T. and Morris, J. A., *J. Biol. Chem.*, **242**, 1533 (1967).

120 Lindigkeit, R., *Folia Haematol.*, **74**, 251 (1956).

121 Adachi, K., Nagano, K., Nakao, T. and Nakao, M., *Biochem. Biophys. Acta*, **92**, 59 (1964).

122 Goto, S. and Mizuno, D., *Arch. Biochem. Biophys.*, **145**, 64 (1971).

123 Goto, S. and Mizuno, D., *Arch. Biochem. Biophys.*, **145**, 71 (1971).

124 Burka, E. R., *J. Clin. Invest.*, **50**, 60 (1971).

125 Farkas, W. R. and Marks, P. A., *J. Biol. Chem.*, **243**, 6464 (1968).

126 Smith, T. J. and Schulman, H. M., *Fed. Proc.*, **25**, 798 (1966).

127 Rost, G., *Acta Biol. Med. German.*, **3**, 276 (1959).

128 Traub, P., Zillig, W. and Milette, R. L., *Hoppe Seyler Z. Physiol. Chem.*, **343**, 261 (1966).

129 Priess, H. and Zillig, W., *Hoppe Seyler Z. Physiol. Chem.*, **348**, 817 (1967).

130 Burka, E. R., *Science*, **162**, 1287 (1968).

131 Klaus, B., Diplomarbeit, Mathematisch-Naturwissenschaftliche Fakultät (Berlin, 1968).

132 Prehn, S., Belkner, J. and Rosenthal, S., unpublished.

133 Rapoport, S., Leva, E. and Guest, G. M., *J. Cell Comp. Physiol.*, **19**, 103 (1942).

134 Rosenthal, S., Ruprecht, A. and Zank, W., *Folia Haematol.*, **90**, 142 (1968).

135 Rosenthal, S. and Zank, W., Seventh International Congress of Biochemistry (Tokyo, 1967), J-434.

136 Goetze, E., Lindigkeit, R. and Rapoport, S., *Biochem. Z.*, **326**, 48 (1954).

137 Goetze, E. and Rapoport, S., *Biochem. Z.*, **326**, 53 (1954).

138 Goetze, E. and Rapoport, S., *Biochem. Z.*, **327**, 305 (1955).

139 Schulz, K., *Folia Haematol.*, **79**, 455 (1962).

140 Haschen, R. J., Farr, W. and Groh, F., *Acta Biol. Med. German.*, **14**, 205 (1965).

141 Künzel, W., *Folia Haematol.*, **78**, 94 (1961).

142 Künzel, W., Wagenknecht, C. and Rapoport, S., *Acta Biol. Med. German.*, **7**, 609 (1961).

143a Reichelt, D., Jacobsohn, E. and Haschen, R. J., VI. Internationales Symposium über Struktur und Funktion der Erythrozyten, Berlin;

in: Abhandlungen der Deutschen Akademie der Wissenschaften zu Berlin (Akademie-Verlag, Berlin, 1972), p. 505.
143b Haschen, R. J., *Acta Biol. Med. German.*, **9**, 15 (1962).
143c Haschen, R. J., Farr, W. and Groth, F., *Acta Biol. Med. German.*, **14**, 205 (1965).
144 Schweiger, H. G., Rapoport, S. and Schölzel, E., *Hoppe Seyler Z. Physiol. Chem.*, **306**, 33 (1957).
145 Schweiger, H. G. and Rapoport, S., *Hoppe Seyler Z. Physiol. Chem.*, **313**, 97 (1956).
146 Dobilasova, M., Pokorna, V. and Drahota, Z., *Physiol. Bohemoslov.*, **20**, 173 (1971).
147 Waite, M., *Fed. Proc.*, **28**, 596 (1969).
148 Delbauffe, D., Paysant, M. and Polonowski, S., *Bull. Soc. Chim. Biol.*, **50**, 1431 (1968).
149 Ferber, E., Munder, P. G., Kohlschütter, A. and Fischer, H., *Europ. J. Biochem.*, **5**, 395 (1968).
150 Rapoport, S. and Gerischer-Mothes, W., *Hoppe Seyler Z. Physiol. Chem.*, **302**, 167 (1955).
151 Rapoport, S. and Nieradt, Ch., *Hoppe Seyler Z. Physiol. Chem.*, **302**, 179 (1955).
152 Augustin, H. W. and Rapoport, S., *Acta Biol. Med. German.*, **3**, 433 (1959).
153 Rapoport, S. and Schewe, T., unpublished results.
154 Rapoport, S. and Gerischer-Mothes, W., *Hoppe Seyler Z. Physiol. Chem.*, **304**, 213 (1956).
155 Wiesner, R., Rosenthal, S. and Hicbsch, Ch., *Acta Biol. Med. German.*, **30**, 631 (1973).
156 Rapoport, S. and Gerischer-Mothes, W., *Acta Biol. Med. German.*, **3**, 450 (1959).
157 Rapoport, S., Gerischer-Mothes, W. and Nieradt-Hiebsch, Ch., *Hoppe Seyler Z. Physiol. Chem.*, **304**, 207 (1956).
158 Rapoport, S. and Gerischer-Mothes, W., *Hoppe Seyler Z. Physiol. Chem.*, **315**, 38 (1959).
159 Scheme, T., Hiebsch, Ch. and Rapoport, S., *Acta Biol. Med. German.*, **29**, 189 (1972).
160 Rapoport, S. and Wagenknecht, C., *Naturwissenschaften*, **43**, 582 (1956).
161 Wagenknecht, C. and Rapoport, S., *Hoppe Seyler Z. Physiol. Chem.*, **308**, 127 (1957).
162 Schewe, T. and Rapoport, S., 7th meeting FEBS, Varna 1971, Abstracts.
163 Altenbrunn, H. J. and Rapoport, S., *Acta Biol. Med. German.*, **2**, 599 (1959).

164 Wiesner, R. and Rapoport, S., *Acta Biol. Med. German.*, **31**, 289 (1973).

165 Konopatzki, H., Scharfschwerdt, H., Friedemann, H., Hinterberger, U., Scheuch, D., Haase, B., Ramshorn, E., Jagemann, K. and Arend, A., *Acta Biol. Med. German.*, Suppl. III, 325 (1964).

166 Scheuch, D. and Rapoport, S., *Acta Biol. Med. German.*, **6**, 23 (1961).

167 Scheuch, D. and Rapoport, S., *Acta Biol. Med. German.*, **8**, 31 (1962).

168 Rapoport, S. and Scheuch, D., *Nature*, **186**, 967 (1960).

169 Shrago, E., *Arch. Biochem. Biophys.*, **109**, 57 (1965).

170 Lajtha, L. G. and Oliver, R., *in*: Ciba Foundation Symposium on Haemopoiesis Cell Production and its regulation; ed. by G. E. W. Wolstenholme and O'Connor, M. (Churchill Ltd., London, 1960).

171 Davidson, J. N., Leslie, J. and White, J. C., *Lancet*, **I**, 1287 (1951).

172 Weicker, H., *Folia Haematol.*, **76**, 225 (1959).

173 Asakura, H., *Acta Med. Okayama*, **19**, 217 (1965).

174 Ganzoni, A. S., Hillman, R. S. and Finch, C. A., *Brit. J. Haematol.*, **16**, 119 (1969).

175 Becker, H. J., Knecht, L. H. and Straschil, F., *Acta Haematol.*, **43**, 144 (1970).

176 Stohlman, F., Jr., *Proc. Soc. Exptl. Biol. Med.*, **107**, 884 (1961).

177 Hershko, Ch., Schwartz, R. and Izak, G., *Brit. J. Haematol.*, **17**, 569 (1969).

178 Bohne, F., Haas, R. J., Fliedner, T. M. and Fache, I., *Brit. J. Haematol.*, **19**, 533 (1970).

179 Coutelle, Ch., Reineke, H. H., Meurach, W., Steindamm, E., Grieger, M. and Rosenthal, S., Manuscript submitted.

180a Rosenthal, S., Gross, J., Grauel, E. L., Papies, B., Schulz, W., Belkner, J., *et al.*, VI. Internationales Symposium über Struktur und Funktion der Erythrozyten; Abhandlungen der Deutschen Akademie der Wissenschaften zu Berlin (Akademie-Verlag, Berlin, 1971), p. 513.

180b Gross, J., Papies, Bl, Grauel, E. L., Hartwig, A. and Rosenthal, S., *Acta Biol. Med. German.*, **30**, 617 (1973).

180c Wiesner, R., Rosenthal, S., Hiebsch, Chr., *Acta Biol. Med. German.*, **30**, 631 (1973).

180d Gerber, G., Schröder, K. and Rosenthal, S., *Acta Biol. Med. German.*, **30**, 773 (1973).

180e Gross, J., Staak, R. and Rosenthal, S., *Acta Biol. Med. German.*, **30**, 781 (1973).

180f Papies, B., Gross, J., Coutelle, Ch. and Rosenthal, S., *Acta Biol. Med. German.* (in the press).

180g Gross, J., Pietsch, L. and Rosenthal, S., *Folia Haematol.* (Leipzig),

100, 82 (1973).
180h Müller, M., Rosenthal, S. and Botscherowa, L. *Acta Biol. Med. German.* (in the press).
181 Coutelle, Ch., Papies, B. and Müller, M., 7th FEBS Meeting, Varna, Abstract No. 924 (1971).
182 Lord, B. J., *Nature*, **217**, 1026 (1968).
183 Rapoport, S., *Folia Haematol.*, **78**, 96 (1962).
184 Rapoport, S., Ababei, L., Hinterberger, U., Kahrig, C., Künzel, W., Gerischer-Mothes, W., Raderecht, H. J., Scheuch, D. and Viereck, G., *Acta Biol. Med. German.*, **7**, 589 (1961).
185 Ababei, L., *Acta Biol. Med. German.*, **5**, 630 (1960).
186 Scheuch, D. and Viereck, G., *Acta Biol. Med. German.*, **7**, 589 589 (1961).
187 Sarkar, R., *Acta Biol. Med. German.*, **12**, 67 (1964).
188 Loeb, J. N., Howell, R. R. and Tomkins, G. M., *Science*, **169**, 1093 (1965).
189 Hirsch, C. A. and Hiatt, H. H., *J. Biol. Chem.*, **241**, 5936 (1966).
190 Fletscher, M. J. and Sanadi, D. R., *Biochim. Biophys. Acta*, **51**, 356 (1961).
191 Menzies, R. A. and Gold, P. H., *J. Biol. Chem.*, **246**, 2425 (1971).
192 Omura, T., Siekewitz, P. and Palade, G. E., *J. Biol. Chem.*, **242**, 2389 (1967).
193 Prujan, R., De Bernard, B. and Rabinowitz, M., *J. Biol. Chem.*, **244**, 5874 (1969).
194 De Bernhard, J. B., Getz, G. S. and Rabinowitz, M., *Biochim. Biophys. Acta*, **193**, 58 (1959).
195 Schewe, T., Krause, W., Rosenthal, S. and Rapoport, S., Symposium on "Intracellular Protein Catabolism", GDR, Reinhardsbrunn, May 7–11, 1973 (in the press).
196a Müller, M., Dissertation Mathematisch-Naturwissenschaftliche Fakultät der Humboldt-Universität (Berlin, 1970).
196b Müller, M., Hartwig, A. and Rapoport, S., VII. Internationales Berliner Symposium über Struktur und Funktion der Erythrozyten, in: Abhandlungen der Akademie der Wissenschaften der DDR (Akademie-Verlag, Berlin, 1974).
197 Ababei, L. and Rapoport, S., *Acta Biol. Med. German.*, **5**, 636 (1960).
198 Rapoport, S. and Wagenknecht, C., *Hoppe Seyler, Z. Physiol. Chem.*, **309**, 196 (1957).
199 Syllm-Rapoport, I., Reichelt, E., Remitschka, M. E., Gerber, G., Nieradt-Hiebsch, Ch., Thamm, R. and Rapoport, S., VI. Internationales Symposium über Struktur und Funktion der Erythrozyten Berlin (1970). *in*: Abhandlungen der Deutschen Akademie der Wissenschaften zu Berlin (Akademie-Verlag, Berlin, 1971), p. 487.

200 Augustin, H. W. and Rapoport, S., *Acta Biol. Med. German.*, **3**, 433 (1959).
201 Jacobasch, G. and Rapoport, S., *Folia Haematol.*, **83**, 284 (1965).
202 Dunsing, M., Diplomarbeit Sektion Biologie der Humboldt-Universität (Berlin, 1969).
203 Rapoport, S. and Ababei, L., *Acta Biol. Med. German.*, **7**, 533 (1961).
204 Schweiger, H. G. and Rapoport, S., *Acta Biol. Med. German.*, **1**, 422 (1958).
205 Rapoport, S., Hinterberger, U., *et al. Acta Biol. Med. German.*, **7**, 528 (1961).
206 Rapoport, S., Nieradt-Hiebsch, Ch. and Thamm, R., *Acta Biol. Med. German.*, **21**, 291 (1968).
207 Hinterberger, U., Dissertation Mathematisch-Naturwissenschaftliche Fakultät der Humboldt-Universität (Berlin, 1964).
208 Newsholme, E. A. and Randle, P. J., *Biochem. J.*, **80**, 655 (1961).
209 Passonneau, J. V. and Lowry, O. H., *Biochem. Biophys. Res. Comm.*, **7**, 10 (1962).
210 Vinuela, E., Salas, M. L. and Sols, A., *Biochem. Biophys. Res. Comm.*, **12**, 140 (1963).
211 Salas, M. L., Vinuela, E., Salas, M. and Sols, A., *Biochem. Biophys. Res. Comm.*, **19**, 371 (1965).
212 Rapoport, S. and Jacobasch, G., 1. Internationales Symposium, Wien (1968). Stoffwechsel und Membranpermeabilität von Erythrozyten und Thrombocyten, S. 1; ed. by Deutsch, E., Gerlach, E., Moser, K., Georg Thieme Verlag (Stuttgart, 1968).
213 Warburg, O., Kubowitz, F. and Christian, W., *Biochem. Z.*, **242**, 170 (1931).
214 Brandt, H. and Rapoport, S., *Acta Biol. Med. German.*, **2**, 290 (1959).
215 Schultze, M., Scholz, I. *et al.*, *Folia Haematol.*, **78**, 183 (1962).
216 Rapoport, S., Rost, J. and Schultze, M., *Europ. J. Biochem.*, **23**, 166 (1971).
217 Buchmann, R. and Rapoport, S., *Acta Biol. Med. German.*, **13**, 819 (1964).
218 Schultze, M., Rapoport, S. and Scholz, I., *Folia Haematol.*, **83**, 361 (1965).
219 Rapoport, S. and Schultze, M., unpublished.
220 Rapoport, S., *Folia Haematol.*, **89**, 105 (1968).
221 Rost, J. and Rapoport, S., *Europ. J. Biochem.*, **26**, 106 (1972).
222 Heinz, E., Pichler, A. G. and Pfeifer, B., *Biochem. Z.*, **342**, 542 (1965).
223 Bertino, J. R., Semmons, B. and Donohue D. M., *J. Biol. Chem.*, **237**, 1314 (1962).
224 Wilmanns, W. and Jaenicke, L., *Klin. Wschr.*, **41**, 1077, 1027 (1963).
225 Rapoport, S., Müller, M. and Knöfel, R., *Europ. J. Biochem.*, **10**, 207

(1969).
226 Jänig, G. and Schultze, M., *Folia Haematol.* (Leipzig), **89**, 212 (1968).
227 Gregor, U., Diplomarbeit, Mathematisch-Naturwissenschaftliche Fakultät der Humboldt-Universität (Berlin, 1968).
228 Shemin, D., *Ergeb. Physiol.*, **49**, 299 (1957).
229 Weinhouse, S., A Symposion on Amino Acid Metabolism (Baltimore, 1955), p. 637.
230 Urbahn, H. and Rapoport, S., *Acta Biol. Med. German.*, **6**, 16 (1961).
231 Schultze, M. and Rapoport, S. M., *Acta Biol. Med. German.*, **13**, 310 (1964).
232 Jacobasch, G., Mattusch, J., Schönian, G., Gerth, Ch. and Rapoport, S., VII. Internationales Berliner Symposium über Struktur und Funktion der Erythrozyten, in Abhandlungen der Akademie der Wissenschaften der DDR (Akademie Verlag, Berlin, 1974).
233 Müller, M., Dumdey, R., Scholz, M., Schultze, M. and Rapoport, S., 8. Jahrestagung, Biochemische Gesellschaft der DDR, Oberhof, Thüringer (1972).
234 Rapoport, S. and Schultze, M., *Acta Biol. Med. German.*, **13**, 847 (1964).
235 Roigas, H., Zöllner, E., Jacobasch, G., Schultze, M. and Rapoport, S., *Europ. J. Biochem.*, **12**, 24 (1970).
236 Hofmann, E. C. G., v. Krepl, H. and Peschke, R., *Folia Haematol.*, **78**, 213 (1962).
237 Schultze, M., Rapoport, S. and Lach, A., *Folia Haematol.*, **83**, 371 (1965).
238 Rapoport, S. and Schultze, M., *Acta Biol. Med. German.*, **20**, 553 (1968).
239 Schultze, M., Rost, J., Augustin, W., Gellerich, F. and Rapoport, S., *Europ. J. Biochem.*, **27**, 43 (1972).
240 Ramadan, M. E. D. and Greenberg, D. M., *Anal. Biochem.*, **6**, 144 (1963).
241 Benson, J. V., Gordon, M. J. and Patterson, J. A., *Anal. Biochem.*, **18**, 228 (1967).
242 Stein, H. W. and Moore, St., *J. Biol. Chem.*, **211**, 915 (1954).
243 Goodman, D. S., *J. Amer. Chem. Soc.*, **80**, 3892 (1958).
244 Tsuboi, K. K. and Hudson, P. B., *Arch. Biochem. Biophys.*, **43**, 339 (1953).
245 Ababei, L. and Rapoport, S., *Acta Biol. Med. German.*, **6**, 288 (1961).
246 Rubinstein, D. and Denstedt, O. F., *Canad. J. Biochem. Physiol.*, **34**, 927 (1956).

Pentose Phosphate Pathway in Human Erythrocytes

F. J. LIONETTI

Center for Blood Research, 800 Huntington Avenue, Boston, Massachusetts 02115, U.S.A.

The pentose phosphate pathway in human erythrocytes converts approximately 10% of glucose utilized into CO_2 and pentose phosphates. The oxidation of glucose-6-P helps maintain the reduced state of ferroheme and SH-dependent functions. Pentose phosphates produced from 6-phosphogluconate supply parts of the pentose of red-cell ATP while transketolase-transaldolase (TK-TA) mediated conversion of fructose-6-P supplies an additional large fraction. The decarboxylation of C-1 of [1-^{14}C]-glucose is a cyclic process with C-2 and C-3 being successively converted to C-1 of glucose and decarboxylated. Ribulose-5-P, the product, isomerizes to ribose-5-P and epimerizes to xylulose-5-P. These are substrates for red-cell TK and TA, whose activity leads to accumulation in ghosts of hexose phosphates and triose phosphates. The inactivation of TA of hemolysates causes accumulation of sedoheptulose-7-P from ribose-5-P. Nucleosides are a readily metabolized source of ribose-5-P. Ribulose diphosphate is produced in ghosts from inosine. It is degraded by hemolysates to pyruvate and 3-PG. ^{14}C-Bicarbonate is simultaneously incorporated into acid-stable compounds.

Deoxynucleosides are metabolized by red-cell deoxyriboaldolase to produce triose phosphates (glyceraldehyde-3-P and DHAP) and acetaldehyde. The triose phosphates combine to form fructose diphosphate which is converted in hemolysates to fructose-6-P. By means of TK, xylulose-5-P is formed. Pentoses and hexoses are thus seen to be readily interconverted by red cells. PRPP is formed from ribose-5-P and ATP. By means of it, red cells are able to incorporate adenine into ATP and nicotinic acid into precursors of NADP$^+$.

INTRODUCTION

The pentose phosphate pathway in human erythrocytes may be described as an aerobic means to convert glucose, the normal substrate of the cell, into lactate by means of reactions which liberate CO_3 and involve pentose phosphates as intermediates. At the hexose level of the sequence, celled the hexose monophosphate shunt, glucose is phosphorylated to form glucose-6-P oxidized to 6-phosphogluconate, and decarboxylated. Pentose phosphates are formed which isomerize and dismutate to produce 3 to 8 carbon carbohydrate phosphates. Principal among these are fructose-6-P and GAP which are further metabolized glycolytically to lactate. About 10% of the carbon of glucose is metabolized by means of the phosphogluconate pathway under aerobic conditions.[1,2] This is nevertheless quantitatively significant, as the hexose monophosphate shunt and pentose phosphate pathways exercise several red-cell regulatory functions. The oxidation of glucose-6-P effects the reduction of $NADP^+$ to NADPH, contributing to the reduced state of the red-cell and providing it with a continual source of electrons to maintain cellular sulfhydryl groups and hemoglobin in the ferroheme state. This is a remarkable mechanism since the function of red cells is the transport of molecular oxygen, from which the cellular redox systems are effectively insulated.

Although the amounts of pentose phosphates arising in red cells through the hexose monophosphate shunt are quantitatively small, pentoses are produced from several other reactions and the capacity to metabolize these is relatively large. Pentose phosphates may be derived from nucleosides, the hydrolysis of nucleotides or from glycolytic intermediates (for instance, by the TK-catalyzed reaction of fructose-6-P and GAP). The red-cell content of 2,3-DPG, an important regulator of hemoglobin function, may be supported by the metabolism of pentoses from nucleosides while the synthesis of nucleotides (AMP, ATP) depends on the availability of PRPP. The metabolism of pentose phosphates is thus related ultimately to the important functions of ionic regulation, oxygen transport and membrane integrity.

OXYGEN UTILIZATION AND CO_2 EVOLUTION

The hexose monophosphate aspect of the pentose phosphate pathway was elucidated at the time when the Embden-Meyerhof glycolytic sequence was being established as the major pathway for the conversion of monosaccharides to lactate in yeasts and other tissues. In the early 1900's, Warburg described oxygen consumption by avian and mammalian erythrocytes, finding it for man and rabbit to be a small but real respiration, in that oxygen utilization was accompanied by an equivalent evolution of CO_2.[3] The Q_{O_2} was nevertheless so small as to raise doubts that it might be due to platelets and white cells contaminating red-cell suspensions. By freeing rabbit red cells to the maximum extent of other elements and by plotting CO_2 against the percentage of reticulocytes, Ramsay and Warren showed the mature rabbit red-cell to have a minimum oxygen consumption of 8.5 mm^3 per gm cells per hr.[4)] Red cells were shown by Harrop and Barron (1928) to produce CO_2 simultaneously with O_2 uptake and yielded respiratory quotients in the physiological range. They also made the important discovery that an enormous increase in oxygen consumption could be caused by catalytic quantities of methylene blue.[5)] They showed that methylene blue caused a reduction in the ratio of glucose utilized to lactate produced and that its effect depended on the presence of oxygen. They concluded that methylene blue enhanced the oxidation of hexose monophosphate by molecular oxygen. Warburg, on visiting Harrop and Barron, learned of the phenomenon and commenced a series of studies which formed the historical basis for the hexose monophosphate shunt. Warburg and Christian[6)] showed that glucose-6-P was readily oxidized by methylene blue in red-cell hemolysates. These hemolysates could not oxidize glucose. Therefore, the intact cell, but not the lysates, contained a phosphorylating system (HK) required to initiate oxygen consumption. They succeeded in isolating from hemolysates the enzyme "zwischenferment" (GPD) and isolated and described a dialyzable heat-stable cozymase ($NADP^+$), and showed that it was required for the aerobic oxidation of glucose-6-P.[7)] The discovery was highly significant because of the ubiquitous distribution of pyridine nucleotide-linked dehydrogenases and because it defined the molecular function of a vitamin (nicotinamide) as a constituent of a coenzyme. When intact cells plus glucose or hemolysates plus glucose-6-P take up oxygen in the presence or absence of methylene blue, the dye is reduced by NADPH. In order to function catalytically it must be repeatedly oxidized and reduced. In red cells several mechanisms exist for oxidation of NADPH but the most probable involves reduction of the flavoprotein enzyme, "yellow enzyme", obtained by Warburg and Christian in small amounts from red cells and in large yields from yeast.[8)] This enzyme is reduced by NADPH and is oxidized by methylene blue, the latter then combining with molecular oxygen. The product of oxidation of glucose-6-P was identified as 6-phosphogluconate.[9)] Its conversion to pentose phosphate was first described by Dickens.[10)] Ribulose-5-P was identified as the product of oxidative decarboxylation of 6-phosphogluconate in yeast and animal tissues by Horecker *et al.*[11)]

The current concept of the hexose monophosphate pathway is

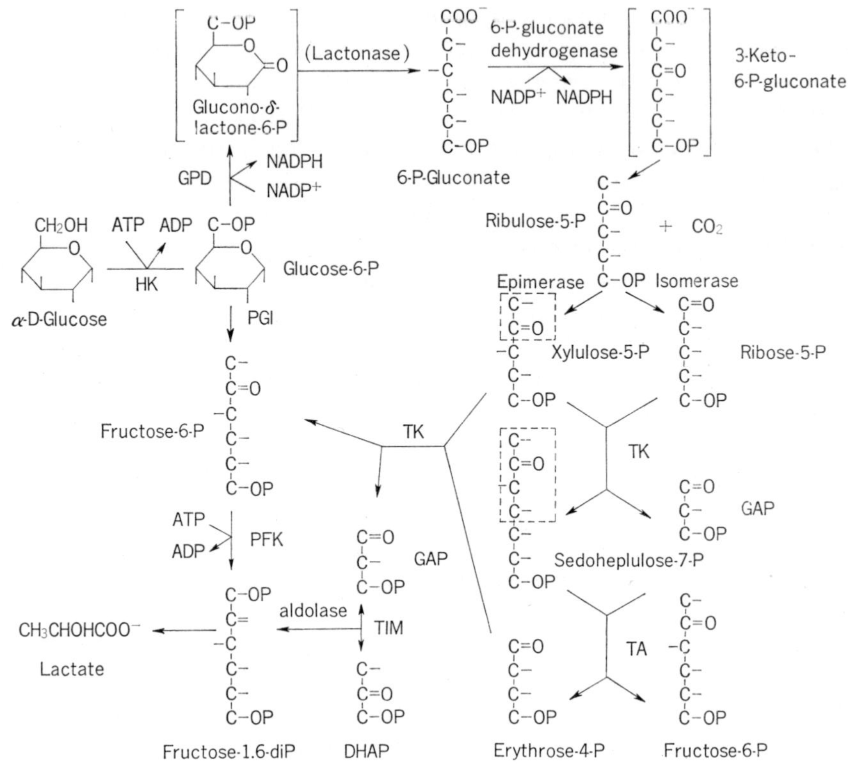

Fig. 1. Relationship of hexose shunt and pentose phosphate pathways to glycolysis in human erythrocytes. The dotted boxes represent the "glycolaldehyde" moiety transferred by TK and the "dihydroxyacetone" moiety transferred by TA. All formulae represent the D family of carbohydrates. Components presumed to be present in human red cells are indicated by brackets.

given in Fig. 1. It represents the reaction sequence from glucose through the decarboxylation of 6-phosphogluconate. Lactonases have been described in plants and bacteria which cause rapid hydrolysis of glucono-δ-lactone-6-P to 6-phosphogluconate. Neither the lactonase nor lactone have been described in red cells and their presence is implied.

The evolution of CO_2 from glucose in red cells has been demonstrated with ^{14}C-glucose. With red cells from a relatively large sampling of individuals, about 10% of the glucose utilized (0.23 μg per ml per minute) at pH 7.5, was aerobically converted to $^{14}CO_2$.[1)] A similar magnitude of decarboxylation of the C-1 position of [1-^{14}C]-glucose was observed by DeLoecker and Prankerd.[2] In both studies, methylene blue stimulated the shunt pathway. Brin and Yonemoto studied the methylene blue effect on human red cells both with glucose uniformly labeled and at carbons 1, 2, and 6. They concluded that the oxidation was confined to the upper half of the glucose molecule.[12] No $^{14}CO_2$ was obtained from ^{14}C[6-^{14}C]-glucose and the total activity obtained from C-1 and C-2 was about equal to that from uniformly labeled glucose. The recovery of C-2 as $^{14}CO_2$ was about half that from C-1 labeled glucose. Assuming that 6-phosphogluconic dehydrogenase selectively removed C-1 from glucose, the relatively high conversion of C-2 carbon to $^{14}CO_2$ suggested that pentose phosphates produced by decarboxylation were recycled to form glucose-6-P, exposing successive carbons in glucose to oxidation. An oxidation cycle by which all 6 carbons of glucose are selectively removed at C-1 and the pentose phosphates recycled to reform glucose-6-P has been described by Racker and Gatt.[13]

PENTOSE PHOSPHATES IN ERYTHROCYTES

Under normal conditions pentose phosphates of human erythrocytes are produced in part from blood-plasma glucose which is transported into and oxidized by the cells. A relatively small but significant synthesis takes place, as a significant amount of this pentose is incorporated into red-cell ATP.[14] Denstedt and co-workers found a little less than half of the pentose of ATP was derived from glucose in human and rabbit erythrocytes. Pentose phosphates may also be produced from hexose phosphates by means of TK and TA (see Fig. 2). The pentose phosphates of major importance in red cells are ribose-5-P, ribose-1-P, ribulose-1, 5-diP, xylulose-5-P and PRPP. A small amount of ribose-1, 5-diP has been found which may be a cofactor in the conversion of ribose-1-P to ribose-5-P.[15] The reduction of xylitol to xylulose has been thought to occur in human red cells but its significance is obscure, as the substrate does not normally occur in blood.[16] Addition of 10 m*M* xylitol to erythrocytes produced a large increase in DHAP and a decrease in pyruvate in all probability due to its effect on NADH L-xylulose dehydrogenase. Xylitol is of special interest because it is an intermediate in the glucuronic acid pathway whereby L-xylulose is reduced to xylitol which is in turn oxidized to D-xylulose.[17] A ribokinase for D-ribose and 2-deoxyribose in non-nucleated red cells has been described but its contribution to erythrocyte pentose content must presently be judged to be insignificant.[18] Erythrocytes do, however, possess considerable capacity for the metabolism of ribose phosphates. An oxidative pathway from glucose-6-P to ribose-5-P was suggested by Dickens, who found that when glucose-6-P was oxidized by GPD from yeasts, orcinolreactive pentoses were produced.[19,20] Later, with extracts of horse erythrocytes, Dickens and Williamson[21] demonstrated the presence of ribose-5-P isomerase and ribulose-5-P-3-epimerase by which ribulose-5-P and xylulose-5-P respectively are synthesized (see Fig. 1). An equilibrated mixture of ribose-5-P, xylulose-5-P and ribulose-5-P was produced. This equilibrium has been studied in hemolysates of human erythrocytes by Dische and Shiguera,[22] by Bruns *et al.*[23,24] and in ghosts by Lionetti and Fortier.[25]

Many of the relationships among ketopentose phosphates in erythrocytes have been elucidated by Dische and co-workers. By application of color reactions for carbohydrates and inhibition of glycolytic and pentose phosphate pathway enzymes, they were able to identify and study intermediate pentoses and deduce the pathway of conversion of pentose to hexoses in erythrocytes.[26] They used 6-fold diluted hemolysates of human red cells, dialyzed to remove ATP, containing fluoride to inhibit phosphatases, and incubated at 43°C for 4 hours at pH 8.4 to inactivate TA. Dische and Shiguera[22] showed that 60% of ribose-5-P was metabolized and an equilibrium mixture was produced containing 60% xylulose-5-P and ribulose-5-P and 40% of residual ribose-5-P. Xylulose-5-P and ribulose-5-P were present in the ratio of 2.65, while Bruns *et al.*,[23] with very dilute hemolysates, observed 3.0. The proportion of xylulose-5-P to ribulose-5-P was variable, depending on the species of red-cell, the incubation, and the mode of identification, *i.e.*, as free sugars. Dickens and Williamson[21] found xylulose-5-P to be 0.1 of ribulose-5-P with isolated isomerase and epimerase from horse erythrocytes. Lionetti and Fortier[25] incubated ghosts depleted by about 90% of ATP, NAD^+, and $NADP^+$, with inosine and inorganic phosphate. Xylulose-5-P and ribulose-5-P were identified with purified yeast TK and ribulose-5-P-3-epimerase (Fig. 2). In a 6-hour incubation xylulose-5-P accumulated and reached a maximum value (100 μmoles per 10^{12} ghosts). There was no ribulose-5-P until 2 hours (15 μmoles). Thereafter both ketopentose phosphates remained in a steady state at a ratio of xylulose-5-P to ribulose-5-P of 1.7–1.8 for 3–5 hours. The equilibrium among the ketopentose phosphates and

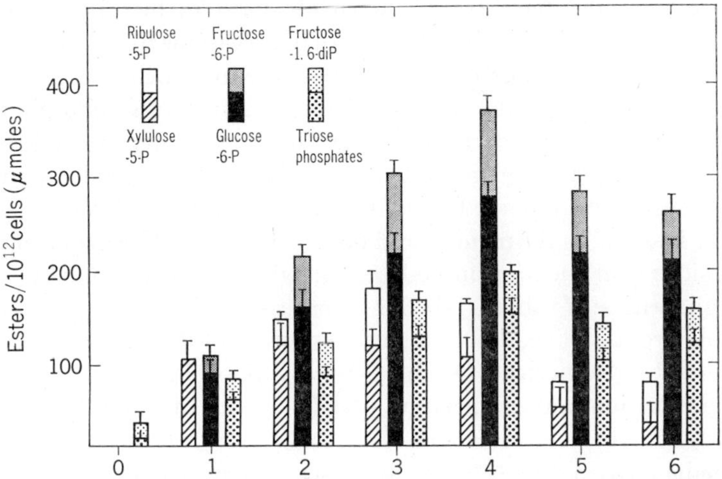

Fig. 2. Pentose and Hexose phosphates from inosine in ghosts. Human erythrocyte ghost were incubated in physiological buffer with inosine (10.0 mM) and P_i (4.0 mM) at a cell count of 4.0×10^6 cells per mm^3 of suspension. The average pH was 7.2. At the intervals shown extracts were prepared and assayed for the components indicated. Values are corrected to a cell count of 5.0×10^6 per mm^3. The bars indicate positive deviations from the means of 4 experiments on different samples of blood.

ribose-5-P has been studied with ribose-5-P isomerase purified from spinach and with xylulose-5-P epimerase from rabbit muscle by Tabachnick *et al.*[27)] Whether approached from ribulose-5-P or xylulose-5-P, the equilibrium mixture contained ribose-5-P, ribulose-5-P, and xylulose-5-P in the proportion of 3: 1: 3. In this, as in most red-cell studies, at equilibrium about equal quantities of ribose-5-P and xylulose-5-P are found while the ribulose-5-P amounts to 30–50% of either.

1) *Nucleosides as Sources of Pentose Phosphates*

Human erythrocytes accumulate and utilize purine ribosides with the production of lactic acid.[28)] Adenosine, xanthosine and guanosine undergo esterification with inorganic phosphate and produce lactate from the pentose of the nucleoside.[29,30)] Purine nucleoside phosphorylase, present in the water-soluble cytoplasm of anucleated red cells causes phosphorolysis of inosine with production of ribose-1-P and hypoxanthine.[31,32)] This reaction has both practical and theoretical significance in that nucleosides have been extensively used in blood preservation studies. Such work had its inception with observations by Dische in 1938, that human hemolysates contained enzymes by which the pentose of adenosine was converted to hexose phosphates and triose phosphates.[33] Subsequently, significant improvement in the viability of erythrocytes and extension of the storage time of red cells of whole blood stored with nucleosides has been made by Denstedt, DeVerdier, Yoshikawa, Nakao, Gabrio, Bartlett, and Strumias and their colleagues. The major effect of nucleosides like inosine on red-cell metabolism is a contribution of large quantities of ribose-1-P, far in excess of the pentose ordinarily available from the oxidative decarboxylation of 6-phosphogluconate. Ribose-1-P is isomerized to ribose-5-P by phosphoribomutase,[34] and on isomerization and epimerization yields a pool of ketopentose phosphates from which hexoses and trioses may be synthesized in TK- and TA-mediated reactions[25,33] (to be discussed in a later section). The inosine pathway is energy-conserving in that esters are produced without reaction with ATP and the utility of nucleosides in blood storage is especially advantageous when ATP is low or depleted, or at acidic pH of stored blood.

2) *Ribulose Diphosphate Metabolism in Ghosts. CO_2 Fixation*

The observation that ribulose-5-P was absent from incubations of ghosts with inosine and phosphate for more than an hour althrough xylulose-5-P accumulated rapidly and exhibited precurser kinetics to hexose phosphates led to the observation that ribulose-5-P is metabolized rapidly to ribulose diphosphate by hemolysates.[35] In the presence of ATP it was found that ribulose-5-P reacted with ^{14}C-bicarbonate to produce acid-stable compounds. Ribulose diphosphate was also shown to be metabolized to nearly equivalent quantities of 3-PG and pyruvate (Fig. 3). Phosphoribulokinase and ribulosediphosphate carboxylase (carboxydismutase) were shown to be present in erythrocytes and were partially purified. It was speculated that the synthesis of 3-PG from bicarbonate in a nonglycolytic pathway, although small, may influence the synthesis of red-cell 2,3-DPG due to the catalytic role of 3-PG on 2,3-DPG mutase. Although the effect of bicarbonate may be to raise the pH which enhances synthesis of 2,3-DPG,[36] bicarbonate *per se* has a stimulatory effect on the synthesis of 2,3-DPG in hemolysates.[37]

3) *Conversion of Pentoses to Hexoses with TA and TK*

Human erythrocytes possess a well-defined chemical pathway by

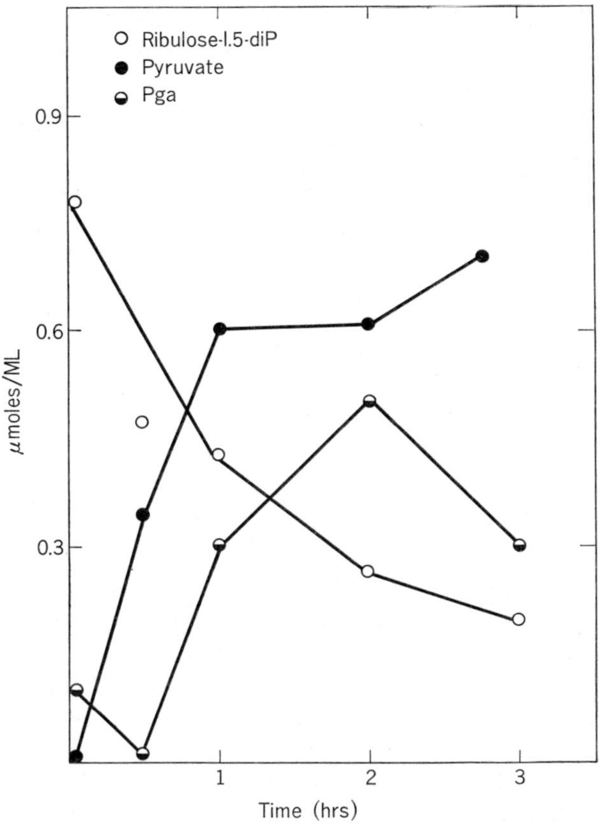

Fig. 3. Metabolism of ribulosediphosphate by hemolysates. Hemolysates (13 ml) were incubated with ribulose-1,5-diP (0.8 mM) open circles, in Tris buffer, pH 7.4 at 37°C. At the times indicated 2.0 ml. were deproteinized with perchloric acid (1.0 ml 15%) the precipitate extracted with 1.0 ml 5% perchloric acid and the supernatant solution neutralized (pH 6.8) with KOH. Hemolysates without ribulose-1,5-diP were also incubated and endogenous values for pyruvate (closed circles) and 3-PG (half open circles) were subtracted.

which hexose phosphates are synthesized from pentose phosphates. Numerous studies implicate the presence of TA and TK, the purification and properties of which have been elucidated by Horecker and Racker and their colleagues from studies with muscle, liver, yeast, and spinach. Horecker and Smyrniotis demonstrated the conversion of ribose-5-P to sedoheptulose-P by liver extracts.[38)] This was shown to be a transketol reaction in that 2 carbons were transferred to acceptor ribose.[39] The enzyme was called transketolase.[40] The reaction mechanism is illustrated in Fig. 1. The reaction catalyzed is the reversible transfer of a glycolaldehyde group from a donor ketose to an acceptor aldose. Xylulose-5-P is the donor of the 2-carbon keto configuration and ribose-5-P is the acceptor.[41] Sedoheptulose-7-P and GAP are products in this reaction. TK is not specific, as other keto donors and aldo acceptors with similar configurations also react, *i.e.*, fructose-6-P and erythrose-4-P. Sedoheptulose-7-P was shown by Horecker and Smyrniotis to react with the enzyme TA, which affected the transfer of the top 3 carbons to 6AP.[42] D-fructose-6-P and D-erythrose-4-P were the products (see Fig. 1). TA catalyzes the transfer of DHAP from a donor ketose to an acceptor aldose. It has been crystallized from yeast by Horecker and colleagues[43] and has properties and a similar mechanism to fructosediphosphate aldolase.[44]

TK activity has been described in mammalian red cells by Bruns *et al.*[23] and by Brownstone and Denstedt[45] measuring sedoheptulose-7-P formation in diluted hemolysates from ribose-5-P. Dische *et al.* demonstrated an approximate stoichiometric conversion of ribose-5-P into sedoheptulose-7-P and triose phosphates in hemolysates under conditions in which TA was inactivated.[46] TK is thiamine dependent, requiring thiamine pyrophosphate as a coenzyme.[40,47] This dependence was also shown for red-cell TK. When rats were maintained for 5 days or more on a thiamine-free diet, TK in their red cells was inactivated.[24] The recycling of glucose through the hexose monophosphate shunt and pentose phosphate pathway was also inhibited with red cells from thiamine-deficient rats.[12] Pentose accumulated within the cells and less $^{14}CO_2$ was evolved from [2-^{14}C]-glucose. TA activity has been estimated by Dische *et al.* in human hemolysates inactivated at 43°C and pH 8.4 by measuring hexose phosphates formed from ribose-5-P assuming steadystate levels of sedoheptulose-7-P and erythrose-4-P.[46]

The overall reaction of TK and TA may be summarized:

$$\text{Xylulose-5-P} + \text{ribose-5-P} \overset{\text{TK}}{\rightleftharpoons} \text{sedoheptulose-7-P} + \text{G-3-P} \quad (1)$$

$$\text{Sedoheptulose-7-P} + \text{G-3-P} \overset{\text{TA}}{\rightleftharpoons} \text{fructose-6-P} + \text{erythrose-4-P} \quad (2)$$

$$\text{Erythrose-4-P} + \text{xylulose-5-P} \overset{\text{TK}}{\rightleftharpoons} \text{fructose-6-P} + \text{G-3-P} \quad (3)$$

Sum

$$2\ \text{xylulose-5-P} + \text{ribose-5-P} \rightleftharpoons 2\ \text{fructose} + \text{G-3-P} \quad (4)$$

In the red-cell, the combined activity of TK and TA provides an active system for the interconversion of pentoses and hexoses. In the hexose shunt, decarboxylation of 6-phosphogluconate yields ribulose-5-P which is epimerized to xylulose-5-P or isomerized to ribose-5-P. These are substrates for TK, which initiates the sequence giving fructose-6-P and GAP, which are further metabolized via glycolysis. In intact cells the end product is lactate[28] and amounts of the intermediates accumulate. If TA of hemolysates is heat inactivated, or the hemolysates greatly diluted, or ghosts made, the enzyme rates are sufficiently diminished to permit kinetic study of some intermediates. Mention has been made above of the techniques applied by Dische, and by Bruns and co-workers to identify intermediates and estimate pentose isomerases, TK, and TA. In ghosts utilizing inosine as substrate, the kinetic turnover of hexose phosphates and triose phosphates was studied[25] (see Fig. 2). Inosine was metabolized according to the scheme:

$$\text{Inosine}+\text{Pi}\ \xrightarrow[\substack{\text{Phosphorylase}\\ \text{(fast)}}]{\text{nucleoside}}\ \text{hypoxanthine}$$

$$+\ \text{ribose-1-P}\ \xrightarrow[\substack{\text{Mutase}\\ \text{(slow)}}]{\text{ribose-1-P}}\ \text{ribose-5-P} \qquad (5)$$

The synthesis of hypoxanthine was much faster than the metabolism of ribose-5-P, suggesting that ribose-1-P mutase limited the rate of utilization of inosine. Reaction 5 depicts extracellular inosine and inorganic phosphate which is rapidly assimilated and converted more slowly into ribose-5-P within the red cells or ghosts. The ghosts retained approximately 10% of intracellular enzymes, the rates of which were sufficiently slow to permit evaluation of the turnover of esters. The ketopentose relationships have been discussed above. Also evident is the accumulation of equilibrated hexose monophosphates fructose-6-P and glucose-6-P and triose phosphates GAP and DHAP, including fructose diphosphate. These remained in a ratio of almost 2: 1 for 2–6 hours of incubation. Dische,[33] with hemolysates, found the ratio of hexose phosphates to triose phosphates from adenosine to be of similar magnitude (1.5–2.1). We did not test for erythrose-4-P but it is unlikely to have accumulated if the sequence of reactions 1–4 operative. It is a strong inhibitor of glucose-6-P isomerase[48] which was very active in ghosts as glucose-6-P and fructose-6-P remained equilibrated at around 80% of glucose-6-P. It is of interest that human hemolysates can form sedoheptulose-P from glucose-6-P without an exogenous acceptor.[49] This is because the fructose-6-P formed is a substrate for both TK and TA present. The TK-glycolaldehyde complex provides erythrose-4-P, an acceptor for TA, while the TA-DHAP complex leaves GAP as an acceptor for TK.[50] Although reaction 4 is written in the forward direction, the K_M's for the enzymes are near unity and their ready reversibility also allows the reverse sequence to occur, that is, the conversion of hexoses to pentoses.[51] An important example of the hexose to pentose conversion is the observation that ^{14}C-glucose was incorporated into the pentose of ATP by human and rabbit red cells.[14] Although a portion of ATP arose via oxidation in the hexose monophosphate shunt, more than half of ATP pentose was derived from glucose by a mechanism consistent with the reverse of reactions.[1-3]

DEOXYNUCLEOSIDE METABOLISM

1) *Conversion of Deoxyribose-5-P to Ribose-5-P*

Nucleoside pathways in human erythrocytes have been discussed above in terms of pathways of ribose metabolism in which pentose isomerases, TK and TA converted pentose carbon chains into hexoses, heptoses, erythroses, trioses and lactate. A critical factor in the conversion of pentoses is the alcoholic (OH) group in the C-2 of ribose-5-P. This is required for isomerization and epimerization to produce ribose-5-P and xylulose-5-P respectively. Both inosine and deoxyinosine were utilized by erythrocytes at comparable rates and produced similar magnitudes of lactate.[28,52] Deoxyinosine was converted to deoxyribose-5-P with purine deoxynucleoside phosphorylase[53] and phosphoribomutase[34] analagous to the phosphorolysis of inosine to form ribose-1-P[31] and then ribose-5-P.[33] Although nucleoside phosphorylases exist in red cells capable of acting on either inosine[31] or deoxyinosine[53] it is not known whether a specific deoxyphosphoribomutase is required. The deoxyribose-5-P is incapable of reaction with ribose-5-P isomerase or ribulose-5-P-3-epimerase due to the absence of an OH group on C-2. Therefore it is incapable of synthesis of xylulose-5-P required for reaction with TK to produce triose phosphates. Thus it was surprising to observe that deoxyinosine in ghosts produced triose phosphates and xylulose-5-P[54] (see Fig. 4 and Table I). Rates of substrate utilization and hypoxanthine production were similar to those previously observed for inosine.[25] The major differences were in the nature and amounts of glycolytic intermediates synthesized as lesser quantities of esters accumulated. These included GAP, DHAP, PG, and xylulose-5-P (Table I). No hexose phosphates were found. However, muscle aldolase added to the ghost extracts caused

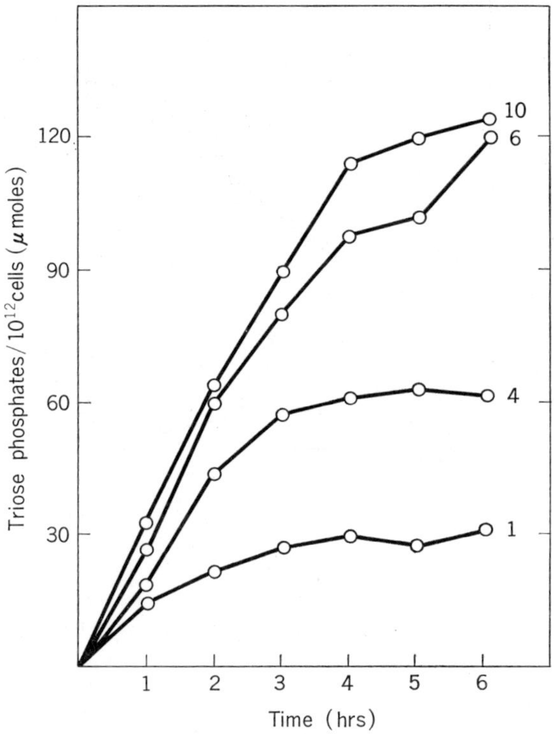

Fig. 4 (a)

TABLE I. Products of deoxyinosine metabolism in ghosts.

Time (h)	Phosphate esters (μ moles/10^{12} cells)				Nonphosphate products (μ moles per 10^{12} cells)			
	3-PG	2,3-DPG	Xylulose-5-P		Acetaldehyde	Pyruvate	Lactate	
			pH 6.8	pH 7.4			pH 6.8	pH 7.4
0	4	60	0	0	0.0	0.0	0	0
2	12	80	14	<1	24	3.0	120	90
4	16	90	20	<1	48	1.0	240	150

Deoxyinosine was 10 m*M* and P 1 m*M*. Conditions were the same as in Fig. 4 except that part of the suspension was incubated at pH 6.8.

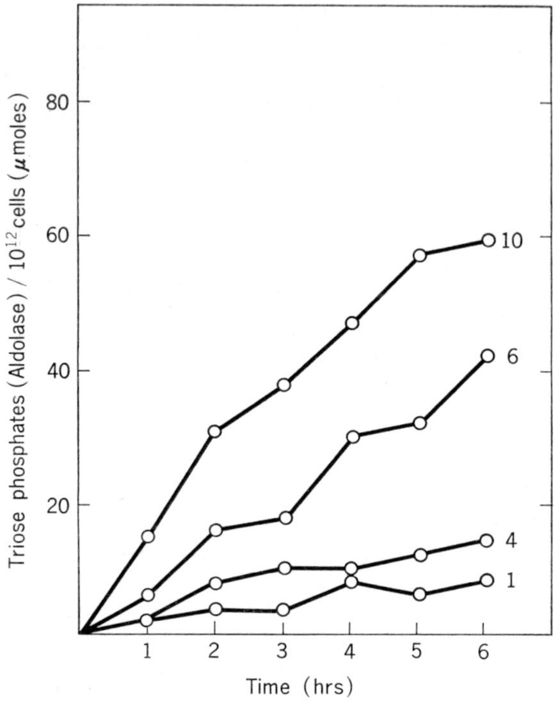

(b)

Fig. 4a, b. Triose phosphates from deoxyinosine in ghosts. Ghosts were incubated at 37°C in physiological buffer at pH 7.4±0.2 containing P_i (4 m*M*) and deoxyinosine at the concentrations shown (m*M*). Cell counts were 4.0×10^6—5.0×10^6 per mm^3 and values are corrected to 5.0×10^6 per mm^3. Fig. 4a (represents triose phosphates (GAP and DHAP) from deoxyinosine). Fig. 4b (Additional triose phosphates released by muscle aldolase).

release of additional DHAP amounting to 0.3–0.5 of that found free (see Fig. 4B, triose phosphate released by aldolase). It was speculated that the principal ester was octulose diphosphate as this has been described to be a product of the reaction between deoxyribose-5-P and DHAP when deoxyinosine was metabolized by erythrocytes.[55] A unique aspect of the deoxynucleoside pathway was the observation that acetaldehyde was synthesized from either deoxyinosine (see Table I) or deoxyribose-5-P.[56] The presence of deoxyriboaldolase in erythrocytes explained the degradation of deoxyribose-5-P to GAP independent of TK. Deoxyriboaldolases were first described by Racker[57] from extracts of *E. coli*, *C. diptheriae* and mouse liver, and later crystallized from *L. plantarum* by Horecker and colleagues.[58,59] Deoxyriboaldolase in red cells could not, however, explain the conversion of deoxyribose-5-P to xylulose-5-P. This was investigated by Fortier, Lionetti and Silva,[60] who explained xylulose-5-P synthesis as the product of triose phosphates (GAP and DHAP) by means of fructosediphosphate aldolase, fructose-6-P phosphatase, and TK according to the reaction sequence 6–10:

$$\text{Deoxyinosine} \xrightarrow[\text{Pi}]{\text{Phosphorylase}} \text{hypoxanthine}$$

$$+\text{deoxyribose-1-P} \xrightarrow{\text{Mutase}} \text{deoxyribose-5-P} \quad (6)$$

$$\text{Deoxyribose-5-P} \xrightarrow{\text{Aldolase I}} \text{acetaldehyde}$$

$$+\text{GAP} \xrightarrow{\text{Isomerase}} \text{DHAP} \quad (7)$$

$$\xrightarrow{\text{Aldolase II}} \text{fructose-1, 6 diP} \xrightarrow{\text{Phosphatase}} \text{fructose-6-P} + \text{Pi} \quad (8)$$

$$\text{Fructose-6-P} + \text{GAP} \xrightarrow{\text{TK}} \text{xylulose-5-P} + \text{erythrose-4-P} \quad (9)$$

$$\text{Xyllulose-5-P} \xrightarrow{\text{Epimerase}} \text{ribulose-5-P} \xrightarrow{\text{Isomerase}} \text{ribose-5-P} \quad (10)$$

In reaction 7) aldolase I is deoxyriboaldolase and in reaction (8) aldolase II is fructosediphosphate aldolase. The significant observations were: (a) Approximately 10% of deoxyribose-5-P was converted to orcinol-reactive compounds by hemolysates (Fig. 5). (b) A non-specific phosphatase capable of reacting with fructose diphosphate to produce fructose-6-P was demonstrated in hemolysates. c) Deoxyribose-5-P labeled with ^{14}C in carbons 3, 4, 5 was synthesized. It was incubated with hemolysates and ^{14}C-ribose-5-P isolated by column and paper chromatography. The specific activity of the labeled ribose-5-P and the free ribose was consistent with all of the carbon originating from the bottom 3 carbons of the substrate deoxyribose-5-P. In the scheme shown, carbons 1 and 2 of deoxyribose-5-P (unlabeled) were cleaved by red-cell deoxyriboaldolase and trapped as acetaldehyde (unlabeled). The uniformly labeled GAP thus became the source of all the carbons of ribose-5-P. The reaction sequence (6–10) for red cells was proposed by Steinbreacht and Hoffman.[61] Data consistent with it have also been obtained by Bartlett[55] and Wiley and Whittam.[62]

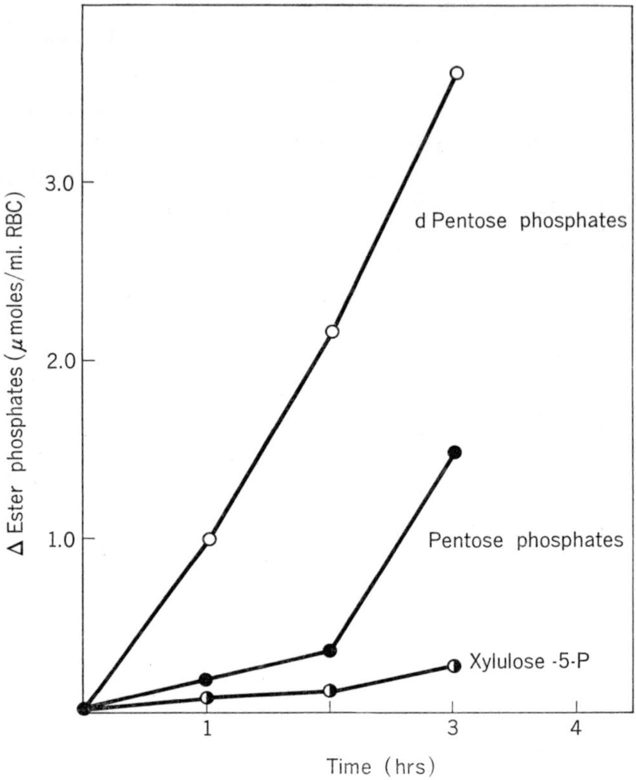

Fig. 5. Conversion of deoxyribose-5-P to pentose phosphates in hemolysates. Hemolysates from washed red cells frozen and thawed twice were incubated (4.0 ml hemolysate with 20 m*M* glycylglycine-HCL, pH 7.0) with deoxyribose-5-P (5.0 m*M*). Open circles, deoxypentose phosphates; closed circles, pentose phosphates; and half open circles. xylulose-5-P.

PHOSPHORIBOSYLPYROPHOSPHATE

1) Synthesis and Reactions

A pentose phosphate of great biological significance and of particular importance in red-cell metabolism is 5-phospho-α-D-ribosyl-1-pyrophosphate (PRPP). It is formed by the reaction of ribose-5-P and ATP.[63)]

$$\text{ribose–5–P+ATP} \longrightarrow \text{PRPP+AMP} \tag{11}$$

The enzyme pyrophosphorylase (pyrophosphotransferase) catalyzes one of few known reactions where the pyrophosphate group is transferred intact from ATP. PRPP is an intermediate of purine biosynthesis contributing the pentose of nucleosides and nucleotides.[64] The amination of PRPP with glutamine to form 5-phosphoribosyl-1-NH_2 is an early step in the biosynthesis of inosinic acid. PRPP may also react with the N-1 position of the purine of ATP or adenine (reactions 12–13). With ATP in bacterial extracts, N-1-(5′-phosphoribosyl)-ATP an intermediate in the synthesis of histidine is formed.[65]

$$\text{PRPP}+\text{ATP} \longrightarrow \text{N-1-(5}'\text{-phosphoribosyl)-ATP}+\text{PP} \qquad (12)$$

The reaction with free purines or pyrimidines produces nucleotides as shown in reactions 13, 14 is the "salvage" reaction for the synthesis of nucleotides.[66]

$$\text{PRPP}+\text{AD} \longrightarrow \text{AMP}+\text{PP} \qquad (13)$$

$$\text{PRPP}+\text{nicotinic acid} \longrightarrow \text{NaRP (Nicotinic acid ribonucleotide)}+\text{PP} \qquad (14)$$

In mammalian red cells the nucleotides (principally adenine nucleotides and pyridine nucleotides—NAD^+, NADP) are constantly being formed and degraded. In human erythrocytes, only reactions (13, 14) have significance as non-nucleated mature cells are unable to undergo *de novo* synthesis of purines from small precursors. Mature rabbit erythrocytes could synthesize both ATP and GTP from labeled formate if preformed 5-amino-1-ribosyl-4-imidazolecarboxyamide was supplied.[67] However immature reticulocytes possessed the capability for total synthesis of purine.[68] Evidently the deficient steps in *de novo* biosynthesis are acquired at the formate activation level of the pathway and are introduced biochemically during the maturation of reticulocytes. Although human and rabbit cells can produce IMP from formate, only rabbit cells can convert IMP to AMP. This makes the reaction of PRPP with free adenine of utmost significance, as it represents the major means of replenishment of the adenine of red-cell ATP (reaction 13). AMP equilibrates rapidly with ATP in red cells by means of adenylate kinase.[69] In a similar way PRPP reacts with nicotinic acid in human red cells to form nicotinic acid ribotide (reaction 14). This reacts further with ATP and glutamine to form NAD^+.[70,71] The synthesis of PRPP in acetone-powder extracts of human red-cell hemolysates was shown by Priess and Handler, who demonstrated its participation in the synthesis of nicotinamide mononucleotide, inosine-5′-P, guanosine-5′-P and adenosine-5′-P.[72] The general rcaction was formulated as:

$$H^+ + \text{N-base} + \text{PRPP} \longrightarrow \text{Nucleotide} + \text{PP} \qquad (15)$$

Similar incorporation of purines into nucleotides of red cells has also been observed by Lowy *et al.*[73)] and Bishop.[74)] By contributing to red-cell ATP the incorporation of adenine into AMP helps sustain red-cell energy-dependent functions, *i.e.*, viability, ionic translocation, regulation of volume, and erythrocyte preservation. Henderson and LePage, studying mice, sugested that purines are incorporated into nucleotides and are transported by blood cells to the tissues.[75)] Rapoport *et al.* in studies of patients with erythrogenesis imperfecta (Diamond-Blackfan) showed that the level of ATP in circulating red cells was determined by an elevated plasma concentration of adenine.[76)] Presumably the liver supplied adenine for this and erythrogenesis in bone marrow. Nakao *et al.* described the loss of biconcavity and progressive shape changes due to ATP depletion of stored erythrocytes, the restoration of which occurred upon regeneration of ATP with adenine and inosine.[77)] Lionetti and McKay observed that adenine serially added to blood at 37°C would facilitate the maintenance of red-cell volume for 50 hr as long as the capacity for ATP regeneration of erythrocytes was sustained.[78)] The capability for synthesis of ATP by means of adenine incorporation into AMP was presumed to be dependent on capability of red cells to synthesize PRPP from ribose-5-P and ATP. Preserved red cells have also been shown to have improved *in vivo* survival when stored with adenine[79)] or adenine plus inosine.[80)] Fundamental to the utilization of adenine for ATP synthesis or nicotinic acid for NAD^+ synthesis is the capability of red cells to sustain biosynthesis of PRPP.

INTERACTION OF THE PENTOSE PHOSPHATE AND THE GLYCOLYTIC PATHWAYS

1) *The Normal Balance of the 2 Pathways*

Erythrocytes in whole blood are in dynamic equilibrium with respect to intermediates of both glycolytic and pentose phosphate pathways. When glucose is the substrate, steady-state levels normally do not flucturate despite transient changes in the glycolytic quotient. In the normal state glycolytic intermediates are low, as are the pentose phosphates or related sugar esters. Only adenylates and 2,3-DPG are present in significant quantities.[81)] The combined operation of both pathways, merging at triose phosphates and ending in the production of lactate, contributes substantially to maintenance of cellular viability. Probably the overall limited metabolism when compared to typical somatic cells is designed to sustain the levels of ATP for maintenance of red-cell dimensions and elasticity, to support the state of hemoglobin (Fe^{2+}) and its function through adequate 2,3-DPG content, and to provide electrons to maintain cellular sulfhydryl groups. ATP formed in glycolysis is required for translocation of ions[82,83] the regulation of volume and shape[77,84–86] and to maintain the integral composition of the membrane. For instance, the lytic substance lysolecithin synthesized in plasma is converted in red-cell membranes to lecithin by ATP-activated fatty acids.[87] In preserved blood the "detoxification" of lysolecithin through acylation depends on the storage-dependent level of ATP in the cells.[88] ATP prevents Ca^{2+}-induced shrinkage of the membrane[86] as well as Ca^{2+}-induced loss of elasticity.[85] The red-cell possesses the capacity for synthesis of a small fraction of red-cell ATP within or on the membrane[89] which may be substrate for Na^+, K^+-ATPase located there.[90] Glycolytically produced NADH (from the oxidation of GAP) is important in the reduction of methemoglobin[91] as is NADPH produced in the hexose shunt by oxidation of glucose-6-P. However, the NADPH-dependent methemoglobin reductase appears to be a reserve system.[92] In steady-state glycolysis the rate of oxidation of glucose-6-P is also an adequate source of electrons for the maintenance of cellular glutathione in the reduced state,[93] while the pentose phosphate pathway to lactate provides PRPP for the biosynthesis of ATP from adenine and of NAD^+ from nicotinamide.

2) Conditions which Favor the Pentose Phosphate Pathway

When other substrates, *i.e.*, nucleosides, are present, however, or when red-cell enzyme activity is reduced by dilution as in hemolysates or ghosts, or enzyme activity is selectively inhibited, the glycolytic pathway may be inhibited in favor of the pentose phosphate pathway. This principle was employed by Dische and co-workers and by Lionetti and co-workers to facilitate the accumulation of intermediates for identification and turnover studies.[33,25] With intact cells, it was shown that inosine interacted competitively with glucose, inhibiting its utilization[1]. High levels of nucleosides (ca. 10 mM) exercised several controls on glycolysis at the hexose and triose levels. The suppression of glycolysis was attributed to a lowered intracellular Pi caused by nucleoside phosphorylase.[94] More probably the effect was due to inhibition of HK by glucose-6-P,[95] as in methylene blue-treated cells the level of glucose-6-P decreased and HK activity increased. Rapaport has postulated a pacemaker role of HK in red-cell glycolysis due to its having a *V*max about 25% of the glycolytic rate and an effective activity which correlated best with glycolytic rate.[96] He cited the ATP concentration in red cells as a regulating factor of HK since its intracellular concentration is close to its K_m for the enzyme (2×10^{-3} *M*), and there is normally about half the amount of ATP present required for saturation (ca. 1 m*M*). This effective activity of HK is further reduced by a pH-dependent inhibition by glucose-6-P.[95] Thus for a system where HK activity approximates 3–4 times the glycolytic rate, the rate decreases due to insufficient ATP to saturate HK and inhibition due to increased glucose-6-P could effectively stop glycolysis.

The intracellular pH of red cells is an important factor in regulating the activity of the glycolytic or pentose phosphate pathways. A pH optimum of 7.6 was found for pentose phosphate metabolism, and 8.2 for glycolysis, by Chapman *et al.*[97] At pH 7.4 the glycolytic rate is limited by the activity of HK[96] and or PFK.[98] At a higher pH (7.6–7.7) control of the glycolytic rate shifted to aldolase as fructose diphosphate accumulated.[99,100] In erythrocytes of blood preserved at 4°C in ACD Yoshikawa and Minakami observed detectable increases in glucose 6-P and fructose-6-P in 1 day at the acid pH (6.9–7.0) of ACD-preserved whole blood. Their data was consistent with rate-limiting by PFK. On the other hand, in whole blood stored for 6–18 weeks in ACD at 4°C the accumulated acidity is favorable for the metabolism of intracelular pentose phosphates. That is, the glycolytic rate is inhibited despite high glucose and ATP, organic phosphates are near zero, and inorganic phosphate is increased. When incubated with nucleosides a large resynthesis of hexose phosphates and PG occurred.[101,102] This can be accounted for by TK-TA mediated reactions of pentose phosphates. Although phosphorylation of fructose-6-P may be inhibited, triose phosphates supplied by the pentose pathway can reconstitute the cells intracellular esters. If adenine is also supplied, the cell adenylates are greatly increased[101–103] by the PRPP mechanism described above.

In depleted stored cells the pentose phosphate pathway is a means to replenish the 2,3-DPG content, which has been shown to support the hemoglobin function.[104,105] The relatively large amounts of GAP obtainable this way provide substrate for 2,3-DPG synthesis, the rate of which has been greatly reduced by glycolytic inhibition at the hexose level. As has been pointed out by Dische[26] 2,3-DPG may exercise several controls on red-cell metabolism. HK is inhibited by 2,3-DPG in a feedback mechanism at physiological concentrations.[22] There is also an inhibition of coupled TK-TA reactions, indicating that 2,3-DPG may serve to keep both pathways in balance and to place the red cell in a "resting" state when 2,3-DPG content is normal.

REFERENCES

1 Murphy, J. R., *J. Lab. Clin. Med.*, **55**, 286 (1960).
2 DeLoecker, W. C. J. and Prankerd, T. A. J., *Clin. Chem. Acta*, **6**, 241 (1961).
3 Bishop, C., *in* "The Red Cell", ed. by Surgenor, D. and Bishop, C. (Academic Press, N. Y., 1964), p. 151.
4 Ramsay, R. and Warren, C. D., *Quart. J. Exp. Physiol.*, **20**, 213 (1930).
5 Harrop, G. A., Jr. and Barron, E. S. G., *J. Exptl. Med.*, **48**, 207 (1928).
6 Warburg, O. and Christian, W., *Biochem. Z.*, **238**, 131 (1931).
7 Warburg, O. and Christian, W., *Biochem. Z.*, **242**, 206 (1931).
8 Warburg, O. and Christian, W., *Biochem. Z.*, **254**, 438 (1932).
9 Warburg, O., Christian, W. and Griese, A., *Biochem. Z.*, **282**, 157 (1935).
10 Dickens, F., *Biochem. Z.*, **32**, 1626 (1938).
11 Horecker, B. L., Smyrniotis, P. Z. and Seegmiller, J. E., *J. Biol. Chem.*, **193**, 383 (1951).
12 Brin, M. and Yonemoto, R. H., *J. Biol. Chem.*, **230**, 307 (1958).
13 Racker, E. and Gatt, S., *Ann. N.Y. Acad. Sci.*, **72**, 427 (1958).
14 Manohar, S. V., Denstedt, O. F. and Rubenstein, D., *Canad. J. Biochem.*, **44**, 59 (1966).
15 Vanderheiden, B. S., *Biochem. Biophys. Res. Comm.*, **6**, 117 (1961).
16 Yoshikawa, H. and Minakami, S., *Folia Haematol.*, **89**, 357 (1968).
17 Horecker, B. L. and Hiatt, H. H., *New Eng. J. Med.*, **258**, 177 (1958).
18 Lachhein, L. and Matthies, H., *Acta Biol. Med. Ger.*, **4**, 403 (1960).
19 Dickens, F., *Biochem. J.*, **38**, 1626 (1938).
20 Dickens, F., *Ibid.*, **38**, 1645 (1938).
21 Dickens, F. and Williamson, D. H., *Biochem. J.*, **64**, 5671 (1956).
22 Dische, Z. and Shiguera, H. T., *Biochem. Biophys. Acta*, **24**, 87, (1957).
23 Bruns, F. H., Noltmann, E. and Valhauls, E., *Biochem. Z.*, **330**, 438 (1958).
24 Bruns, F. H., Noltmann, E. and Valhauls, E., *Ibid.*, **330**, 497 (1958).
25 Lionetti, F. J. and Fortier, N. L., *Arch. Biochem. Biophys.*, **103**, 15 (1963).

26 Dische, Z., *in* "The Red Cell", ed. by Bishop, C. and Surgenor, D. M. (Academic Press, N.Y., 1964), p. 189, 208.
27 Tabachnick, M., Srere, P. A. and Cooper, J., *Arch. Biochem. Biophys.*, **74**, 315 (1958).
28 Lowy, B. A., Jaffe, E. R., Vanderhoff, G. A., Crook, L. and London, I. M., *J. Biol. Chem.*, **230**, 409 (1958).
29 Gabrio, B. W. and Huennekens, F. M., *Biochem. Biophys. Acta*, **18**, 585 (1955).
30 Rubenstein, D. and Denstedt, O. F., *Canad. J. Biochem. Physiol.*, **34**, 927 (1956).
31 Tsuboi, K. K. and Hudson, P. B., *J. Biol. Chem.*, **224**, 879 (1957).
32 Huennekens, F. M., Nurk, N. E. and Gabrio, B. W., *J. Biol. Chem.*, **221**, 971 (1956).
33 Dische, Z., *in* "Phosphorus Metabolism" ed. by McElroy, W. D. and Glass, B. (Johns Hopkins Press, Baltimore, Md., 1951), p. 171.
34 Guarino, A. J. and Sable, H. Z., *J. Biol. Chem.*, **215**, 515 (1955).
35 Fortier, N. L., Galland, L. and Lionetti, F. J., *Arch. Biochem. Biophys.*, **119**, 69 (1967).
36 Rapoport, S. and Guest, G. M., *J. Biol. Chem.*, **131**, 675 (1939).
37 Forstner, J. F., Fortier, N. L. and Lionett, F. J., *Biochim. Biophys. Acta*, **158**, 317 (1968).
38 Horecker, B. L. and Smyrniotis, P. Z., *J. Amer. Chem. Soc.*, **74**, 2123 (1952).
39 Horecker, B. L., Smyrniotis, P. Z. and Klenow, H., *J. Biol. Chem.*, **205**, 661 (1953).
40 Racker, E., de La Habe, G. and Leder, I. G., *J. Amer. Chem. Soc.*, **75**, 1010 (1953).
41 Srere, P. A., Cooper, J. R., Klybas, U. and Racker, E., *Arch. Biophys.*, **59**, 535 (1955).
42 Horecker, B. L. and Smyrniotis, P. Z., *J. Biol. Chem.*, **212**, 811 (1955).
43 Pontremoli, S., Prandine, D. B., Bonsignore, A. and Horecker, B. L., *Proc. Natl. Acad. Sci. U.S.*, **47**, 1942 (1961).
44 Lai, C. Y., Tchola, O., Cheng, T. and Horecker, B. L., *J. Biol. Chem.*, **240**, 1347 (1965).
45 Brownstone, Y. S. and Denstedt, O. F., *Canad. J. Biochem. Physiol.*, **39**, 534 (1961).
46 Dische, Z., Shiguera, H. T. and Landsberg, E., *Arch. Biochem. Biophys.*, **89**, 123 (1960).
47 Horecker, B. L. and Smyrniotis, P. A., *J. Amer. Chem. Soc.*, **75**, 1009 (1953).
48 Dische, Z. and Igals, D., *Arch. Biochem. Biophys.*, **93**, 201 (1961).
49 Dische, Z., *Ann. N.Y. Acad. Sci.*, **75**, 129 (1958).
50 Horecker, B. L., Harvey Lecture Series 57 (Academic Press, N. Y., 1962), p. 49.

51 Fortier, N. L., Lionetti, F. J. and Silva, J., *Biochim. Biophys. Acta*, **208**, 181 (1970).
52 Jaffe, E. R., *J. Clin. Invest.*, **38**, 1555 (1959).
53 DeVerdier, C. H. and Gould, B. J., *Biophys. Acta*, **68**, 333 (1963).
54 Lionetti, F. J. and Fortier, N. L., *Biochim. Biophys. Acta*, **119**, 462 (1966).
55 Bartlett, G. R., *Biochim. Biophys. Acta*, **156**, 254 (1968).
56 Jedziniak, J. A. and Lionetti, F. J., *Biochim. Biophys. Acta*, **212**, 478 (1970).
57 Racker, E., *J. Biol. Chem.*, **196**, 347 (1952).
58 Pricer, W. E. and Horecker, B. L., *J. Biol. Chem.*, **235**, 1292 (1960).
59 Hoffee, P., Rosen, D. M. and Horecker, B. L., *J. Biol. Chem.*, **240**, 1512 (1965).
60 Fortier, N. L., Lionetti, F. J. and Silva, J., *Biochim. Biophys. Acta*, **208**, 181 (1970).
61 Steinbrecht, I. and Hoffman, E., *Z. Physiol. Chem.*, **344**, 89 (1966).
62 Wiley, J. S. and Whittam, R., *Biochim. Biophys. Acta*, **115**, 233 (1966).
63 Khorana, H. G., Fernandes, J. F. and Kornberg, A., *J. Biol. Chem.*, **230**, 941 (1958).
64 Buchanan, J. M. and Hartman, S. C., *Adv. Enzymol.*, **21**, 199 (1959).
65 Ames, B. M., Martin, R. G. and Garry, B. J., *J. Biol. Chem.*, **236**, 2018 (1961).
66 Kornberg, A., Lieberman, I. and Simms, E. S., *J. Biol. Chem.*, **215**, 417 (1955).
67 Lowy, B. A. and Williams, M. K., *J. Biol. Chem.*, **235**, 2924 (1960).
68 Lowy, B. A., Cook, J. L. and London, I. M., *J. Biol. Chem.*, **236**, 1442 (1961).
69 Kashket, S. and Denstedt, O. F., *Canad. J. Biochem. Physiol.*, **36**, 1057 (1958).
70 Priess, J. and Handler, P., *J. Amer. Chem. Soc.*, **79**, 1514 (1957).
71 Priess, J. and Handler, P., *Ibid.*, **79**, 4246 (1957).
72 Priess, J. and Handler, P., *J. Biol. Chem.*, **225**, 759 (1957).
73 Lowy, B. A., Williams, M. K. and London, I. M., *J. Biol. Chem.*, **237**, 1623 (1962).
74 Bishop, C., *J. Biol. Chem.*, **235**, 3228 (1960).
75 Henderson, F. J. and LePage, G. A., *J. Biol. Chem.*, **234**, 3219 (1959).
76 Rapoport, I. S., Jacobasch, G., Pren, S. and Rapoport, S., *Blood*, **33**, 617 (1969).
77 Nakao, M., Nakao, T., Yamazoe, S. and Yoshikawa, H., *J. Biochem.*, **49**, 487 (1961).
78 Lionetti, F. J. and McKay, J., *in* "Modern Problems in Blood Preservation", ed. by Spielmann, W. and Seidl, S., G. Fisher Verlag (Stuttgart, 1970), p. 34.

79 Sugita, Y. and Simon, E. R., *J. Clin. Invest.*, **44**, 629 (1965).
80 Yoshikawa, H. and Nakao, M., *Haematologica*, **10**, 48 (1965).
81 Bartlett, G. R., *J. Biol. Chem.*, **234**, 449 (1959).
82 Hoffman, J., *Circulation*, **26**, 1201 (1962).
83 Dunham, E. T., *Physiologist*, **1**, 23 (1957).
84 Lionetti, F. J., McKay, J. and Gendron, H., *Microvascular Res.*, **1**, 196 (1968).
85 Weed, R. I., LaCelle, P., Merrill, E. W., Craig, G., Gregory, A., Karch, F. and Pickens, F., *J. Clin. Invest.*, **48**, 795 (1969).
86 Palek, J., Curby, W. A. and Lionetti, F. J., *Amer. J. Physiol.*, **220**, 19 (1971).
87 DeGier, J., The XI Cong. Int. Soc. Hematol. Plenary Sessions (V. C. N. Blight and Co., Sidney, 1966), p. 384.
88 Ferber, E., Kohlschutter, A., Munder, P. G. and Fisher, H., *in* " Modern Problems of Blood Preservation ", ed. by Spielmann, E. and Seidl, S. (Gustav Fischer, Stuttgart, 1970), p. 14.
89 Ronquist, G., *Forsvarsmedicin*, **5**, 179 (1969).
90 Post, R. L., Merritt, C. R., Kinsolving, C. R. and Albright, C. D., *J. Biol. Chem.*, **235**, 1796 (1960).
91 Scott, E. M. and McGraw, J. C., *J. Biol. Chem.*, **237**, 249 (1962).
92 Jaffe, E. R., *in* " The Red Cell ", ed. by Bishop, C. and Surgenor, D. M. (Academic Press, N.Y., 1964), p. 412.
93 Jacob, H. S. and Jandl, J. H., *J. Biol. Chem.*, **241**, 4243 (1966).
94 Wu, R. and Racker, E., *in* " Control Mechanisms in Respiration and Fermentation ", ed. by Wright, E. G. (Ronald Press, New York, 1963).
95 Rose, I. A. and O'Connell, E. L., *J. Biol. Chem.*, **239**, 12 (1964).
96 Rapoport, S., XIth Cong. Int. Soc. Hematol. Plenary Sessions (V. C. N. Blight and Co., Sidney, 1966), p. 358.
97 Chapman, R. G., Huennekens, F. M. and Gabrio, B. W., *Clin. Res.*, **8**, 127 (1960).
98 Rose, I. A., *Exptl. Eye Res.*, **11**, 264 (1971).
99 Minakami, S., Saito, T., Suzuki, C. and Yoshikawa, H., *Biochem. Biophys. Res. Comm.*, **17**, 748 (1964).
100 Mills, G. C., *Arch. Biochem. Biophys.*, **117**, 487 (1966).
101 Yoshikawa, H. and Minakami, S., XIth Cong. Int. Soc. Hematol. Plenary Sessions (V. C. N. Blight and Co., Sidney, 1966), p. 389.
102 Shafer, A. W. and Bartlett, G. R., *J. Clin. Invest.*, **42**, 690 (1962).
103 Nakao, M., Nakao, T., Tatibana, M. and Yoshikawa, H., *J. Biochem.*, **47**, 661 (1960).
104 Chanutin, A. and Curnish, R. R., *Arch. Biochem. Biophys.*, **121**, 96 (1967).
105 Benesch, R. and Benesch, R. E., *Biochem. Biophys. Res. Comm.*, **26**, 162 (1967).

Catalase and Glutathione Peroxidase

S. M. RAPOPORT and M. MÜLLER

Institute of Physiological and Biological Chemistry, Humboldt University, Berlin, GDR

Catalase and peroxidase are enzymes competing for the removal of H_2O_2. Their distribution in the tissues and their kinetic properties are reviewed. Catalase acts *in vivo* probably only as a peroxidase, with formate as its predominant hydrogen donor. Formate may originate within the body from external sources or be formed in the immature red cell. The possible sources of H_2O_2 are considered. It is estimated that the steady-state level of H_2O_2 is 0.1 μM and that of formate 0.3 mM. Under normal conditions, catalase participates significantly in the removal of H_2O_2. Its function, however, is not essential for the existence of red cells since it can be completely taken over by GSH peroxidase. GSH peroxidase on the other hand acts as an essential protective mechanism, probably because of its ability to react with lipid peroxides.

INTRODUCTION

Catalase was perhaps the first enzyme whose mode of action was described (Thénard, 1818). Even at that time its ubiqitous occurrence in animals and plants, and later also in aerobic microorganisms, was noted. The total amount of catalase in the human body was originally estimated at 5 gm[1] but this now appears to be low. We estimated it to be 20–25 gm, *i.e.*, 80–100 μmoles. It accounts for much more of the total body iron than the cytochromes. Its concentration is highest in the liver with 30–45 μM, and about one-tenth as much in red cells (3–4.5 μM), white cells and kidney.[2] The catalase activity in the red cells of different species varies greatly over a range of 3 orders of magnitude, being highest in those of man, monkeys and the cat and lowest in those of the duck. Among mammals, the dog erythrocyte has the lowest catalase activity, about one-fiftieth that of the human red cell (Table I).[3] These differences are not reflected in the catalase concentration of the liver and other tissues.[4] The biological variability of the red cells would suggest that catalase is not of primary importance for the mature erythrocyte. On the other hand one might expect higher values in the immature cells of birds and the dog if catalase

TABLE I. Catalase activity in erythrocytes.

Species	Activity* mmoles H_2O_2/ml cells per min
Cat	95.0±11.2
Monkey	87.0± 3.7
Man	80.5± 7.5
Rabbit	55.5± 4.8
Rat	22.5± 1.1
Chicken	3.0± 1.0
Dog	2.2± 2.2
Pigeon	0.5± 0.4
Duck	0.1± 0.05

* calculated from ref. [3].

were of importance for the immature stages of their cells, with a secondary decline during maturation. In keeping with these assumptions, the catalase content of reticulocytes of man and rabbit is little higher, if at all, than in their mature erythrocytes, which maintain high catalase concentrations.[5–7] Recently we studied the catalase in red cells, bone marrow and liver of ducks during anemia. The catalase of reticulocyte rich blood cells was tenfold higher than of mature erythrocytes, but still only 1–2% of the value in the liver. The catalase content of bone marrow did not exceed that of the streaming blood. There was no difference between erythroid and myeloid cells. From these data one may conclude that there exist two levels of control of catalase content. One, a repression, which includes all elements of erythropoiesies and myelopoiesis, and is particularly pronounced in ducks, and secondly, a maturational decline by one order of magnitude.[7a]

Catalase in the liver is localized largely in peroxisomes,[8] with some species differences,[9] while it is found entirely in the cytosol of red cells. This also may be a secondary development. In the liver cell, catalase has a high rate of turnover, with a biological half-life of 1–4 days, while it is as stable as hemoglobin in the red cell.

THE MOLECULAR AND CATALYTIC PROPERTIES OF CATALASE

Catalase is one of the best-studied enzymes, as regards to its molecular and kinetic properties. Most of the work has been performed on the enzyme from beef and horse liver. It has been crystallized from liver, erythrocytes and various other sources.[10,11] It is a tetramer with a molecular weight of about 250,000,[12] consisting of 4 identical subunits in a tetrahedral arrangement.[13,14] The elucidation of its sequence and 3-dimensional structure are under way. The data so far available indicate that substitutions in the amino acid sequences of the enzymes from liver and red cells will be less than 20%.[15]

The question of isoenzymes of catalase appears not to have been settled definitely as yet. The chromatographic and electrophoretic heterogeneity found in preparations from both liver and erythrocytes may well be due to a varying degree of oxidation or disulfide formation by the SH groups.[16,17] Some reports would suggest however that there remains a genuine molecular heterogeneity which is not an artifact.[18] Catalase reacts consecutively with H_2O_2 and hydrogen donors in bimolecular reactions without change of the valence of the trivalent iron in the heme. The events could be studied by spectrophotometric methods.[19] (See simplified scheme, Fig. 1). In the first, at very fast bimolecular reaction the enzyme-H_2O_2 complex (complex I) is formed, which reacts subsequently with hydrogen donors or other agents, with the possible formation of other complexes (II and III). All of these reactions with the exception of those with formate, methanol and ethanol arc probably without any physiological significance.

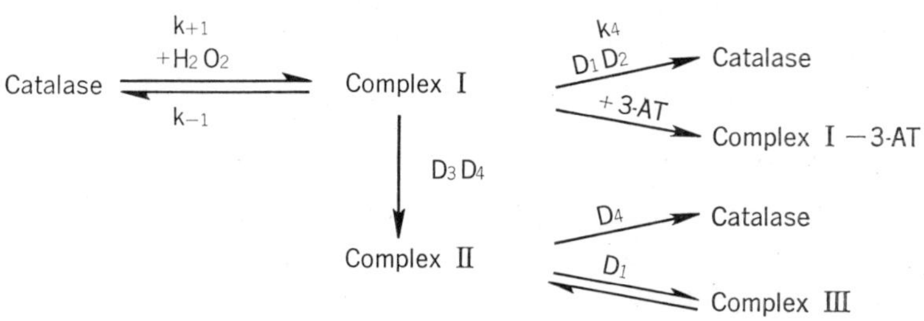

Hydrogen donors:

D_1 — H_2O_2 | D_3 — ascorbate, ferrocyanide
D_2 — alcohols, formate | D_4 — phenols

Kinetic constants:

k_{+1} — $3.10^7\ M^{-1}\ sec^{-1}$; k_{-1} — $0,02\ sec^{-1}$; k_4 — methanol $1000\ M^{-1}\ sec^{-1}$
— ethanol $1000\ M^{-1}\ sec^{-1}$
— formate $470\ M^{-1}\ sec^{-1}$

Fig. 1. Simplified scheme of the reactions of catalase and their kinetic constants.

Catalase is highly selective in its affinity for H_2O_2, the reaction rate for methyl and ethyl peroxide being 2 and 3 orders of magnitude, respectively, lower than that with H_2O_2.[20] Thus, it will not react with lipid peroxides. There is also a strong preference with respect to hydrogen donors. The reaction rate with formate, methanol and ethanol, is about 500 times greater than with acetaldehyde and acetate, and 50 times that with propanol.[20] The low concentration of H_2O_2 in the red cells and in other tissues, as compared with other hydrogen donors make it practically certain that the catalatic activity of the enzyme is a laboratory phenomenon without physiological significance. Thus, the peroxidative action of the enzyme is its true function, as proposed by Keilin and Hartree.[21] Catalase would then differ from other peroxidases mainly in that a side reaction with a second molecule of H_2O_2 can be observed under highly nonphysiological conditions *in vitro*. It is of significance that under such conditions the enzyme is rapidly inactivated.

Mention may be made of the highly selective inhibitory action of 3-amino-1,2,4-triazole (3-AT), a herbicide, which has become a most useful tool for the investigation of the physiological role of catalase. It competes with hydrogen donors for complex I and forms a non-dissociable complex with it; thereby, an irreversible inhibition is produced. Catalase is only inhibited if sufficient H_2O_2 for the formation of complex I is available.[22–24] For this reason one finds after intravenous application of 3-AT that 96–98% of the catalase of liver and leucocytes is inhibited, but practically none of that of red cells.[25]

1) *Sources and Steady-State Levels of Formate and H_2O_2*

As indicated before, the most important hydrogen donor for catalase may be formate, the concentration of which has only rarely been measured. Data on man, dog, sheep and cattle indicate[26–29] a steady-state level in the blood plasma of 0.1 m*M*. Accumulation in the cells may be higher. The sources of this formate have not been studied extensively. It originates, presumably endogenously, from the metabolism of the hydroxymethyl group of serine and possibly other C_1 donors. Another source may be methanol from the pectins of vegetable foods, as suggested by Aebi.[29] In ruminants at least, fermentation in the digestive tract is an important source. There is also some formate formation from serine within the red cell.[30] This is very sizeable in the reticulocyte but is still present in the erythrocyte, which is able to convert the hydroxymethyl group of serine into CO_2

by means of FH_4-dependent reactions and catalase. The methylene-FH_4 dehydrogenase and the FH_4 formylase are indeed still present in the erythrocyte in a concentration about one-tenth that in the reticulocyte.[31] CO_2 formation from formate in the red cell proceeds exclusively by means of the catalase, since inhibition with 3-AT will completely suppress $^{14}CO_2$ formation from formate.[32,33]

The sources of H_2O_2 and its role in cell metabolism are largely unclarified. There exist a multitude of enzymatic and nonenzymatic H_2O_2-forming processes which have to be considered. The enzymes forming H_2O_2 are mostly extramitochondrially located flavoproteins, among them NAD(P)H oxidases, xanthine oxidase, uricase, D-aminoacid oxidase. The most important nonenzymatic reactions are the oxidation of ascorbic acid and of thiols, and autoxidations of lipids, which also may be catalyzed by hemin. Lately, the possible formation of H_2O_2 by heart mitochondria within the respiratory chain from succinate has been demonstrated under special conditions.[34]

The relative role of these reactions, however, cannot be assessed at present. In rat liver homogenates, uric acid and to a lesser degree other substrates of the flavoenzymes mentioned may increase the catalase-dependent oxidation of formate.[35] However, the addition of cysteine and glutathione may yield even more H_2O_2 than the substrates of xanthine oxidase.[36] In erythrocytes most of the enzymes mentioned except for the NAD(P)H oxidases[37] are absent, but all the nonenzymatic reactions are possible and have been partly described.[38,39] We have estimated that with a glucose consumption of 2 μmoles per ml of cells per hr and a proportion of the oxidative pentose phosphate pathway (OPP) of 10%, 0.4μmoles of H_2O_2 per ml of cells per hr are formed, which corresponds fairly well with an oxygen consumption of leucocyte-free red cells of 0.3–0.4 μmoles of O_2 per ml of cells per hr and a rate of oxidation of formate calculated to be 0.36 μmoles.[33] For the mature erythrocyte in the circulating blood, both the supply of formate and of H_2O_2 is in the nonsaturating range. When incubated under substrate-free conditions, formate is exhausted rapidly while the formation of H_2O_2 continues. From a knowledge of the kinetic constants and by employing either formate or H_2O_2 in excess, an approximate estimate of the steady-state concentrations of both formate and H_2O_2 has been possible (Fig. 2). Values of about 0.1 μM for the steady-state concentration of H_2O_2 and 0.3 mM for formate were calculated.[33,40]

In reticulocytes the extent of both H_2O_2 formation and consumption, as well as that of formate, is much greater than in the erythro-

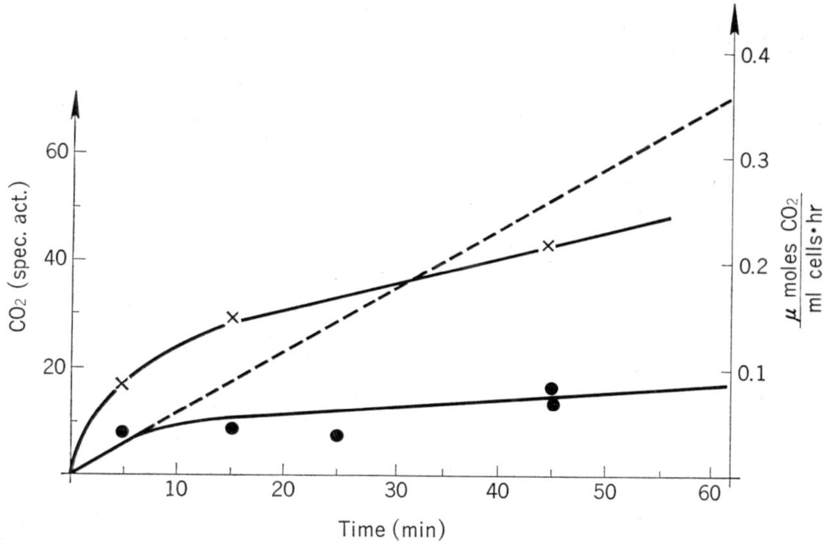

Fig. 2. $^{14}CO_2$ Formation from formate in erythrocytes of man. ●: Formate (4 m*M*); × formate+methylene blue (0.2 m*M*).

cyte. It has been estimated on the basis of the 3-AT inhibition of oxygen consumption that catalase-dependent respiration amounts to about one-fifth of the total.[33] A similar estimate was derived from the percentage of cyanide-resistent respiration.[40a~c] However it was found that cyanide is not suitable, since its effects are both concentration- and time-dependent, without any plateau. On the other hand stable values of a non-respiratory-chain respiration were observed when antimycin A was used. The antimycin-resistent respiration amounts to 15–18% for the reticulocyte of the rabbit and twice as much for that of the duck. It may be assumed that the oxygen consumption yields H_2O_2 by the action of flavoenzymes. The organic substrates of this respiration are serine, glycine, glucose and ribose. The common feature of these reactions is their NADP dependence.[40d] On incubation under substrate-free conditions, formate production continues and its oxidation is limited by the available concentration of H_2O_2. Neither the sources of H_2O_2 nor the character of the hydrogen donors other than serine and C-2 of glycine have been explored. In keeping with the assumed importance of NADPH oxidation is the predominance of the OPP pathway for the oxidation of glucose in the reticulocyte. Summarizing the preceding discussion one may state that one biological function of catalase, namely the oxidation of formate, has been demonstrated. This reaction participates in the removal of H_2O_2. It is doubtful, however, whether this reaction is essential. This is indicated by the fact that human acatalasia in Switzerland and Israel is asymptomatic, although only 0.5–2.0% of the normal enzymatic activity remains.[41,42] The same is true for 5 strains of mice with acatalasia[43] and for acatalatic guinea pigs[44] and dogs.[45] As mentioned before, erythrocytes (but not liver) of the duck are extremely low in catalase.[4] Acatalatic human cells exhibit a 3-fold increase of the OPP pathway compared with normal cells. If challenged with H_2O_2-producing agents they will increase this pathway nearly 20-fold.[46] Cells low in catalase are, however, highly sensitive to peroxides.[47,48] Inhibition of catalase will also produce increased formation of Heinz bodies as an expression of cellular damage of hemoglobin.[49] Thus it would appear that catalase contributes to some extent in the protective mechanism of the red cell against H_2O_2.

What effect acatalasia may have on the metabolism of formate is uncertain. It has been assumed that bacterial enzymes may compensate the enzyme deficiency.[42] It appears possible that the erythrocytes of such individuals may have increased utilization of formate for purine synthesis from 5-amino-1-ribosyl-4-imidazolecarboxamide.[33]

2) *Pathophysiology of Catalase*

There have been a multitude of studies on catalase of the blood. Most of them are vitiated by the lack of consideration of the packed volume of cells. Dramatic changes of catalase activity under pathological conditions have not been found. There is a significant tendency to increased values in hemolytic anemias, and the reverse in polycythemia and panmyelopathy.[50] Various oxidants will decrease the catalase activity, and thus low values have been observed in patients with GPD deficiency.[51,52]

GLUTATHIONE PEROXIDASE

Mills discovered in 1957 that beef erythrocytes contain a second enzyme besides catalase which can inhibit the decomposition of hemoglobin by H_2O_2.[53] In 1970 Flohè *et al.* succeeded in purifying the enzyme.[54] The enzyme has been found so far only in animal tissues. There exist differences in the activity of the enzyme among different tissues and among various species (Table II).[55] The enzyme catalyses the following reaction:

TABLE II. GSH peroxidase activity in various tissues.[55]

	Activity units/gm tissue
Rat liver	261 (84–414)
heart	41 (23– 52)
kidney	46 (30– 57)
lung	62 (25–114)
intestine	13 (0– 26)
leg muscle	17 (0– 34)
blood	407 (378–445)*
Human blood	72 (70– 73)*

* units/ml blood.

$$2GSH + ROOH \longrightarrow GSSG + ROH + H_2O$$

where ROOH indicates a peroxide, including H_2O_2. The enzyme is, surprisingly enough, neither a hemo- nor a flavoprotein.[56] It has a molecular weight of 84,000 and consists of 4 subunits of identical molecular weight.[54] The enzyme exhibits a very high specificity for thiols, GSH being practically the only physiologically significant substrate.[57,58] On the other hand, and in contrast to catalase, GSH peroxidase is much less selective with respect to peroxides. The hydroperoxides of linolenic acid, and its ethyl ester, among others, react nearly as rapidly as hydrogen peroxide.[59] The affinity of enzyme for peroxides is high. On the other hand saturation cannot be achieved with respect to glutathione. A linear dependence of reaction rate on the GSH concentration in the range between 0.05 and 2.25 m*M* GSH has been observed for the enzyme from erythrocytes of beef and rats.[60–62] The apparent K_M for H_2O_2 is a function of GSH concentration.[63] It is approximately 0.025 m*M* at the GSH concentration in erythrocytes (3 m*M*).[64]

Somewhat divergent results were obtained with the GSH peroxidase of pig erythrocytes. Here a K_M of about 3 m*M* was extrapolated for GSH, while it was not possible to estimate the K_M for H_2O_2 since the Lineweaver-Burk plots were not linear.[65] The following formal mechanism of the reaction has been proposed[60]:

$$E_{red} + H_2O_2 \underset{k_{-1}}{\overset{k_{+1}}{\rightleftharpoons}} E_{OX}- + H_2O \qquad (1)$$

$$E_{OX}- + GSH \underset{k_{-2}}{\overset{k_{+2}}{\rightleftharpoons}} E_{OX} - GSH \qquad (2)$$

It is assumed that k_{+2} is limiting and that the apparent K_M does not represent a K_S but approximately the ratio of k_{+2}/k_{+1}. From this relation it would follow that the K_M for H_2O_2 is a function of the GSH concentration. The preceding pair of reactions are presumably followed by a second pair:

$$E_{OX} - GSH + GSH \underset{k_{-3}}{\overset{k_{+3}}{\rightleftharpoons}} E_{OX} - (GSH)_2 \tag{3}$$

$$E_{OX} - (GSH)_2 \underset{k_{-4}}{\overset{k_{+4}}{\rightleftharpoons}} E_{red} + GSSG \tag{4}$$

It is presumed that the intermediate product E_{OX}-GSH represents a mixed disulfide between a thiol group of the enzyme and GSH. The proposed intermediates have so far not been isolated or identified in an unambiguous manner.[56)]

THE FUNCTION OF GSH PEROXIDASE

Under the conditions *in vivo* the concentration of GSH in the red cell amounts to about 3 m*M*, while that of GSSG is vanishingly small.[66,67)] Thus, the enzyme finds excellent conditions for its optimal function. Since it reacts with organic peroxides, *e.g.*, of fatty acids, nearly as well as with H_2O_2, it should be capable of protecting both hemoglobin, enzymes with essential and sensitive SH groups, and membrane constituents from the deleterious effects of peroxidation.[68–73)] It is dependent for its function on continuous regeneration of GSH by way of NADPH-GSSG reductase. In turn, a continuous supply of NADPH is dependent on the integrity of the OPP pathway of glucose.

THE INTERRELATION BETWEEN CATALASE AND GSH PEROXIDASE

Both glutathione peroxidase and catalase participate in the removal of H_2O_2. Their relative share will depend in the steady-state concentration of H_2O_2[74,47)] in such a manner that below 3.5 μM H_2O_2 the contribution of GSH peroxidase predominates. In principle, the relative share will also depend on the GSH concentration in the erythrocyte. One would therefore expect a higher share of the catalase in individuals with inborn low GSH levels, and also in patients with G6PD

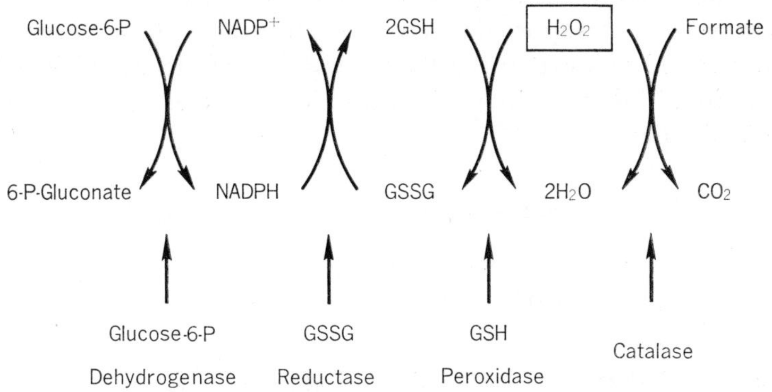

Fig. 3. Scheme of competition of GSH peroxidase and catalase for H_2O_2.

deficiency. A higher concentration of H_2O_2 has indeed been observed in GPD-deficient erythrocytes in the presence of acetyl phenylhydrazine.[75] In most reports the functional significance of catalase is underestimated, since the coupled oxidation of formate is not considered. We could demonstrate that it is possible, by increasing the formate concentration, to reduce the $^{14}CO_2$ formation from [1-^{14}C]-glucose by more than one-half. The mechanism of this effect is probably a decreased steady-state concentration of H_2O_2 due to the formate, by which the oxidation of GSH and consequently the formation of $NADP^+$ is reduced.[76] (Fig. 3). It is also possible by addition of formate to decrease the extent of oxidation of GSH by exogenous H_2O_2.[76] However catalase cannot protect the cell from the consequences of a functional deficiency of GSH peroxidase, probably because H_2O_2 is not the only, and may not even be the most important, toxic agent. Presumably other autoxidation products such as lipid peroxides are responsible for the well-known deleterious effects of disturbances of GSH metabolism, such as formation of Heinz bodies, and hemolysis.[68] GSH peroxidase on the other hand is fully able to protect the red cells from the effects of catalase deficiency, as discussed before.

REFERENCES

1 Drabkin, D. L., *Physiol. Rev.*, **31**, 362 (1951).
2 Rechcigl, M., Jr. and Evans, W. H., *Nature*, **199**, 1001 (1963).
3 Paniker, N. V. and Iyer, G. Y. N., *Canad. J. Biochem.*, **43**, 1029 (1965).
4 Kaziro, K., Kikuchi, G., Nakamura, H. and Yoshida, M., *Chem.*

Ber., **85**, 886 (1952).
5 Sass, M. D., *Nature*, **197**, 503 (1963).
6 Thorup, O. A., Carpenter, J. T. and Howard, P., *Brit. J. Haematol.*, **10**, 542 (1964).
7 Bracci, R., Corvaglia, E., Princi, P., Bettini, F. and Pindinelli, C., *Ital. J. Biochem.*, **18**, 100 (1969).
7a Rapoport, S., Hartwig, A. and Gross, H., *Acta Biol. Med. German.* (in the press).
8 De Duve, C. and Baudhuin, P., *Physiol. Rev.*, **46**, 323 (1966).
9 Makar, A. B. and Mannering, G. J., *Mol. Pharmacol.*, **4**, 484 (1968).
10 Laskowski, M. and Sumner, J. B., *Science*, **94**, 615 (1941).
11 Herbert, D. and Pinsent, J., *Biochem. J.*, **43**, 203 (1948).
12 Deisseroth, A. and Dounce, A. L., *Physiol. Rev.*, **50**, 319 (1970).
13 Sund, H., Weber, K. and Mölbert, E., *Europ. J. Biochem.*, **1**, 400 (1967).
14 Kiselev, N. A., De Rosier, D. J. and Klug, A., *J. Mol. Biol.*, **35**, 561 (1968).
15 Schroeder, W. A., Shelton, J. R., Shelton, J. B., Robberson, B. and Apell, G., *Arch. Biochem. Biophys.*, **131**, 653 (1969).
16 Cantz, M., Mörikofer-Zwez, S., Bossi, E., Kaufmann, H., von Wartburg, J. P. and Aebi, H., *Experientia*, **24**, 119 (1968).
17 Heidrich, H. G., *Hoppe Seyler Z. Physiol. Chem.*, **349**, 873 (1968).
18 Feinstein, R. N., Savol, R. and Howard, J. B., *Enzymologia*, **41**, 345 (1971).
19 Keilin, D. and Nicholls, P., *Biochim. Biophys. Acta*, **29**, 302 (1958).
20 Chance, B., "The Enzymes", 1st ed., Vol. II, New York, Academic Press Inc., 428 (1951).
21 Keilin, D. and Hartree, E. F., *Biochem. J.*, **39**, 293 (1945).
22 Margoliash, E. and Novogrodsky, A., *Biochem. J.*, **68**, 468 (1958).
23 Margoliash, E., Novogrodsky, A. and Schejter, A., *Biochem. J.*, **74**, 339 (1960).
24 Nicholls, P., *Biochim. Biophys. Acta*, **59**, 415 (1962).
25 cf. (2)
26 Annison, E. A., *Biochem. J.*, **58**, 670 (1954).
27 Rietbrock, N. and Hinrichs, W. D., *Klin. Wschr.*, **42**, 981 (1964).
28 Rietbrock, N., Herken, W. and Abshagen, U., *Biochem. Pharmacol.*, **20**, 2613 (1971).
29 Aebi, H., *in* Müller, M., Rapoport, S. and Knöfel, R., *Folia Haematol.* (Leipzig), **89**, 228 (1968).
30 Rapoport, S., Müller, M. and Knöfel, R., *Europ. J. Biochem.*, **10**, 207 (1969).
31 Wilmanns, W. and Jaenicke, L., *Klin. Wschr.*, **41**, 1077 (1963).
32 Rapoport, S. and Müller, M., *Acta Biochim. Pol.*, **14**, 143 (1967).
33 Müller, M., Dissertation, Mathematisch-Naturwissenschaftliche Fa-

kultät (Humboldt-Universität Berlin, 1970).
34 Loschen, G., Flohé, L. and Chance, B., *FEBS Letters*, **18**, 261 (1971).
35 Aebi, H., Quitt, J. and Hassan, A., *Helv. Physiol. Pharmacol. Acta*, **20**, 148 (1962).
36 Aebi, H., Frei, E., Knab, R. and Siegenthaler, P., *Helv. Physiol. Pharmacol. Acta*, **15**, 150 (1957).
37 Rapoport, S. and Ababei, L., *Acta Biol. Med. German.*, **13**, 852 (1964).
38 Rappaport, A., Green, J. A. and Gast, J. H., *Arch. Biochem. Biophys.*, **63**, 343 (1956).
39 Jacob, H. S. and Jandl, J. H., *J. Biol. Chem.*, **241**, 4243 (1966).
40 Müller, M., Rapoport, S. and Knöfel, R., *Folia Haemtol.* (Leipzig), **89**, 228 (1968).
40a Warburg, O., *Hoppe Seyler Z. Physiol. Chem.*, **76**, 331 (1911).
40b Ramsey, R. and Warren, C. O., *Quartern J. Exp. Physiol.*, **24**, 153 (1934).
40c Rapoport, S. and Ababei, L., *Acta Biol. Med. German.*, **7**, 533 (1961).
40d Müller, M., Hartwig, A. and Rapoport, S., VIIth International Berlin Symposium on Structure and Function of Erythrocytes, Berlin, GDR, 1973.
41 Matsubara, S., Suter, H. and Aebi, H., *Humangenetik*, **4**, 29 (1967).
42 Aebi, H., Baggiolini, M., Dewald, B., Lauber, E., Suter, H., Micheli, A. and Frei, J., *Enzymol. Biol. Clin.*, **4**, 121 (1964).
43 Feinstein, R. N., Braun, J. T. and Howard, J. B., *Arch. Biochem. Biophys.*, **120**, 165 (1967).
44 Radev, T., *J. Genetics*, **57**, 169 (1960).
45 Feinstein, R. N., Faulhaber, J. T. and Howard, J. B., *Proc. Soc. Exptl. Biol. Med.*, **127**, 1051 (1968).
46 Jacob, H. S., Ingbar, S. H. and Jandl, J. H., *J. Clin. Invest.*, **44**, 1187 (1965).
47 Aebi, H., Heiniger, J. P. and Lauber, E., *Helv. Chim. Acta*, **47**, 1428 (1964).
48 Aebi, H. and Suter, H., *Humangenetik*, **2**, 328 (1966).
49 Tudhope, G. R. and Leece, S. P., *Acta Haematol.*, **45**, 290 (1971).
50 Klaus, D., Hennemann, H. H. and Bethmann, L., *Klin. Wschr.*, **38**, 291 (1960).
51 Tarlow, A. R. and Kellermeyer, R. W., *J. Lab. Clin. Med.*, **58**, 204 (1961).
52 Tarlow, A. R., Brewer, G. J., Carson, P. E. and Alving, A. S., *Arch. Int. Med.*, **109**, 209 (1962).
53 Mills, G. C., *J. Biol. Chem.*, **229**, 189 (1957).
54 Flohé, L., Eisele, B. and Wendel, A., *Hoppe Seyler Z. Physiol. Chem.*, **352**, 151 (1971).
55 Mills, G. C., *Arch. Biochem. Biophys.*, **86**, 1 (1960).
56 Flohé, L., Schaich, E., Voelter, W. and Wendel, A., *Hoppe Seyler*

Z. Physiol. Chem., **352**, 170 (1971).
57 Flohé, L., Günzler, W., Jung, G., Schaich, E. and Schneider, F., *Hoppe Seyler Z. Physiol. Chem.*, **352**, 159 (1971).
58 Mills, G. C., *J. Biol. Chem.*, **234**, 502 (1959).
59 Little, C. and O'Brien, P. J., *Biochem. Biophys. Res. Comm.*, **31**, 145 (1968).
60 Flohé, L. and Brand, I., *Biochim. Biophys. Acta*, **191**, 541 (1969).
61 Flohé, L. and Brand, I., *Z. Klin. Chem.*, **8**, 156 (1970).
62 Flohé, L., Schlegel, W. and Schaich, E., *Z. Klin. Chem.*, **8**, 149 (1970).
63 Flohé, L., *Hoppe Seyler Z. Physiol. Chem.*, **350**, 1181 (1969).
64 Paglia, D. E. and Valentine, W. N., *J. Lab. Clin. Med.*, **70**, 158 (1967).
65 Little, C., Olinescu, R., Reid, K. G. and O'Brien, P. J., *J. Biol. Chem.*, **245**, 3632 (1970).
66 Güntherberg, H. and Rost, J., *Anal. Biochem*, **15**, 205 (1966).
67 Srivastava, S. K. and Beutler, E., *J. Biol. Chem.*, **244**, 9 (1969).
68 Stocks, J. and Dormandy, T. L., *Brit. J. Haematol.*, **20**, 95 (1971).
69 Mills, G. C. and Randall, H. P., *J. Biol. Chem.*, **232**, 589 (1958).
70 Little, C. and O'Brien, P. J., *Biochem. J.*, **101**, 13 p (1966).
71 Jacob, H. S. and Lux, S. E., *Blood*, **32**, 549 (1968).
72 Miller, A. and Smith, H. C., *Brit. J. Haematol.*, **19**, 417 (1970).
73 Scheuch, D. and Rapoport, S., *Acta Biol. Med. German.*, **8**, 31 (1962).
74 Cohen, G. and Hochstein, P., *Biochemistry*, **2**, 1420 (1963).
75 Liebowitz, J. and Cohen, G., *Biochem. Pharmacol.*, **17**, 983 (1968).
76 Müller, M. and Rapoport, S., VI. Internationales Symposium über Struktur und Funktion der Erythrozyten, *in*: Abhandlungen der Deutschen Akademie der Wissenschaften zu Berlin Akademie-Verlag, Berlin, 255 (1971).

Enzymes of the Red Cell; A Critical Catalogue

H. FRIEDEMANN and S. M. RAPOPORT

Institute of Physiological and Biological Chemistry, Humboldt University, Berlin, GDR

A critical catalogue of more than 140 enzymes of the red cell is compiled. It includes normal values of mature erythrocytes of man and other species as well as maturation changes in particular of reticulocyte. In addition, electrophoretic studies of multiple molecular forms are surveyd.

The widespread interest in the enzymes of red cells has resulted in a continuously growing literature, which is widely dispersed. References to enzymes of red cells may be found not only in biochemical and hematological journals, but also in those devoted to genetics, pharmacology, experimental, clinical or veterinary medicine. In addition to the heterogenous nature of the literature, the manner of reporting, which includes qualitative statements and a variety of units and bases of reference, also provides problems. Therefore it seemed to us of general interest to provide a critical review of the enzymes of the red cell which would comprise a sort of inventory of present knowledge in this field. The only previous attempt to present a comprehensive survey appeared in 1964.[189] The present catalogue covers the literature up to the end of 1973. Older references were omitted if methods were used which are no longer acceptable, particularly if better data were found. This review includes 140 enzymes or enzyme systems, with the exception of membrane transport and metabolism which were not considered. It was decided to list the enzymes in alphabetical order rather than by metabolic pathways in order to avoid ambiguities or duplications. The commonly used "trivial" appelations of the enzymes as listed in the report of the commission on Enzymes of the International Union of Biochemistry were used. If possible, *i.e.*, when the type of reaction could be defined, the number according to the enzyme catalogue of the International Union of Biochemistry (EC) was supplied. In cases where the present knowledge and nomenclature does not permit precise appellation, comprehensive groups are listed.

TABLE (Supplementary Table p. 230∼236)

Enzyme name (Trivial name)	Species or group	Normal value (range) μmoles/ml cells/hr	Ref.	Properties and other remarks	Ref.
Acetylcholineesterase	man, adult	240–330	4, 5, 6, 49	Partially purified, soluble enzyme	1
		714	3, 7		
(E. C. 3.1.1.7)	„ , newborn	80–116	8a	2 components (I, II) with	2
	„ , newborn reti.	105–175		identical molecular weight (∼180,000)	8b-d
	„ , newborn ery.	52–78		I K_m acetylcholine=$1.25\times10^{-4}M$	
				II K_m acetylcholine=$1.7\times10^{-4}M$	
				Inhibitors:	
				Diisopropyl-phosphate $K_i=1.2\times10^{-7}M$ (I, II)	
				Eserin $K_i=9\times10^{-8}M$ (I, II)	
Acid: CoA ligase (E. C. 6.2.1.3)	man, reti.	0.7	9	localisation: particle-bound substrate: oleic acid (activities as ligase (6.2.1.3)-transferase (2.3.1))	9
	„ , ery.	0.4			
Acid phosphatase (E. C. 3.1.3.2)				Partially purified (1,500-fold) from human erythrocytes turnover number	10
				≃450 from horse erythrocytes	11
				pH (opt.)=5.5	
				K_m *nitrophenylphosphate* 2.5×10^{-3} *M* inhibitors: Hg, Cu, Ag, Zn, pCMB Mol. wt.: 30,000–60,000 localisation: cytosol	
				Multiple molecular forms	
	man (pH 5.5)	40–60 (phenyl-phosphate)	18, 19	man, polymorphism: 5 distinct enzymes (A, BA, CA, CB, C) 3 allelic genes;	12
		24 (Glycerine-1-p)		purification and properties of phenotypes	13, 14, 15 16a, 39
		2.1 (AMP)		AA-enzyme	

		153 (extremely)	20	K_m phenyl-P=$8.7\times10^{-4}M$	
	rabbit, ery.	15	21	K_m nitrophenyl-P=$1.2\times10^{-4}M$	
	„ , reti.	35		K_m glycerine-1-P=$5.8\times10^{-3}M$ BB-enzyme	
				K_m phenyl-P=$7.5\times10^{-4}M$	
				K_m nitrophenyl-P=$1.2\times10^{-4}M$	
				K_m glycerine-1-P=$5.5\times10^{-3}M$	
				Mol. wt.: 14,000 to 15,000, type A and B do not differ significantly	
Aconitase (E. C. 4.2.1.3)	man	present	22		
	rabbit	absent in normocytes	23		
Acylase (Glycerol-phosphate acyl-transferase) (E. C. 2.3.1.15)	man	present	24		
Acyl-CoA : lysolecithine-O-acyl-transferase (E. C. 2.3.1)	man	present	9	Further characterisation under Acid: CoA ligase (6.2.1.3)	
Adenosinedeaminase (E. C. 3.5.4.4)	man	9	29	Multiple molecular forms; two autosomale alleles, (ADA-1, ADA-2)	25, 26, 27
	rabbit, ery.	80–90	28, 29, 30		
	„ , reti.	209			
	chicken	426			
Adenylosuccinase (E. C. 4.3.2.2)	man	present	31	localisation: cytosol	
	rabbit				
Adenylate deaminase (E. C. 3.5.4.6)	man	20–75	34, 35	Partially purified, activation by ATP and monovalent cations, pH (opt.)=7.8	32
				K_m AMP = $2.1\times10^{-3}M$, inhibitors:	33a

Enzyme name (Trivial name)	Species or group	Normal value (range) μmoles/ml cells/hr	Ref.	Properties and other remarks	Ref.
				Phosphate, arsenate, p-CMB (see also suppl. table)	
Adenylate kinase (E. C. 2.7.4.3)	man, adults	1,800–2,600	40, 42	man, partially purified, pH (opt.)=7–9	36, 37, 41
		3,400–4,500	43	localisation: cytosol	
		7,200 (extreme value)	44a	Multiple molecular forms:	38, 39a∼c
	man, newborn	2,050	42	Polymorphism, 2 codominant autosomal alleles, common phenotypes AK^1, AK^{2-1}, rare AK^2 (see also suppl. table)	
	sheep, duck	present	36		
Adenylo-succinate synthetase (E. C. 6.3.4.4)	man	absent	31		
	rabbit			erythrocyte can convert hypoxanthine, inosine or adenosine to AMP via IMP	45, 46
Alanine aminopeptidase (E. C. 3.4.1.1)	man	50	47		
Aldolase (E. C. 4.1.2.7b)	man, adults	25–35	34, 42, 48 50–54	Multiple molecular forms: rabbit, reticulocytes present hybride forms of aldolase A (muscle type) and aldolase C (brain type)	55a∼c
		40–75	19, 43, 56–62		
	„ , newborn	103	57		
		48	42		
	rabbit, ery.	18–25	56, 60a, 63, 64		
	„ , reti.	60	63, 64		
	rat	35	56, 60a		
	dog	30–50	56, 60a, b		

	sheep	12–15	56, 60a, b		
	pig	8	60a		
	horse	11	60a		
	monkey	27	60b		
	beef	12–15	60a, b		
	guinea pig	23	60a		
	chicken	30	60a		
	mouse	44	60a		
	goose	93	62		
Aldose reductase (E. C. 1.1.1.21)	rat	present	65	galactose-fed rats, accumulation of galactitol, (intracellular level 0.67 μ moles/ml cells) at high glucose concentration accumulation of sorbitol	17
Alkaline phosphatase (E. C. 3.1.3.1)	man	present	66		
AMP pyrophosphorylase (E. C. 2.4.2.7)	man	8–13	53, 67		
5-Amino-4-imidazole carboxamide ribotide transformylase	man	present	68, 69, 70, 71		
δ-Aminolevulinic acid dehydratase (E. C. 4.2.1.24)	man	0.18–1.13	72–77	partially purified from rabbit reti. and chicken ery., pH (opt.)=6.1	78a, b
	(30°C)	0.7–1.2	454c, 454d		454c
	(37°C)	1.9	450a,b, 451,	SH enzyme	75
		0.09	452, 453a,b		
	man, adults	108–299 units+	79	+units/ml cells/hr (38°C) (unit : activity at 555 nm, color development from Ehrlich's reagent)	
	„ , children	124–260 units+			

Enzyme name (Trivial name)	Species or group	Normal value (range) μmoles/ml cells/hr	Ref.	Properties and other remarks	Ref.
	man, men	0.121±32		activity in diminished is lead poisoning	
	„ , women	0.143±3	454a		
δ-Aminolevulinic acid synthetase (E. C. 2.3.1.37)	human erythroblasts	250×10^{-3}	83	identification in duck ery.	80a, b
				purification from chicken ery.	78
	man, reti.	$200–1.200\times10^{-3}$ (7=640)	84		
	rabbit, reti.	1.100×10^{-3}	84, 85	from rabbit reti.	81
	„ , ery.	0	85	pH (opt.)=7.6	
				IP =5.9	
				Cofactors: Pyridoxal-P	
				Inhibitors: Iron, Hemin	
				K_m succ. CoA=$6.0\times10^{-5}M$	
				K_m glycine=$1.0\times10^{-2}M$	
				rabbit, bone marrow cell mitochondria	82
				K_m glycine=$5\times10^{-3}M$	
				K_m α-ketoglut.=$1\times10^{-4}M$	
				K_m CoA=$6\times10^{-4}M$	
Amino acid-activating enzyme	man	present	86		
Aminotripeptidase (E. C. 3.4.1.3)	man, reti.	1,063	87		
	„ , ery.	1,025			
	rabbit, reti.	900	88	(Phenylhydrazine anemia)	
	„ , ery.	845			
Amylase	man	4.7 starch unit	66		

Arginase (E. C. 3.5.3.1)	man, adults	12–84	89–92	Activation by Mn^{2+}	92
		1,372⁺	93	⁺extreme value	
	„ , with Mn^{2+}	220–370	92		
	„ , newborn	3,800	93	partially purified	94, 95
				Isoenzyme was not found	95, 96
	dog				
	guinea pig	not detectable	94		
	rat				
	hen				
	frog				
ATPase (E. C. 3.6.1.4)	man, adults	150–180	19, 40, 42, 99	partially purified, (500-fold), soluble enzyme,	
		220	51	Activators: Mg^{2+}, cysteine	98
	„ , newborn	170–190	42, 97, 99	K_m ATP$=7.64\times10^{-4}M$	
	„ , fetus (12 th-28 th week of pregnancy)	350	97	K_m ADP$=3.6\times10^{-3}M$ pH (opt.)=7.3–7.6	
	rabbit, ery.	52–80	100		
	„ , reti.	160–190			
	rabbit, bleeding anemia 2d. (10% reti.)	54			
	10d. (40% reti.)	135			
	30d. (10% reti.)	72			
Aspartate carbamoyltransferase (E. C. 2.1.3.2)	man	1.2–1.8	101, 102	soluble enzyme,	101
	duck	0.9		pH (opt.)=9.2–9.3 substrate saturation: $1\times10^{-2}M$ aspartate $5\times10^{-3}M$ carbamoyl-P	
Catechol-O-methyltransferase (E. C. 2.1.1.6)	rat, soluble	0.203	449a-c	2 types	
	„ , membrane	0.224		localisation: soluble and ghost fraction	448
				soluble activity:	449a
				pH (opt.)=7.8–8.2	

Enzyme name (Trivial name)	Species or group	Normal value (range) μmoles/ml cells/hr	Ref.	Properties and other remarks	Ref.
				K_m S-adenosyl-methionine $=3.3\times10^{-6}M$ K_m epinephrine$=2.2\times10^{-4}M$ K_m norepinephrine$=3.7\times10^{-4}M$ K_m dopamine$=4.0\times10^{-4}M$ activation: Mg^{2+}, (divalent ions) inhibition: Tropolone pCMB (3–40%) membrane activity: pH (opt.)=7.0 (with Triton X-100) K_m S-adenosyl-methionine $=3.3\times10^{-6}M$ K_m epinephrine$=3.3\times10^{-6}M$ K_m norepinephrine$=6.0\times10^{-6}M$ K_m dopamine$=5.7\times10^{-6}M$ activation: Mg^{2+}, (divalent ions) inhibition: Tropolone pCMB (20–100%)	
Carbonic anhydrase (E. C. 4.2.1.1)	man (as Carboxyl-esterase activity)			Multiple molecular forms: electrophoretic studies, Polymorphism (variants A, B, C, D, E, F, G, H)	106, 107, 108a, 110
	type A (β-naphthyl)	1,890	103, 104	purification, crystallisation of β-type variant, substitution of aspartic acid by valine, porcine erythrocytes 2 forms, Mol. wt: 3×10^4 (both forms);	108b, 104
	type B (β-naphthyl)	1,850			
	type C (β-naphthyl)	1,225			
	type A (nitrophenyl-acetate)	13,860		enzyme with high (hydrase) activity-type C, low activity-type B	
	type B	33,600			
	porcine (as Carboxyl-esterase activity)			bovine erythrocytes type A, B, the physical constants are very similiar to the human B form constants	105

	type B (β-naphthyl) type C (β-naphthyl)	6,120 1,295		Enzyme deficiency of B and C type possible (see also suppl. table)	111, 112
Carnitine palmityl-transferase	man	present		localisation : membrane K_m D, L-carnitine$=1\times10^{-4}M$ K_i palmitylcarnitine$=2.1\times10^{-4}M$	113
Catalase (E. C. 1.11.1.6)	man	$3,200–7,500\times10^3$	114–117a, 118a, b	Purification and crystallisation Mol. wt. : 222,800 Hemin yield : 1.1%, IP : 5.8	121
	rabbit	$3,300–3,900\times10^3$	116, 117b	Multiple molecular forms : erythrocytes from horse and man show electrophorectically and chromatographically 3 fractions : A, B, C. In presence of oxygen fraction A converted to C, inhibited by SH reagents.	122
	rat	$1,350–2,850\times10^3$	116, 117a, b		
	cat	$5,700\times10^3$	116		
	monkey	$5,200\times10^3$	116		
	dog	$130–1,956\times10^3$	116, 117a, b		
	guinea pig	$2,000\times10^3$	117a, b		
	chicken	180×10^3	116	Reticulocytes show a higher A/C ratio than old cells.	
	duck	$6–12\times10^3$	116, 117b		
	pigeon	30×10^3	116	Enzyme activity in (human) reticulocytes and erythrocytes the same	123, 124
	house mouse	1,400–1,700	117a, b		
	mouse (hypocatalatic)	320×10^3	117b		
	mouse (acatalatic)	36×10^3	117b		
Cholesterol esterase (E. C. 3.1.1.12)	man	present	125		
Coproporphyrinogen oxidase	chicken	present	126, 127	particulate, soluble	
Cyclohydrolase	man	present	71, 128		
Cytochrome oxidase	man, adults	<0.05	120	localisation : stroma, inactivation by an	109, 129

Enzyme name (Trivial name)	Species or group	Normal value (range) μmoles/ml cells/hr	Ref.	Properties and other remarks	Ref.
(E. C. 1.9.3.1)	„ , newborn (28% reti.)	1.4	120	inhibitor protein in the hemolysate (inhibitor C)	
	rabbit, reti.	16	28, 109, 119, 120, 129		
Cysteine aminopeptidase	man	present	47		
Deoxyriboaldolase (E. C. 4.1.2.4)	man	present (ghosts)	130		
Diglyceride kinase	man	present	131	in membranes, activated by K^+	
Dihydroorotase (E. C. 3.5.2.3)	man	40–55	101	soluble, substrate saturation at $1\times 10^{-3}M$ dihydroorotate pH (opt.)=8.2	101
	duck	65	135		
Dihydroorotic dehydrogenase (E. C. 1.3.3.1)	duck	160		localisation: sedimented with nuclei and larger particles	135
				substrate saturation $5\times 10^{-4}M$ dihydroorotate, pH (opt.)=8.4–8.6 not in human erythrocytes	
Diphosphoglycerate mutase (E. C. 2.7.5.4)	man, adults	214–260	99, 136	partially purified, localisation: soluble fraction	138
		86	137	K_m 1,3-DPG=0.53 μM	
	„ , newborn	266	99	K_m 3-PG=1–1.5 μM	
				Inhibitors: 1,3-DPG, 3-PG, sulfhydryl reagents, 3 electrophoretic bands, polymorphism	139
Diphosphoglycerate phosphatase	man	0.82^+	140	$^+$activated with phosphate and chloride	
		0.06	141		

(E. C. 3.1.3.13)	rabbit, reti.	1.19	140		
	rabbit, ery.	0.75		partially purified	141–145
	rat	0.92		pH (opt.)=6.5–7.5	
	dog	0.49		K_m 2,3-DPG$=4\times10^{-5}$	
	pig	0.50		Activators: Phosphate, chloride	
	horse	0.43		Inhibitors: 3-PG, 2-PG	
	sheep	0.35			
	cat	0.34			
	bovine	0.20			
	chicken	0.76			
DNase (E. C. 3.1.4.5)	snake and bull frog	present	147		
	frog (fed)		148	activity masked	
	frog (starving)	present		localisation: stroma 4 enzymes present: 1. pH 5–7, 2. pH 5–7, Mg^{2+}-dependent, 3. pH 8–9, 4. at extremly acid pH	148
	rabbit		149, 150		
	10–40% reti.	$3.5\text{–}4.3\times10^{-2}$			
	rabbit, ery.	0			
DOPA decarboxylase (E. C. 4.1.1.26)	man	70×10^{-8}	146		
Enolase (E. C. 4.2.1.11)	man, adult	120–230	40, 42, 43, 53, 57, 59, 62, 99, 151, 152		
	„ , newborn	270–340	42, 57, 97, 99, 151		
	„ , fetus 12 th–28 th week of pregnancy	626	97		

Enzyme name (Trivial name)	Species or group	Normal value (range) μmoles/ml cells/hr	Ref.	Properties and other remarks	Ref.
Enolose	man, preservation				
(E. C. 4.2.1.11)	1st day	146	61		
	7 th day	112 (76%)			
	goose	195	62		
	rat	158	56		
	horse	270	464		
Fructose-1,6-diphosphatase (E. C. 3.1.3.11)	man, adult	18	42	specifity not proven	
	„ , newborn	29			
Fumarase	rabbit	15	23, 154		
(E. C. 4.2.1.2)	rabbit, ratio ery. : reti.	1 : 1.8	155		
Galactokinase (E. C. 2.7.1.6)	man, adult	0.1–0.7	43, 156–159a, b	partially purified	
				K_m galactose $=1.36\times10^{-4}M$ cordblood	160
	„ , newborn	0.4–1.2	158, 159a, b	K_m galactose $=2.25\times10^{-4}M$	
	rat	0.5	465	inhibitors: galactose-1-P, 2-deoxygalactose, partially purified (3,300–3,900-fold)	
	rabbit	0.6		K_m galactose $=1\text{–}1.5\times10^{-4}M$	161
				K_m ATP $=2\text{–}5\times10^{-4}M$	
				pH (opt.) = 7.7–7.9, IP = 5.7	
				Mol. wt.: 53,000–57,000, dimeric structure, monomer Mol. wt.: 25,000–27,000	
				Multiple molecular forms:	
				adult blood: a single strip	162
				cord blood: a single strip with increased mobility	

Galactose-1-phosphate uridyltransferase (E. C. 2.7.7.10)	man, adult	6–10	43, 158, 163, 164	pH (opt.)=8.5 K_m UDPG=0.233 mM (galactose-1-P =6.45 mM)	165
	„ , newborn	8–12	158, 164	K_m galactose-1-P=0.390 mM(UDPG= 0.6 mM) increasing the concentration of either substrate increased the K_m for the other substrate. Multiple molecular forms: Polymorphism, normal: 1 band, Duarte variant: 3 bands Los Angeles variant: similiar to Duarte variant	43, 158
Glucosamine-6-phosphate deaminase (E. C. 4.3.1)	rabbit			partially purified (560-fold) pH (opt.)=7.8–8.2 activator: N-acetylglucosamine-6-*P* K_m glucosamine-6-P=$2.5\times10^{-4}M$ K_m fructose-6-P=$5.5\times10^{-3}M$ K_m $(NH_4)_2CO_3=4.3\times10^{-2}M$ (data in presence of N-acetylglucosamine-6-P) localisation: cytosol	166
Glucose-6-phosphatase (E. C. 3.1.3.9)	man rat rabbit, ery. „ , reti.	4.1 3.5 4.2 6.7	167	specifity not proven	
Glucose-6-phosphate dehydrogenase (E. C. 1.1.1.49)	man, adult	90–150	42, 50, 53, 57, 59, 99, 61, 151, 170, 171, 174	25°C inhibitor: dehydroepianolrosterone	467
		140–220	56, 152, 168, 169, 172, 174	37°C hormones may influence in the form of a seasonal variation	174, 186a, b
		270	43	Polymorphism	

Enzyme name (Trivial name)	Species or group	Normal value (range) μmoles/ml cells/hr	Ref.	Properties and other remarks	Ref.
	„ , newborn	190–225	42, 57, 99, 151, 171		
	„ , fetus 19th week of gestation	260	171		
	man, preservation				
	1st day	99	61		
	7th day	9 (10%)			
	„ , ery.+	60–100	173, 175–177	+density gradient centrifugation	
	„ , reti.+	90–280	170, 173, 175–177		
	rabbit (25°C)	70–100	178, 179		
	(37°C)	220	175		
	dog	234	180		
	goat	37	181		
	deer	125			
	rat (37°C)	620	182		
	mouse (several strains)	95–248	183		
	sheep, fetal	107	184		
	„ , newborn	98			
	„ , adults	33			
	sheep	(7.9)+	185+	+may be low	
	goat	(13.8)+			
	cattle	(70.4)+			
		230	456	(37°C)	
	pig	(122)+			
	horse	(187)+			
		540	464		
Glutamate dehydro-	man	23	187	partially purified	

genase (E. C. 1.4.1.2)	rabbit, ery. „ , reti.	25 38		pH (opt.)=8 K_m α-Ketoglutarate=$3.5\times10^{-2}M$ K_m Ammonium=$5.5\times10^{-2}M$ (with NADH) Inhibitors: ATP ($10^{-4}M$, 75%), AMP ($5\times10^{-4}M$, 90%), ADP ($1\times10^{-5}M$, 70%)	187
Glutamate formiminotransferase (E. C. 2.1.2.5)	man	present	71, 153		
Glutaminase I (E. C. 3.5.1.2)	chicken duck rabbit, reti.	3.8 4.7 16.0^{+}	196	stroma-free hemolysates: man, horse, bovine, sheep, dog, rabbit, rat erythrocytes. After removal of leucocytes no activity was detectable $^{+}$stromabound activity, with phosphate, no activity in stroma-free hemolysate of human and rabbit ery., no activity in ghosts of ery. and reti.	196
Glutaminase II (E. C. 2.6.1.15)	rabbit, reti.	9			
Glutamine fructose-6-phosphate aminotransferase (E. C. 2.6.1.16)	rabbit, reti.	95×10^{-3}	188		
Glutamicoxalacetic transaminase (E. C. 2.6.1.1)	man, adults „ , newborn „ , reti. rabbit, ery. „ , reti.	20–40 70 95–140 130 10–40 140	19, 189–191 42, 43, 54 42, 191 54 28, 87 28	Density gradient centrifugation: GOT is the best simple index of mean age of erythrocytes, stimulation with pyridoxal-P Multiple molecular forms: rabbit erythrocytes shows electrophoretically only an anionic band, rabbit reticulocytes (after bleeding) show 2 new bands (1 cationic) (cationic GOT lost during maturation)	151, 170, 192–194 43, 191 195a, b

Enzyme name (Trivial name)	Species or group	Normal value (range) μmoles/ml cells/hr	Ref.	Properties and other remarks	Ref.
				man, polymorphism, phenotypes S-GOT 1, S-GOT 2–1, S-GOT 3–1	197
Glutamicpyruvic transaminase (E. C. 2.6.1.2)	man	9–15	19, 42, 190	$^{+}$no difference in reticulocytes	
	rabbit	10^{+}	28	Multiple molecular forms: Polymorphismus, 3 phenotypes (S-G / PT-1, S-GPT 2–1, S-GPT-2) 2 alleles, autosomol locus, dimeric structure, 2 identical subunits	199
	rat, ery.	7–11	198		
	rat, reti.	10.8–14.2	198		
γ-Glutamylcysteine synthetase (E. C. 6.3.2.2)	man	8.1	200	partially purified inhibitors: SH reagents	201
γ-Glutamyl transpeptidase (E. C. 2.3.2)	man	present	202	low activity	
Glutathione peroxidase (E. C. 1.11.1.9)	man, adults	60–146	43, 208	Purification,	209a∼c
	children	210–230	205–207, 468	a selenoenzyme	209d
	„ , newborn fetus	138–218	205–207, 468		
		78^{+}	205–207	$^{+}$20th week of pregnancy	
		237^{+}	205	$^{+}$28th week of pregnancy	
Glutathione reductase (E. C. 1.6.4.2)		NADPH activity			
	man, adults	60–175	19, 34, 42, 43, 51, 57, 171, 172, 208, 210, 211, 214, 216	NADPH activity purification pH (opt.)=5–8 K_m GSSG=$25–96\times10^{-6}M$ K_m NADPH=$11–16\times10^{-6}M$	216–223
	„ , newborn	120–210	42, 57, 171, 211	NADH activity pH (opt.)=6.1–6.3	216–119, 222, 223

Enzyme	Species	Activity	Ref.	Properties	Ref.
	man, fetus	146	171	K_m GSSG=17–48×$10^{-6}M$	
	beef	85	216	K_m NADH=190–270×$10^{-6}M$	
	sheep	80		Mol. wt.: 115,000	
	pig	80			
	dog	80			
	rabbit	60			
	horse	56	464		
		NADH activity			
	man, adults	60–110	57, 172, 211, 216	Multiple molecular forms: 2 distinct isoenzymes	214, 215
	„ , newborn	110–190	57, 211	Erythrocytes fractionated by serial osmotic hemolysis	217
	beef	120	216	affinity constants are affected by sodium concentration	
	sheep	95		Na phosphate 0.03M	
	pig	45		K_m GSSG: fraction 1=7.6×$10^{-6}M$, fraction 7=52×$10^{-6}M$	
	dog, rabbit	>5		Na phosphate 0.3M fraction 1=42×$10^{-6}M$, fraction 7=170×$10^{-6}M$	
				Na phosphate 0.03M	
				K_m NADPH: fraction 1=5.3×$10^{-6}M$, fraction 7=32×$10^{-6}M$	
				Na phosphate 0.03M	
				K_m NADH: fraction 1=81×$10^{-6}M$, fraction 7=370×$10^{-6}M$	
Gluthatione synthetase (E. C. 6.3.2.3)	man	2.4	200	partially purified (man, beef)	201
		12.6	202	Mol. wt.: 150,000, 122,000	469a, b
			224		
Glyceraldehyde-3-phosphate dehydrogenase	man, adults (25°C)	500–800	48, 51, 54, 151	pH (opt.)=7.4	
				K_m GAP=21×$10^{-6}M$	228
		1,070–2,280	19, 57, 225,	K_m NAD$^+$=140×$10^{-6}M$	

Enzyme name (Trivial name)	Species or group	Normal value (range) μmoles/ml cells/hr	Ref.	Properties and other remarks	Ref.
(E. C. 1.2.1.12)			226, 230	$K_m P_i = 6.6\,mM$ K_i NADH$=9.1\times10^{-6}M$	
				localisation: membrane activity present, ratio membrane to hemolysate 1 : 6	52, 229, 231–233
		2,890+	237b 40–43	+under optimal conditions (pH 8.5, 10 mM Arsenate, 1 mM NADH, start: 1.25 mM GAP)	
	(37°C)	900–3,020	40–43 59, 152, 227	purification (hemolysate with stroma) and crystallization	234–236
	man, newborn (25°C)	530–2,980	57, 151		
	(37°C)	3,046	42, 97		
	man, fetus 12th–28th week of pregnancy	3,866	97		
	man, preservation				
	1st day	280	61		
	7th day (25°C)	11			
	rat (25°C)	1,380	230		
	rabbit (25°C)	1,390	230		
	„ , reti. (30%)	3,600	237		
	„ , ery.	1,430	237		
	goose (25°C)	213	62		
Glycine aminopeptidase (E. C. 3.4.1.1)	man	present	129		
Glycogen phosphorylase (E. C. 2.4.1.1)	man	15 mg glycogen/ml cells/hr	239		

Glycoprotein synthesis	man rabbit	present	238a, b	incorporation of ^{14}C-glucosamine, localisation: membrane, incorporation in human reticulocyte stroma is greatly increased in thalassemia	238b
Glycylglycine dipeptidase (E. C. 3.4.3.1)	man rabbit, ery. „ , reti.	325 360 1,280	87 88 88		
Glycyl-leucine dipeptidase (E. C. 3.4.3.2)	man rabbit, ery. „ , reti.	1,075–1,800 1,330 8,500	87, 240, 241 88 88	activation by Zn^{2+}	240
Glyoxalase (E. C. 4.4.1.5)	man	800–1,900	242, 243	(see also suppl. table)	
Guanase	man	present	244		
Hemesynthetase (E. C. 4.99.1.1)	man, (whole blood)	14–31+ pmoles/ml cells/hr	245	(+hemolysate from whole blood with 5.1×10^3 white blood cells/μl) soluble enzyme in red blood cell precursors, which is stimulated by ether	245
	„ , reti.	10 pmoles/ml cells/hr	127		
	„ , erythroblasts	8 μmoles/ml cells/hr	83		
	„ , rabbit+	present	82	+bone marrow mitochondria partially purified duck erythrocytes pH (opt.)=8.2 K_m $Fe^{2+}=8\times10^{-5}M$ K_m Protoporph.$=7\times10^{-5}M$	 246, 247
Hexokinase (E. C. 2.7.1.1)	man, adults (37°C)	10–23	40, 42, 43, 48, 51, 53, 54, 57–59,	in rabbit reticulocytes high K_m enzyme with K_m deoxyglucose$=63\,mM$, Multiple molecular forms: starch gel	255

Enzyme name (Trivial name)	Species or group	Normal value (range) μmoles/ml cells/hr	Ref.	Properties and other remarks	Ref.
			99, 151, 152, 173, 248, 249, 255	electrophoresis man, adults: 2 bands type I, III	257–259
	,, , newborn	20–36	42, 57, 97, 99, 151, 255	man, newborns: 2 bands type I, III and a third band type II (associated with Hb_F)	
	man, fetus 12th–28th week of pregnancy	46	97	rat: only 1 band (equivalent type I of human erythrocytes)	260
	preservation ACD				
	day zero	10	250		
	30th day	2–4	251		
	60th day	1.8			
	rabbit, ery.	12–17	23, 253–255		
	,, , reti.	30–160	23, 253, 254		
	rat	12 (pH 7.5)	252		
		24 (pH 8.1)	253		
	dog	4.2	253		
	goat	4.5			
	deer	2.0			
	horse	4.9	464		
	man⁺, ery.	0	255	⁺high-K_m enzyme (calculated from the data from 255)	
	,, , reti.	0			
	rabbit⁺, reti.	180			
	,, , ery.	0			
Hexose-1-phosphate uridyltransferase (E. C. 2.7.7.12)	man	0.6–1.3	157, 261, 262	partially purified	263
Hydroxysteroid (17 β-estradiol)	man			ˣsubstrate: 17-β-estradiol	
	rat			substrate: 17α-estradiol only in cow,	264

dehydrogenase (E. C. 1.1.1.51)	syrian hamster mouse guinea pig rabbit pigeon chicken goat sheep bovine pig cat dog frog	 present[×] present	 264a, b–266	sheep, goat	
Hypoxanthine-guanine phosphoribosyl-transferase (E. C. 2.4.2.8)	man, substrate : xanthine	0.109	269		
	,, , substrate : hypoxanthine	30–35	53, 67, 267–269		
	,, , substrate : guanine	35–45	53, 67, 268, 269	with substrate : hypoxanthine K_m PRPP$=2.4\times10^{-4}M$ K_m hypoxanthine$=9.9\times10^{-6}M$ K_i PP$=2.1\times10^{-2}M$ K_i guanylate$=1.25\times10^{-6}M$	270
	chicken, ery. substrute hypoxanthine	0.9	466	K_i inosinate$=2.5\times10^{-5}M$ substrate : guanine	
	substrate guanine	1.6		K_m PRPP$=2.4\times10^{-4}M$ K_m guanine$=4.0\times10^{-6}M$ K_i PP$=2.1\times10^{-3}M$ K_i guanylate$=1.5\times10^{-6}M$ K_i inosinate$=2.5\times10^{-6}M$	
	substrate adenine	5.1		Mutant from with 10-fold higher substrate saturation, sigmoidal kinetics (see also suppl. table)	271

Enzyme name (Trivial name)	Species or group	Normal value (range) μmoles/ml cells/hr	Ref.	Properties and other remarks	Ref.
Imidodipeptidase	man	480	87, 272, 273		
(E. C. 3.4.3.7)	rabbit, ery.	300	88		
	„ , reti.	270	88		
Iminodipeptidase	man	300	87		
(E. C. 3.4.6)	rabbit, ery.	400	88		
	„ , reti.	1,073	88		
Inosine kinase (E. C. 2.7.1.73)	man	present		pH (opt.)=7.7 K_m ATP=$8.6\times10^{-4}M$ K_m Inosine=$7.1\times10^{-4}M$	274
ITPase (E. C. 3.6.1.8)	man	present		pH (opt.)=8–8.5 K_m ITP=$1\text{–}6\times10^{-4}M$ activation : Mg^{2+}, SH compounds inhibitor : adenine	275–277
	rabbit, ery.	46		partially purified from rabbit reti. (2,000-fold), soluble	278
	„ , reti.	279		pH (opt.)=9.7 activation : Mg^{2+} inhibitor : IDP	
Isocitric dehydrogenase (E. C. 1.1.1.42)	man, adults	8–10	19, 42, 50, 57, 59, 62, 280		
	man, newborn	13–15	42, 57		
	„ , reti.	23×	194	×density gradient centrifugation	
	„ , ery.	17×	194		
	rabbit, ery.	252	282		
		(0.47)	281		
	„ , reti.×	510××	282	××calculated for 100% reticulocytes as	
		41	23	the actual maximal capacity at the	

				$NADP^+$ saturation localisation : stroma	
				SH enzyme	282, 283
				activation : Mn^{2+}, Mg^{2+}	
				K_m NADP$=2\times10^{-5}M$	
	density gradient centrifugation				
	rabbit, 50% reti.	153	194		
	„ , 20% reti.	86			
	„ , 0% reti.	30			
Lactic acid dehydrogenase (E. C. 1.1.1.28)	man, adults	1,000–1,200	19, 48, 50, 151, 285	Multiple molecular forms: electrophoretically 5 bands, activity of whole activity :	287–289
		1,400–1,900	40, 42, 51, 57, 284, 286	LDH-1 about 30–40%	
	(37°C)	2,155–3,530	43, 59	LDH-2 about 40–45%	
				LDH-3 about 14–16%	
				LDH-4 about 3–5%	
	man, newborns	1,600–2,500	42, 57, 97, 151	LDH-5 about 2%	
	man, fetus 12th–28th week of pregnancy	4,380	97		
	preservation				
	1st day	1,187	61		
	7th day	628			
	rat	3,626	286		
	rabbit	2,100	28, 286, 284		
	goose	734	62		
	dog	500–800	286, 60b		
	sheep	300–400	286, 284, 60b		
	pig	540	284, 60b		
	beef	180–190	284, 60b		
	horse	350	60b		

Enzyme name (Trivial name)	Species or group	Normal value (range) μmoles/ml cells/hr	Ref.	Properties and other remarks	Ref.
	calf	180	284		
	monkey	1400	60b		
Leucine aminopeptidase (E. C. 3.4.1.1)	man	15–28	87, 241, 290		
	rabbit, ery	172	88		
	,, , reti.	208	88		
Lipase (E. C. 3.1.1.3)	man	present	66		
Lipid synthesis	man			Incorporation studies: ^{14}C-acetate in human reticulocytes and erythrocytes into mixed and neutral lipids	294, 295, 300
	rabbit			^{14}C-acetate into cholesterol, localisation: stroma	279, 292, 293, 296–298
				^{14}C-glycerol into glycerides and glycerophosphatides. Ratio of erythrocytes to reticulocytes 1 : 70, no incorporation in stored blood.	
				Linoleate, ratio of erythrocytes to reticulocytes 1 : 5	291
				[2-^{14}C]-Mevalonic acid into squalene (3%) and cholesterol (70%) and cholesteryl ester (1%).	299
				32p incorporation into phospholipids	301
Lysophospholipase (E. C. 3.1.1.5)	man, reti.	1.1	9	density gradient centrifugation localisation: particle-bound	
	,, , ery.	0.7			
	preservation (ACD medium) day zero	0.4			

	25th day	0.5			
	61st day	0.37			
Malate dehydrogenase (decarboxylating) (E. C. 1.1.1.40)	man	0.03	302	partially purified pH (opt.)=7.5–8.5 K_m malate=$96\times10^{-6}M$ K_m NADP$^+$=$2.2\times10^{-6}M$ K_m NADPH=$2.0\times10^{-6}M$ K_m pyruvate=$0.75\times10^{-3}M$ K_m bicarbonate=$12.5\times10^{-3}M$	302
	rabbit, reti.	no activity detectable	303		
Malate dehydrogenase (E. C. 1.1.1.37)	man, adults	800–1,300	19, 42, 306	partially purified (3,000-fold) human erythrocytes	
		2,200–3,300	50, 57, 59	pH (opt.)=7.6 (substrate oxalacetate)	305
	„ , newborn	2,800–3,000	42, 57	pH (opt.)=7.8–9.9 (substrate malate)	
	rabbit, reti. (20°C)	740	23, 304	K_m oxalacetate=$9.5\times10^{-6}M$ K_m NADH=$3.5\times10^{-5}M$ K_m malate=$3.8\times10^{-4}M$ K_m NAD$^+$=$9.3\times10^{-5}M$ Inhibitors: $HgCl_2$, $CdCl_2$, ammonium molybdate localisation: cytosol and mitochondria	
				mitochondrial form inhibited by high conc. of oxalacetate; ratio of cytoplasmatic to mitochondrial form mature erythrocytes: 1.1 reticulocyte-rich „ : 2.0 chicken erythrocytes: 2.0 mitochondrial enzyme is lost at full maturity, cytoplasmatic part is unchanged.	306

Enzyme name (Trivial name)	Species or group	Normal value (range) μmoles/ml cells/hr	Ref.	Properties and other remarks	Ref.
				Multiple molecular forms: Starch gel electrophoresis, normal subjects: 1 band, genetic variant: 3 bands	307
Methemoglobin reductase				see NADH: acceptor oxidoreductase (E. C. 1.6.99.3)	
N^5, N^{10}-Methylene-tetrahydrofolate dehydrogenase (E. C. 1.5.1.5)	man, ery.	2–6	71, 128, 132, 134, 153, 308		
	„ , reti	40	132, 134		
NADH-cytochrome c oxidoreductase	man, adults	0.7–1.7	120a, b	electron donor: NADH, electron acceptor: cytochrome c	120a
	„ , newborn	14.4	120a	washed stroma	
	rabbit, reti.	19.8	119, 120a, 310, (28)	washed stroma	
NADH/NADPH acceptor oxidoreductase (E. C. 1.6.99.3(1))	man, adults	15–19	19, 322	electron donor: NADPH	
	„ , newborn	18	322		
	man, adults	60–80	43, 317	electron donor: NADH	
		27	322		
	man, newborn	25–40	317, 322		
	„ , fetus < 18th week of pregnancy	19	317		
	> 18th week of pregnancy	36	317		
				NADH-dependents system (Diaphorase, ferrihemoglobin reductase, NADH. methemoglobin reductase, NADH-dehydrogenase I, II)	455

NADH-dehydrogenase I	318a ~ d
95% of the capacity of normal erythrocyte,	319
contain FAD,	
electron acceptor : oxygen, cyt c ferricyanide, met. Hb or dyes (DCIP)	
purification 50,000-fold	
NADH-dependent diaphorase A, C.	314a, b
purified 129,000-fold.	
Enzyme A forming 90% of the total activity, whih FAD, no heme.	
Mol. wt. 33,000–34,400, only 3% of normal in methemoglobinemic red cells.	
enzyme A : K_m 2,3-DPIP$=3,3\times10^{-4}M$, in 1,0M sodium phosphate buffer, diaphorase B is seen,	
enzyme B : K_m dye$=2\times10^{-5}M$ K_m NADH$=9\times10^{-5}M$	
cytochrome-b_5-reductase, soluble, appeared to be identical with $NADH_2$-dehydrogenase I	326, 462, 475
NADH-dehydrogenase II	
different chromatographic behavior and kinetic properties, lacked flavin.	
purified (20,000-fold), enzyme without	317a ~ d
flavin, hemoprotein, pH (opt.) 5.2	320
electron donor : $NADH_2$ (specific)	

Enzyme name (Trivial name)	Species or group	Normal value (range) μmoles/ml cells/hr	Ref.	Properties and other remarks	Ref.
				electron acceptor: cyt c, Met. Hb, dues, ferricyanide,	
				Mol. wt. 30,000,	
				enzyme did not reduce pure Met. Hb, only with activation by ferrocyanide,	
				K_m Met. Hb=8μM,	
				pure enzyme catalyzed the reduction of cyt c diectly (cyt c-reductase),	
				electrophoretic pattern: two bands	
				NADH-enzyme (from rabbit ery.)	310, 321
				pH (opt.)=6.2 (first, second fraction) =7.7 (third fraction)	
				electron acceptors: Ferricyanide, 2,6-Dichlorphenol-indophenol, cyt b_5	
				K_m Ferri=$1.35\times10^{-5}M$	
				K_m NADH=$2\times10^{-5}M$	
				Inhibitors: pCMB, Antimycin A, Rotenon,	
				SH-enzyme,	
				NADPH-dependent system (hemiglobin reductase)	
				contain FAD	34, 313, 314
				partially purified, human erythrocytes (900–1,800-fold),	309
				electron donor: NADPH, NADH,	

electron acceptor : cyt c, Met. Hb,	
activity present without	
methylene blue,	
inhibitor : p CMB,	
human erythrocytes (44,000-fold),	315
enzyme contains no flavine nucleotides,	
no heme.	
Mol. wt. : 28,000,	
electron donor : NADH,	
K_m (Met. Hb)$=3.1\times10^{-4}M$	
K_m (cyt c-ox.)$=8.7\times10^{-5}M$	
K_m (cyt b_5 ox.)$=7.1\times10^{-6}M$	
K_m (2,6-Dichlor$=5.0\times10^{-5}$ phenolindoph.)	
Inhibitors : pCMB	
partially purified, human erythrocytes	323
enzyme is a hemoprotein	
Mol. wt. : 185,000	
electron donator : NADPH	324
electron acceptors : Met Hb,	
cyt c,	
oxygen,	
partially purified, 3 enzymes,	
devoid of flavin, with variable	
amount of heme,	
electron donor : $NADH_2$, $NADPH_2$,	325
(ratio 4 : 1)	
electron acceptors : oxygen,	
Met. Hb,	
cyt c,	
2,6-Dichlorphenol-	327
indophenol,	
Methemoglobin reductase :	447
from human ery. highly purified, two	

Enzyme name (Trivial name)	Species or group	Normal value (range) μmoles/ml cells/hr	Ref.	Properties and other remarks	Ref.
				forms I, II, multiple molecular forms:	
				I, II: both Mol. wt. 22,000,	
				both forms react with $NADH_2$, $NADPH_2$	
				absorption spectra:	
				$I_{\lambda max}=278$ nm	
				$II_{\lambda max}=268$ nm	
				Species	330a, b
				Bovine ery.	
				purification and crystallisation	
				Mol. wt.: 2.9×10^4	
				ratio $NADH_2$: $NADPH_2$-activity=2.9 : 1,	
				pH (opt.)=6.0,	
				enzyme contained neither flavin nor heme.	
				blue white delphin,	
				partially purified (450–1,000-fold)	
				enzyme is not a hemoprotein	316
				electron donor: NADP, NAD (2 : 1)	
				electron acceptor: maximal activity with Met. Hb,	
				Mol. wt.: 20,000–30,000,	
				human ery.	311
				localisation: membrane	312
				pH (opt.)=7.5–8.5	
				electron donor: $NADH_2$,	
				electron acceptors: ferricyanide, 2,6-Dichlorphenolindophenol, cyt c not methylene,	

				blue,	
				not oxygen,	
				with $NADPH_2$ no activity,	
				Multiple molecular froms:	455
				In most electrophoretic studies	320
				(starch gel) a single band with	328a, b
				$NADH_2$-Met. Hb reductase,	329a∼c
				partial purification or prolonged	
				storage of hemolyzate *in vitro* gives	
				an anodic minor band,	
				a representative survey	328a
				(2783 individuals) show one common	
				and five rare variants,	
				incidence of abnormal bands about	
				1/100 in a European, Indian, Negro,	
				Greek unspecified population group.	
NAD^+ nucleosidase (E. C. 3.2.2.6)	man	0.1–1.14	331–333	NAD^+ enzyme in newborn: activity low or absent, adult levels are reached within the first year of life.	
	rabbit, ery.	580	331	locatisation: outer membrane surface	
	„ , reti.	600		purification, pH (opt.)=7.0	334
	beef	280		Inhibitor=Nicotinicamide acid.	
	sheep	260			
	pig	150			
	chicken, ery.	9			
	„ , reti.	28			
	frog (summer)	64			
	frog (winter)	15			
	fish	4			
	rat	2			
	dog	2			

Enzyme name (Trivial name)	Species or group	Normal value (range) μmoles/ml cells/hr	Ref.	Properties and other remarks	Ref.
	man	0.36	331	$NADP^+$ enzyme	
	rabbit, ery.	50			
	„ , reti.	110		purification	
	beef	250		pH (opt.)=6.1	
	sheep	180			
	pig	90			
	chicken, ery.	7.5			
	„ , reti.	7.5			
	rat	4			
	mouse	2			
	dog	2			
	pigeon	2			
	frog (summer)	18			
	frog (winter)	4			
	cat	1			
	fish	1			
NAD^+ pyrophosphorylase (NMN adenylyl-transferase) (E. C. 2.7.7.1)	man	present	335		
NAD^+ synthetase (E. C. 6.3.5.1)	man	present	335b		
NMN nucleosidase (E. C. 3.2.2)	man	1.86	331		
NMN-synthetase (E. C. 2.4.2.12)	man	present	335a, b, 336	purification (600-fold)	335a

Nicotinate phosphoribosyltransferase (E. C. 2.4.2.11)	man	present	335b	(see also suppl. table)	
Nucleosidediphosphate kinase (E. C. 2.7.4.6)	man	present	337	Multiple molecular forms : 6 peaks, each a different enzyme Mol. wt. : 80,000–100,000, differences in temperature dependence and kinetic behaviour	
Nucleoside diphosphatase (E. C. 3.6.1.6)	man	10.5–52.5	275	substrate : IDP	
Orotidine-5'-phosphate decarboxylase (E. C. 4.1.1.23)	man	0.1–0.17	101	pH (opt.)=6.2–6.8 K_m orotidine-5-P=$1.1\times10^{-5}M$, soluble enzyme	101
Orotidine-5-phosphate pyrophosphorylase (E. C. 2.4.2.10)	man	0.07–0.17 0.1–0.6	101 477	pH (opt.)=7.8 K_m orotidine-5-P=$0.4\times10^{-5}M$ K_m PRPP=$1.6\times10^{-5}M$, soluble enzyme	101
α-Oxoglutarate dehydrogenase (E. C. 1.2.4.2)	rabbit, ery. ,, , reti.	0 18	155		
Phosphatidic acid phosphatase (E. C. 3.1.3.4)	man	present	131	2 types, only 1 dependent on Mg^{2+}	131
Phosphatidylglycerol-phospholipase A (E. C. 3.1.1.4)	rat	2.4	338	partially purified, pH (opt.)=6.5–7.5 soluble enzyme $K_m=1.25\times10^{-5}M$, activators : NaCl, Ca^{2+}	338

Enzyme name (Trivial name)	Species or group	Normal value (range) μmoles/ml cells/hr	Ref.	Properties and other remarks	Ref.
Phosphatidyl inositol kinase (E. C. 2.7.1.67)	swine	0.44	339	erythrocyte ghosts	339
				product : diphosphoinositide	
		0.34		product : triphosphoinositide	
				inhibitors : Ca^{2+}, SH reagents	
Phosphofructokinase (E. C. 2.7.1.11)	man, adults (37°C)	210–290	28, 43		
		72–150	152		
	(25°C)	70–170	19, 40, 42, 51, 53, 57, 59 60, 151, 251		
	man, newborn (25°C)	50–330	42, 57, 151		
	Preservation (37°C)		250, 342	ACD medium	
	day zero	175–220			
	10th day	40–70			
	30th day	5–50			
	60th day	10			
	day zero	210		AMD medium	
	10th day	120–160			
	30th day	80			
	60th day (37°C)	20			
	rabbit,	372	343	bleeding anemia	
	„ , reti. (40–50%)	900–1,050			
	„ , top fraction (90% reti.)	1,800		density gradient centrifugation (after bleeding anemia, maximal activity on third day of bleeding)	
	man, bottom fraction (5% reti.)	340		purification studies, partially purified (human erythrocytes)	340, 341
	rat	515	56, 253	Mol. wt.: $3.8–4.3 \times 10^5$, electrophoretically a single band, immunological no distinction from muscle enzyme	
	dog	370			
	goat	25			

	deer	27		human erythrocytes:	345, 346
	horse	70	464	evidence for different oligomeric forms of enzyme (see also suppl. table)	347
Phosphoglucomutase (E. C. 2.7.5.1)	man, adults	25–45	42, 53, 56, 99, 285, 348	Multiple molecular forms: Polymorphism, 3 types	17, 349–352
	(37°C)	50–70	43	PGM-1 (bands a, c, e, f)	
	man, newborn	14–50	42, 99	PGM-2-1 (bands a, b, c, d, e, f)	
	rat	73	56	PGM-2 (bands a, d, e, f)	
	dog	22			
	sheep	18			
	rabbit,	19			
	„ , ratio				
	„ , ery.	1.4	63		
	„ , reti.				
Phosphogluconate dehydrogenase (E. C. 1.1.1.44)	man, adults (25°C)	45–90	19, 42, 50, 51, 53, 57, 58, 59, 61, 99, 171, 185, 194, 208, 353, 354	Multiple molecular forms: 2 autosomale alleles ($6\text{-}PGD^{A}$, $6\text{-}PGD^{B}$), type I=A=usual type, type II=AB=common variant, type III=B or C=canning type,	485
	(37°C)	150–194	43, 172		
		60–102	152		
	man, newborn	90–125	42, 57, 99, 171		
	man, fetus (19th week of pregnancy)	75	171		
	sheep	7	185		
	goat	13			
	cow	8			
	pig	12			
	horse	10–18	185, 464		

Enzyme name (Trivial name)	Species or group	Normal value (range) μmoles/ml cells/hr	Ref.	Properties and other remarks	Ref.
	rabbit, ery.	48	194	density gradient centrifugation	194
	„ , reti.	96			
Phosphoglucose isomerase (E. C. 5.3.1.9)	man, adults (25°C)	400–700	19, 40, 42, 50, 51, 57, 59	K_m fructose-6-P=$5\times10^{-4}M$ (pH 7.5) K_m glucose-6-P=$2.5\times10^{-4}M$ (pH 7.5)	356
		((240))	151	partially purified, human erythrocytes, a major component (a) and 2 minor components (b, c)	357
	man, adults (37°C)	900–1,100	56, 152, 285		
		((400–700))	43	Isomerase a : K_m fructose-6-P=$1.86\times10^{-5}M$	
	man, newborn (25°C)	900–1,400	42, 57, 97	Isomerase b : K_m fructose-6-P=$2.13\times10^{-5}M$	
		((336))	151	Isomerase c :	
	man, fetus (25°C) (12th–28th week of pregnancy)	1,250	97	K_m fructose-6-P=$2.05\times10^{-5}M$ dimeric enzyme structure,	
				wild mice, starch gel electrophoresis, 3 bands	359
	rabbit (37°C)	2,700	358		
	pig	3,100			
	guinea pig	4,900			
	chicken	1,230			
	rat	1,120	56		
	sheep	740			
Phosphoglycerate kinase (E. C. 2.7.2.3)	man, adults (25°C)	1,600–1,900	19, 48, 51, 53, 57, 151 225	Purification, human erythrocytes crystallization, Mol. wt. (50,000) 45,000	360a, b 360d
	(osmolic henolysis)	2,100	360b	Isoelectric point : 7.5–8.0	360b
				pH (opt.)=7.6 to 9.0	361
	(dialysis with glycerol-citrate)	3,360	360b	K_m 3-PG=0.8, 1.1 mM	360b

		3,700	40		
	(backward reaction)	2,240–3,230	227, 237b	K_m 1,3-DPG=2–3μM K_m ADP=12μM (low conc.) 100μM (highconc.) K_m Mg-ATP=0.3–0.4 mM	360d
	man, adults (37°C)	1,128–1,620	152	Multiple molecular forms: Polymorphism, 3 phenotypes PGK-1,2-1,2	362
	(backward reaction)	3,000–4,800	43, 227	localisation: cytosol	52, 231–233
	man, newborn (25°C)	2,800	57, 151	variant enzyme (purification), substitution	360c
		5,833	42	asparagine against threonine,	
Phosphoglycerate mutase (E. C. 2.7.5.3)	man, adult (25°C)	220–450	19, 40, 42, 48, 51, 53, 59, 151, 225		
		((913))	57		
	(37°C)	400–700	43, 152, 363		
	man, newborn (25°C)	600–1,000	42, 97, 151		
		1,400	57		
	man, fetus (12th–28th week of pregnancy)	1,513	97		
	rabbit	140	28, 363		
	rat	167	363		
	dog	583			
	sheep	440			
Phosphoribomutase (ribose-1-P→ ribose-5-P)	man	56–66	52, 364		

Enzyme name (Trivial name)	Species or group	Normal value (range) μmoles/ml cells/hr	Ref.	Properties and other remarks	Ref.
Phosphoribose isomerase	man	3,000–5,500	52, 285, 365	partially purified (1,000-fold)	366
				K_m ribose-5-P $= 2.2 \times 10^{-3} M$	
(E. C. 5.3.1.6)	cat	3,900	365	inhibitor=pCMB	
	rabbit	2,800			
	horse	2,200			
	pig	2,000			
	mouse	1,600			
	rat	1,400			
	guinea pig	1,100			
	chicken	870			
Phosphoribosyl-formylglycine-amidine synthetase (E. C. 6.3.5.3)	mouse	no activity present	367		
Phosphoribosyl-pyrophosphate amidotransferase (E. C. 2.4.2.14)	mouse man	no activity present	367		
Phosphoribosyl-pyrophosphate synthetase (E. C. 2.7.6.1)	man	10–20	267, 368–371	Characterization : pH (opt.)=8.0–8.5 K_m ATP $= 1.7 \times 10^{-4} M$ K_m ribose-5-P $= 6.5 \times 10^{-4} M$ inhibitors : fluorite, PP, borate	33
				partially purified (5,100-fold) human erythrocytes pH (opt.)=7.2–7.4 Isoelectric point : 4.7 K_m ATP $= 14 \mu M$	372

				K_m ribose-5-P=33μM activation : P_i, Mg^{2+}, 2 heavy forms Mol. wt. : 1,200,000 and 720,000 electrophoretically : a single band, Mol. wt. 34,500	
Phosphoribulokinase (E. C. 2.7.1.19)				partially purified	373
Porphobilinogen deaminase	rabbit chicken	present	79		
Proteinases Cathepsin (E. C. 3.4.4)				I. stromal enzyme, activated by Zn^{2+}, Fe^{2+}, reducing agents	374
				pH (opt.)=7.4	
	rabbit, ery.	0	88	Cathepsin A	
	„ , reti.	2.7–2.8		pH (opt.)=5.2	88
				II. stromal enzyme, activated, by Zn^{2+}, Fe^{2+}, not activated by reducing agents	374
				pH (opt.)=7.4	
				III. stromal enzyme, not activated by reducing agents	374
				pH (opt.)=3.2	
	rat	3	198	rat : pH (opt.)=3.9	198
	man	3.5	87	human erythrocytes : pH (opt.)=3.0	87
				rabbit, erythrocytes : pH (opt.)=3.5	375, 376
	rabbit, ery.	3.2	88	inhibitors : ascorbic acid, Zn^{2+} SH enzyme	377
	„ , reti.	14			
	rabbit, (bleeding anemia)		376 377		
	1st day (2% reti.)	8			
	7th day (60%)	32			
	11th day (80%)	40			
	15th day (25%)	28			

Enzyme name (Trivial name)	Species or group	Normal value (range) μmoles/ml cells/hr	Ref.	Properties and other remarks	Ref.
	22nd day (2%)	15			
	man (freezing hemolysate)	12 22	378	human erythrocytes pH (opt.)=10.5 partially purified, human erythrocytes pH (opt.)=2.8 K_m=0.5 gm Hb/100 ml inhibitor: SH reagents, gel chromatography: a single band, Mol. wt.: 50,000–60,000	378
Purine nucleoside phosphorylase (E. C. 2.4.2.1)	man	1,000–1,600	34, 52a	substrate: desoxyinosine, ghosts	388
	,, , substrate inosinc	740–1,200	52b	Purine nucleoside phosphorylase and desoxyribonucleoside phosphorylase are the same,	386 387 380, 381
				purification, crystallization pH (opt.)=6.5–8.0	384
	,, , substrate guanosine	400–700		Mol. wt.: 80(81),000	385
				Multiple molecular forms: 7 distinct isoenzymes from youngest to old cells with a progressive increase in number and intensity of the faster bands, trimeric structure	389 382, 383
Pyridoxal kinase (E. C. 2.7.1.35)	man	0.04	390	K_m pyridoxal=$5\times10^{-6}M$	390
Pyrophosphatase, inorganic (E. C. 3.6.1.1)	man, adults (37°C)	212	391	pH 7.5	
		320–714	396	partially purified (1,800-fold), soluble	395
	man, newborn	245–714	396	pH (opt.)=7.7 activator: Mg^{2+}	

	man, reti. (10%)	1,200	396	inhibitor: pCMB SH enzyme	
	rabbit,	300	28, 30		
	„ , ery.	194–355			
	„ , reti.	2,370–3,300	392, 393		
	beef	0–11	394		
	sheep	25–38			
	pig	42–128			
	dog	90–137			
	cat	96–144			
	horse	32–240			
	chicken	80–270			
Pyruvate kinase (E. C. 2.7.1.40)	man, adults (25°C)	100–180	34, 40, 42, 48, 51, 57, 59, 151, 399, 400	Purification (10,000-fold), FDP addition increase of $V_{max}/2$ electrophoretically: 3 bands (I, II, III) at aging only 1 band density gradient centrifugation	402 401, 403 397
		240–255	61, 62		
		((319))	99	K_m PEP=0.12 mM buoyant cells	
	(37°C)	220–250	53, 172, 398	K_m PEP=0.30 mM dense cells, FDP addition:	
	density gradient centrifugation	74–140 (pH 8)	37		
	man, reti. (90%)	448	175	K_m PEP=0.08 mM buoyant cells	
	„ , ery. (reti. 25%)	224		K_m PEP=0.07 mM dense cells pH (opt.)=6.71 buoyant cells pH (opt.)=7.22 dense cells	
	man, newborn (25°C)	150–290	42, 97, 151		
		350–370	57, 99		
	(37°C)	330	172, 398		
	man, fetus (25°C) 12th–28th week of pregnancy	626	97		
	preservation (25°C) 1st day	240[×]	61	[×]Glucose-P-Ringer medium	

Enzyme name (Trivial name)	Species or group	Normal value (range) μmoles/ml cells/hr	Ref.	Properties and other remarks	Ref.
	7th day	185			
	(37°C)				
	1st day	355××	250	××ACD medium	
	10th day	210–240			
	20th day	190–210			
	40th day	105–150			
	90th day	90			
	rat	474 (708)×××	56, 253, 404	×××probably too high	
	(37°C)				
	rabbit	300 (474)×××			
	dog	180 (534)×××			
	goat	315			
	deer	433			
	cat	(360)×××			
	beef	(260)×××			
	chicken	(5,742)×××			
	goose (25°C)	2,750	62		
	rabbit (37°C)+			+bleeding anemia	
	1st day (8% reti.)	194	175		
	6th day (27%)	465			
	10th day (24%)	495			
	15th day (16%)	485			
	18th day (7%)	243			
	density gradient centrifugation		175		
	rabbit (37°C) (1st day of bleeding)			man, ery. purification (30,000-fold)	488
	whole suspension (8% reti.)	192		IP: 7.1 (4°C), Mol. wt.: 225,000	
	top fraction (80%)	640		Michaelis kinetic at PEP conc. $<5\times10^{-4}M$,	488a~c

	bottom fraction (4%) (4th day of bleeding)	160	at higher conc. sigmoidal activators: FDP, Glc-1,$6P_2$ (transform the sigmoidal in a hyperbolic curve), inhibitors: ATP, coupelt with activation,	
	whole suspension (12% reti.)	405		
	top fraction (63%)	1,084	Multiple molecular form:	
	bottom fraction (7%)	270	enzyme differs electrophoretically from M_1-, M_2- and L-types; hybrid of L and M_2-types?	490
Ribonuclease (E. C. 2.7.7.16)			rabbit reticulocytes (30–40% reti.) hemolysate: substrate: cellular RNS pH (opt.)=7.5 Temperature opt.=50°C stroma: pH (opt.)=6 high thermostability	149
			rabbit, reticulocytes pH (opt.)=7.5 (8.0 ionic strength-dependent) Temperature opt.=65°C Substrate: pyrimidine (5′-esterbound) products: nucleosides (uridine) mono-, oligo-, and polynucleotides activation: monovalent cations, enzyme is dissociated by high molar LiCl, urea, inhibition: bound enzyme by Mg^{2+}	409, 410, 412, 413
			rabbit, reticulocytes ribosomes pH (opt.)=7.5, latent RNase activated by monovalent ions ($Tris^+$, $collidine^+$, K^+, Na^+, Li^+)	405, 406, 411
			rabbit, reticulocytes pH (opt.)=8.2	

Enzyme name (Trivial name)	Species or group	Normal value (range) μmoles/ml cells/hr	Ref.	Properties and other remarks	Ref.
				substrate: poly C	
				low activity in ribosomes and soluble fractions, more activity by extraction with hypertonic sucrose, NaCl-EDTA, Tris pH 8.2	414, 415
				rabbit, reticulocytes (whole-cell lysates and membrane-free hemolysates)	417, 418, 419
				pH (opt.)=7.0	
				Temp. (opt.)=50°C	
				membrane-free hemolysate:	
				K_m total RNA=$16.7\times10^{-8}M$	
				K_m rRNA=$12.5\times10^{-8}M$	
				K_m tRNA=$6.1\times10^{-6}M$	
				K_m ribosomes=$2.0\times10^{-6}M$	
	rabbit ratio ery. (2% reti.) to reti. (96%)	1 : 5	419	inhibitors: hemin, cobaltous ions	
				enzyme exists in active and latent form (majority in the latent state)	
				localisation: membrane (inner side)	
				release of latent RNase: 4M urea	
				Membrane+4M urea:	
				K_m total RNA=$7.7\times10^{-8}M$	
				K_m rRNA=$20\times10^{-8}M$	
				K_m tRNA=$16\times10^{-6}M$	
				K_m ribosomes=$1.0\times10^{-6}M$	
				purification studies, rabbit reticulocytes	416
				substrate: poly U, poly C	
				Localisation: Cytosol, pH (opt.)=6.8	
				partially purified (4,800-fold) pH (opt.)=5.8	
				localisation: 93.5% ghost fraction, 1.5%	408

				ribosomes, 5% soluble fraction	
				rat, reticulocytes partial purification of a latent RNA, activation: SH reagents, 6*M* urea, 0.1*M* H_2SO_4, Cu^{2+}, Zn^{2+}	421, 422
				rat, bone-marrow nuclei, chicken, partial purification	420, 491
				pH: 6.2–7.6	
				Substrate: poly C, poly U, no effect of ions (Na^+, K^+, EDTA)	491
				localisation: 40% of the total enzyme activity is present in the nucleus	
Ribulose diphosphate carboxylase (E. C. 4.1.1.f)	man	present	373	partial purification	373
Ribulose phosphate epimerase (E. C. 5.1.3.1)	horse	present	423		
Serine hydroxymethyl transferase (E. C. 2.1.2.1)	man	present	308	no activity in human erythrocytes lysates	71, 128
Succinate dehydrogenase (E. C. 1.3.99.1)	rabbit, ery.	5	28, 30		
	„ , reti.	40			
Succinate cytochrome c oxidoreductase	man, adults	<0.2	120b	localisation: stroma	
	man, newborn (5–20% reti.)	0.4			
	man, newborn (50% reti.)	3.1			
	rabbit (28% reti.)	6.0	119	localisation: washed stroma	

Enzyme name (Trivial name)	Species or group	Normal value (range) μmoles/ml cells/hr	Ref.	Properties and other remarks	Ref.
Superoxide dismutase (E. C. 1.15.1.1)	beef	present	424, 425	beef erythrocytes produce superoxide anion during oxidation of reduced flavins by molecular oxygen. Superoxide is rapidly destroyed by catalytic quantities of erythrocuprein.	424
				purification, beef erythrocytes, enzyme contains 2 eq. copper/mole enzyme, identical with erythrocuprein (human) and hemocuprein (bovine)	425a∼d 492a, b
Tetrahydrofolate reductase (E. C.1.5.1.3)	man, bone „ , marrow „ , cells	25	132–134	in reticulocytes and in erythrocytes not detectable	
Tetrahydrofolate formylase (E. C. 6.3.3.2)	man, ery.	8–16	34, 132, 134, 308, 426		
	density gradient centrifugation		(71, 128, 153)		
	man, top fraction (40% reti.)	21	132 426	activity shows a relationship to the life span of erythrocytes	
	bottom fraction (18% reti.)	19			
	chicken	100	308		
	mouse	277			
	guinea pig	86			
	rat	53			
	rabbit	29			
	pig	19			
	dog	11			

Thymidylate kinase (E. C. 2.7.4.9)	man, ery.	present	427	substrate : de-TMP	
	rat, ox, rabbit, horse } ery.	no activity detectable			
Thymidine kinase (E. C. 2.7.1.21)	man, bone marrow cells	0.3–0.9	133		
	man, megaloblastic anemia	2.6			
Transaldolase (E. C. 2.2.1.2)	man (37°C)	(14 moles/ml cells/hr)	428		
Transketolase (E. C. 2.2.1.1)	man, adults (37°C)	2–7	52, 285, 430–432, 436	increasing activity after TPP supplementation (about 17%)	436 437a
		9–13	428, 433–435a		
		35	436		
	man, newborn	10–13	432, 434, 435		
	rabbit	12.8	438	human RBC, partial purification (8,200-fold)	437b
	mouse	11.7			
	guinea pig	10.4		Mol. wt. : 136,000,	
	rat	8.1		IP : 8.5,	
	beef	4.6		pH (opt.)=7.5–8.6,	
	pig	4.0		K_m (pentosephosphate)=1.7 mM	
	horse	2.0		inhibitors : sulfate, phosphate Rib-5-p	435b
Triosephosphate isomerase (E. C. 5.3.1.1)	man, adults (25°C)	7,000–18,000	40, 53, 151, 356, 439	partially purified activity in 2 distinct peaks	440
		39,000	51		
	(37°C)	26,100–32,640	43		
		((5,100–8,160))	152		

Enzyme name (Trivial name)	Species or group	Normal value (range) μmoles/ml cells/hr	Ref.	Properties and other remarks	Ref.
	man, newborn (25°C)	17,460	151		
		((4,213))	42		
	goose (25°C)	2,380	62		
Tripeptidase (E. C. 3.4.1.3)	man	719	241	localisation: cytosol pH (opt.)=7.6–7.9	440
				partially purified (500–750-fold), horse erythrocytes pH (opt.)=7.9	272
				inhibitor: cysteine partially purified (1,000-fold) human erythrocytes pH (opt.)=7.0 SH enzyme	441
UDP-Galactose pyrophosphorylase (E. C. 2.7.7.10)	man	1.2	157		
UDP-Glucose-4-epimerase (Galactowaldenase) (E. C. 5.1.3.2)	man, adults	0.32	157	×activation with NAD^+, presence of NAD^+ changes the molecular form of the enzyme,	158
		1.4–5.2×	43, 158, 442		
		2.84×	158		
	man, newborn			Multiple molecular forms: newborn-2 bands, adults-1 band, adult ery. with NAD^+ shows 2 bands	
UDP-Glycogen Glycosyltransferase (E. C. 2.4.1.11)	man, adults	1.2–2.6	443		
	„ , newborn	2.3–2.9			
	„ , premature	2.8			
UDPG-	man	1.1	444	partially purified, human erythrocytes	445

pyrophosphorylase (E. C. 2.7.7.9)				pH (opt.)=8.5 K UDP-glucose$=2.3\times 10^{5}M$ K(i) UDP-glucose$=1.5\times 10^{5}M$ K UTP$=3.3\times 10^{4}M$ K(i) UTP$=1.0\times 10^{4}M$ K (glucose-1-P)$=0.17\times 10^{3}M$ K (PPi)$=0.48\times 10^{3}M$
Uroporphyrino- genase (E. C. 4.1.1.37)	rabbit, reti. chicken, ery.	present present	78b, 446	

SUPPLEMENTARY TABLE

Enzyme name (Trivial name)	Species or group	Normal value (range) μmoles/ml cells/hr	Ref.	Properties and other remarks	Ref.
Adenylate cyclase (E. C. 4.6.1.1)	rat, ery. (ghosts)		457	stimulation by isoproterenol and NaF	457
	11. day	2.8 nmoles cycl. AMP/mg protein/hr			
	25. day	1.2 ,,			
	74. day	0.8 ,,			
	with NaF (1 mM)				
	11. day	9.4 nmoles cycl. AMP/mg protein/hr			
	25. day	7.2 ,,			
	74. day	2.0 ,,			
Adenylate deaminase (E. C. 3.5.4.6)				chicken ery., purification (1,400-fold), pH (opt.)=7.1 activators: ATP, ADP, GTP, alkali metal ions, reaction kinetic sigmoidal with AMP, hyperbolic with AMP and ATP or alkali metal ions	33b
Adenylate kinase (E. C. 2.7.4.3)				partial purification of two forms, Mol. wt.: 21,000	41a
				kinetic properties: *type 1* / *type 2* K_m (AMP)=0.33 mM / 0.27 mM K_m $(MgATP)^{2-}$=0.95 mM / 0.40 mM	41b

				K_m (ADP)=0.12 mM K_m $(MgADP)^-$=0.22 mM	0.08 mM 0.20 mM	
3′,5′-Cycl. AMP-phosphodiesterase (E. C. 3.1.4.17)	rat	present	459	soluble enzyme, age dependent changes		457
Amylo-1,6-glucosidase (debranching enzyme) (E. C. 3.2.1.9)	man	present	458			
Carbonic anhydrase (E. C. 4.2.1.1)				adults: 7 isoenzymes, newborns: 5 isoenzymes CA increases during the last trimester of pregnancy from 5% to 20–30% of adult level, CA is a good maturity index		460 461
Cytochrome-b_5 reductase (E. C. 1.6.2.2)				(see also NADH/NADPH acceptor oxidoreductase) man, ery. purification (1,000-fold), prosthetic group: EAD, K_m NADH=$1.6\times10^{-6}M$ K_m DCIP=$4.8\times10^{-7}M$, Mol. wt.: <40,000 substrate specifity: ferricyanide, DCIP, cyt b_5 (8:2:1), high specific for NADH, suggestion, that reductase is the same enzyme as NADH-DH I.		462 475
2′,3′-Cyclic	man, ery.	present	463	localisation: membrane		463

Enzyme name (Trivial name)	Species or group	Normal value (range) μmoles/ml cells/hr	Ref.	Properties and other remarks	Ref.
nucleotide 3′-phosphohydrolase (E. C. 3.1.4)					
α-Glucan: α-1,4 glucan 6-glycosyl transferase (brancher enzyme) (E. C. 2.4.1.18)	man, ery.	present	458		
Glycogen synthetase (E. C. 2.4.1.11)	man, adults „ , newborns „ , children (3–10 year)	1.3–6.4 2.5–3.2 1.2–1.8	470a, b	(37°C) pH (opt.)=7.6 K_m UDPG=0.21 mM K_m G6P=6.6 mM Inhibitors: ATP (5 mM=50%), P_i and SO_4^{2-}, the main factor limiting the activity is the low intracellular conc. of G6P.	 470a, b 458, 471a~c
Glyoxalase (E. C. 4.4.1.5)				porcine ery., purification (2,000-fold), IP=5, Mol. wt.: 52,000, K_m=0.19 mM, inhibitors: chelating agents, reactivators: Mg^{2+}, Mn^{2+}, Ca^{2+}, K (Diss.) Mg-enzyme-complex =0.6 mM.	472a, b
Hypoxanthineguanine				Multiple molecular forms:	

Enzyme	Source	Activity	Ref.	Properties	Ref.
phosphoribosyl-transferase (E. C. 2.4.2.8)				partially purified (300-fold), Mol. wt.: 68,000, two subunits with identical Mol. wt., with preparative isoelectric focusing: 3 isoenzymes, Mol. wt.: ~34,000, no significant differences between I, II, III	459
				in polyacrylamide gel: 4 isoenzymes, immunological identity	473a, b
Methionine synthetase (E. C. 2.1.2)	man, bone marrow	1.7	474		
	„ , ery.	no activity detectable			
Nicotinate phosphoribosyl-transferase (E. C. 2.4.2.11)				man, ery. purification (30,000-fold), single protein, pH (opt.)=6.5–8.0 Mol. Wt.: 86,000 K_m nicotinate=24 μM, K_m PRPP =100 μM, in presence of ATP: K_m nicotinate=0.5 μM K_m PRPP =5 μM	476
Peptidase (E. C. 3.4.1.3)				man, ery., polymorphism, electrophoretic studies, *Peptidase A:* substrate: dipeptides (except Leu-Pro) no hydrolysis of tripeptides, 3 electrophoretically distinct zones of activity	478

Enzyme name (Trivial name)	Species or group	Normal value (range) μmoles/ml cells/hr	Ref.	Properties and other remarks	Ref.
				Peptidase B: substrate: tripeptides also dipeptides, four or more distinct electrophoretic components	
				Peptidase C: substrate: dipeptides, substrate specifity is different from that of peptidase A, two distinct zones.	
				Peptidase D: substrate: only Leu-Pro.	
				Peptidase E: substrate: Leu-Leu, Lys-Leu, Phe-Leu, Phe-Tyr, Leucyl-β-naphtylamide sheep, ery., partially purified (4,000-fold, about 75% pure)	479
				specifity: N-formylmethionylvaline to give N-formylmethionine+valine, Mol. wt.: 340,000, contains sex identical subunits, pH (opt.)= ~7, K_m N-formyl-Met-Val=2 mM K_m Gly-Met-Gly =2 mM	

	Inhibitor : Disopropylfluorophosphate ($10^{-5}M$).	
Phosphofructokinase (E. C. 2.7.1.11)	rat, ery., purification (2,000-fold),	344a, b
	pH (opt.)=8.0–8.4	
	at pH 7 : substrate dependence (F6P) : sigmoidal kinetics, (T-dependent), allosteric enzyme,	
	activation : K^+, NH_4^+,	
	positive effectors : AMP, G1, 6P, P_i, SO_4^{2-} ; NH_4^+	
	negative effectors : ATP (pH, F6P-dependent), PEP, 2,3-DPG, Citrate,	
	rabbit, ery. purification	480
	(25,000-fold), Mol. wt. : 500,000	
	four identical subunits possible, (Mol. wt. $enzyme_{Diss.}$ in Guanine=53,000)	
	Amino acid composition is different from skeletal PFK,	
	Inhibition :	
	2,3-PGA (5 mM)=48%	
	2,3-PGA+AMP (5 mM)=80%	
	ADP=67%	
	inhibition is released by P_i,	483
	rabbit enzyme type B (liver)	484
	man, ery.,	
	purification (15,000-fold)	481a,
	electrophoretic studies :	482
	1 single band, 4 subunits (not identical),	
	allosteric properties at pH 7.0 :	481a~c

Enzyme name (Trivial name)	Species or group	Normal value (range) μmoles/ml cells/hr	Ref.	Properties and other remarks	Ref.
				influenced by ATP, ADP, P_i, AMP, cycl. AMP, not by 2,3-DPG.	
Phosphoribosyl-pyrophosphate synthetase (E. C. 2.7.6.1)	man, ery.			man, ery. partially purified, K_m (Rib-6-P)=33 μM K_m (Mg-ATP)=14 μM K_m (Mg)=0.2 μM Inhibitors: ADP, GMP, GDP, GTP, IDP, ITP, 2,3-DPG, XDP, CDP, CTP, TDP, TTP, $NADH_2$, $NADPH_2$, FAD	486
Glycogen phosphorylase (E. C. 2.4.1.1)	man, ery.	1.6–2.4	487a, b		
Triokinase (E. C. 2.7.1.28)	man, ery.	2.8–3.2	493	partially, purified (50-fold) substrate: dihydroxyacetone, glyceraldehyde, pH (opt.)=6.6 K_m (DHA)=0.5 μM K_m (GA)=11 μM K_m $(ATP\text{-}Mg)^{2-}$=1.45 mM	
Uroporphyrinogen III cosynthetase (E. C. 4.3.1.(8))	man	present	494	diminished in porphyria patients	

One instance is particularly controversial, that of the methemoglobin reductases, diaphorases, etc. All data pertaining to these enzyme activities have been listed as NADH-oxidoreductases; the actual electron acceptors used have been listed. As far as possible, all values in the literature have been recalculated on a common basis of μmoles of substrate transformed per ml cells per hr. Temperature and other experimental conditions are given if the original literature contains the relevant data. The "normal" values are given as means, ranges or as individual values, as the case may be. The authors have been grouped according to the coincidence of their normal ranges. The age of the data has been taken into consideration, and grouped accordingly. Maturational changes including data on the reticulocytes are listed, as well as data on red cells from different species. Furthermore pains have been taken to assess the localisation of the enzymes, note purification and crystallisation studies and to present as fully as possible the properties of the enzymes, including kinetic constants, pH optima, activators and inhibitors. In addition, electrophoretic studies on isoenzymes and polymorphism have been surveyed. They are listed as "multiple molecular forms" since not in all a genetic causation has been established in other hand purely population genetic studies of which they are now multitude have not been included. An assessment of the data collected indicates the great advances which have been made in recent years in the purification and characterisation of enzymes and in the detection of multiple molecular forms. The remarkably close agreement among different authors in the values for the normal ranges for many enzymes is perhaps a pleasant surprise. On the other hand, it is apparent that only a few enzymes have been studied from various aspects and that in many cases, only preliminary data are available. There is particularly a lack of modern data on intraspecies differences. It is very much hoped that this compilation will be an incentive to fill the gaps and avoid unnecessary repetitious work.

REFERENCES

1 Pevsner, D. L., *Biokhimia* (Moskva), **30**, No. 5, 980 (1965).
2 Shafai, T. and Cortner, J. A., *Biochim. Biophys. Acta*, **236**, 612 (1971).
3 Sawitsky, A., Fitch, H. and Meyer, L. M., *J. Lab. Clin. Med.*, **33**, 203 (1948).
4 Calloway, S., Davies, D. R. and Rutland, J. P., *Brit. Med. J.*, **2**, 812 (1951).

5 Sabine, J. C., *J. Clin. Invest.*, **19**, 833 (1940).

6 Palek, J., Brabek, V., Vopatova, M., Michalec, C. and Mirčevova, L., *Clin. Chim. Acta.*, **23**, 133 (1969).

7 Sabine, J. C., *Blood*, **10**, 1132 (1955).

8a Herz, F., Kaplan, E. and Scheye, E. S., *Clin. Chim. Acta*, **36**, 537 (1972).

8b Wright, D. L., Plummer, D. T., *Biochem. J.*, **153**, 521 (1973).

8c Burns Bellhorn, M., Blumfeld, O. O. and Gallop, P. M., *Biochem. Biophys. Res. Comm.*, **39**, 267 (1970).

8d Jackson, P. and Whittacker, M., *Enzymologia*, **43**, 359 (1972).

9 Ferber, E., Munder, P. G., Kohlschütter, A. and Fischer, H., *Europ. J. Biochem.*, **5**, 395 (1968).

10 Tsuboi, K. K. and Hudson, P. B., *Arch. Biochem. Biophys.*, **53**, 341 (1954).

11 Iio, M., Hashimoto, T. and Yoshikawa, H., *J. Biochem.*, **55**, 321 (1964).

12 Hopkinson, D. A., Spencer, N. and Harris, H., *Nature*, **199**, 969 (1963).

13 Scott, E. M., *J. Biol. Chem.*, **241**, 3049 (1966).

14 Fischer, R. A. and Harris, H., *Ann. Hum. Genet.*, **34**, 431 (1971).

15 Fischer, R. A. and Harris, H., *Ann. Hum. Genet.*, **34**, 439 (1971).

16 Fischer, R. A. and Harris, H., *Ann. Hum. Genet.*, **34**, 449 (1971).

17 Travis, S. F., Morrison, A. D., Clements, R. S., Jr., Vinegrad, A. J. and Oski, F. A., *J. Clin. Invest.*, **50**, 2104 (1971).

18 Tsuboi, K. K. and Hudson, P. B., *Arch. Biochem. Biophys.*, **43**, 339 (1953).

19 Löhr, G. W. and Waller, H. D., *Folia Haematol.* (Leipzig), **78**, 384 (1962).

20 Valentine, W. M., Tanaka, K. R. and Fredericke, R. E., *Amer. J. Clin. Path.*, **36**, 328 (1961).

21 Berry, D. H. and Hochstein, P., *Arch. Biochem. Biophys.*, **131**, 170 (1969).

22 Beutler, E. and Yeh, K. Y., *J. Lab. Clin. Med.*, **54**, 456 (1959).

23 Rubinstein, D., Ottolenghi, P. and Denstedt, O. F., *Canad. J. Biochem. Physiol.*, **34**, 222 (1965).

24 Shohet, S. B., *J. Clin. Invest.*, **49**, 1668 (1970).

25 Spencer, N., Hopkinson, D. A. and Harris, H., *Ann. Hum. Genet.*, **32**, 9 (1968).

26 Harris, H., *Brit. Med. Bull.*, **25**, 5 (1969).

27 Hopkinson, D. A., Cook, P. J. L. and Harris, H., *Ann. Hum. Genet.*, **32**, 361 (1969).

28 Rapoport, S., *Folia Haematol.* (Leipzig), **78**, 364 (1962).

29 Ababei, L. and Rapoport, S., *Acta Biol. Med. German.*, **6**, 288 (1961).

30 Rapoport, S., Ababei, L., Hinterberger, U., Kahrig, C., Künzel, M.,

Gerischer-Mothes, W., Raderecht, H. J., Scheuch, D. and Viereck, D., *Acta Biol. Med. German.*, **7**, 589 (1961).
31 Lowy, B. A., Ramot, B. and London, I. M., *J. Biol. Chem.*, **235**, 2920 (1960).
32 Askari, A. and Franklin, J. E., Jr., *Biochim. Biophys. Acta*, **110**, 162 (1965).
33a Banaschak, H., *Acta Biol. Med. German.*, **17**, 261 (1966).
33b Kawamura, Y., *J. Biochem.*, **72**, 21 (1972).
34 Hennessey, M. A., Waltersdorph, A. M., Huennekens, F. M. and Gabrio, B. W., *J. Clin. Invest.*, **41**, 1257 (1962).
35 Askari, A. and Rao, S. N., *Biochim. Biophys. Acta*, **151**, 198 (1968).
36 Tatibana, M., Nakao, M. and Yoshikawa, H., *J. Biochem.*, **45**, 1037 (1958).
37a Carletti, P. and Marchesini, B. M., *Ital. J. Biochem.*, **10**, 156 (1961).
37b Carletti, P. and De Ritis, G., *Clin. Chim. Acta*, **7**, 402 (1962).
38 Fildes, R. A. and Harris, H., *Nature*, **209**, 261 (1966).
39a Harris, H., Hopkinson, D. A., Luffman, J. E. and Rapley, S., *in*: Beutler, E., Hereditary Disorders of Erythrocyte Metabolism (New York, London: Grune & Stratton, 1968).
39b Rapley, S. and Harris, H., *Ann. Hum. Genet.*, **33**, 361 (1970).
39c Modiano, G., Scozzari, R., Gigliani, F., Santolamazza, C., Spinnati, G. F. and Saini, P., *Amer. J. Hum. Genet.*, **22**, 292 (1970).
40 Arnold, H., Blume, K. G., Busch, D., Lenkeit, U., Löhr, G. W. and Lübbs, E., *Klin. Wochenschr.*, **48**, 1299 (1970).
41a Brownson, C. and Spencer, N., *Biochem. J.*, **130**, 797 (1972).
41b Brownson, C. and Spencer, N., *Biochem. J.*, **130**, 805 (1972).
42 Barthelmai, W., *Monatsschr. Kinderheilk.*, **116**, 410 (1968).
43 Beutler, E., Red Cell Metabolism (New York, London: Grune & Statton, 1971).
44a Haslam, R. J. and Mills, D. C. B., *Biochem. J.*, **103**, 773 (1967).
44b Heller, M. and Hanahan, D. J., *Biochim. Biophys. Acta*, **255**, 239 (1972).
45 Lowy, B. A., Cook, J. L. and London, I. M., *J. Biol. Chem.*, **236**, 1442, (1961).
46 Lowy, B. A. and Dorfman, B.-Z., *J. Biol. Chem.*, **245**, 3043 (1970).
47 Klaus, D., *Ärztliche Forsch.*, **15**, 548 (1961).
48 Chapman, J., Hennessey, M. A., Waltersdorph, A. M., Huennekens, F. M. and Gabrio, B. W., *J. Clin. Invest.*, **41**, 1249 (1962).
49 De Sandre, G. and Chiotto, G., *Brit. J. Haematol.*, **6**, 39 (1960).
50 Heller, P., Weinstein, H. G., West, M. and Zimmerman, H. J., *Ann. Intern. Med.*, **53**, 898 (1960).
51 Streiff, F., Stoltz, J.-F. and Vigneron, C., *Rev. Franc. Transfus.*, **14**, 335 (1971).
52a Schrier, S. L. and Doak, L. S., *J. Clin. Invest.*, **42**, 756 (1963).

52b Ramachandran, M. and Jyer, G.Y.N., *Clin. Chim. Acta*, **40**, 276 (1972).
53 Cartier, P., Habibi, B., Leroux, J.-P. and Marchand, J.-C., *Nouv. Rev. Fr. Hematol.*, **11**, 565 (1971).
54 Chapman, R. G. and Schaumburg, L., *Brit. J. Haematol.*, **13**, 665 (1967).
55a Hatzfeld, A., Schapira, F. and Debré, M. R., *C. R. Akad. Sci. Ser.* D., **269**, 1799 (1969).
55b Schapira, F., *Bull. Soc. Chim. Biol.*, **43**, 1357 (1961).
55c Schapira, F., *Bull. Soc. Chim. Biol.*, **43**, 1367 (1961).
56 Jacobasch, G., Thesis, Dr. Sc., Humboldt-Universität (Berlin, 1970).
57 Witt, J., Müller, H. and Künzer, W., *Klin. Wochenschr.*, **45**, 262 (1967).
58 Brok, F., Ramot, B., Zwang, E. and Danon, D., *Isr. J. Med. Sci.*, **2**, 291 (1966).
59 Kübler, W., Kuhn, H., Mertens, H.-M. and Seipel, L., *Klin. Wochenschr.*, **49**, 1294 (1971).
60a Bruns, F., *Biochem. Z.*, **325**, 429 (1954).
60b Smith, J., Barnes, J. K., Kaneko, J. J. and Freedland, R. A., *Nature* (London), **205**, 298 (1965).
61 Löhr, G. W., Waller, H. D., Karges, O., Schlegel, B. and Müller, H. A., *Klin. Wochenschr.*, **36**, 1008 (1958).
62 Löhr, G. W. and Waller, H. D., *Klin. Wochenschr.*, **37**, 833 (1959).
63 Coltorti, M., Di Simone, A. and Budillon, G., *Boll. Soc. Ital. Biol. Sper.* (Napoli), **35**, 1630 (1959).
64 Schapira, F., *Rev. Franc. Etud. Clin. Biol.*, **4**, 151 (1959).
65 Quan-Ma, R. and Wells, W. W., *Biochem. Biophys. Res. Comm.*, **20**, 486 (1965).
66 Cacciari, E., Corsini, F., Manfredi, G. and Pintozzi, P., *Boll. Soc. Ital. Biol. Sper.* (Napoli), **35**, 395 (1959).
67 Kelley, W. N., Rosenbloom, F. M., Henderson, I. F. and Seegmiller, J. E., *Proc. Nat. Acad. Sci. U.S.*, (Washington), **57**, 1735 (1967).
68 Hartman, S. C. and Buchanan, J. M., *J. Biol. Chem.*, **234**, 1812 (1959).
69 Bishop, Ch., *J. Biol. Chem.*, **235**, 3228 (1960).
70 Lowy, B. A., Williams, M. K. and London, I. M., *J. Biol. Chem.*, **237**, 1622 (1962).
71 Arakawa, T., Fujii, M., Ohara, K., Watanabe, S., Karahashi, M., Kobayashi, M. and Hirono, H., *Tohoku J. Exp. Med.*, **88**, 341 (1966).
72 Rubino, G. F., Teso, G. and Rosetti, L., *Acta Haematol*, **24**, 300 (1960).
73 Rimington, C. and Booji, H. L., *J. Biol. Chem.*, **3**, 65 (1957).
74 Fallot, P., Canivet, J., Moudet, M. and Poidaz, J., Comptes Rendus, **242**, 2668 (1956), cited *in*: Bishop, Ch. and Surgenor, D. M., The Red Blood Cell (Academic Press, N.Y. London, 1964), p. 29.
75 Lichtman, H. C. and Feldman, F., *J. Clin. Invest.*, **42**, 830 (1963).
76 Nakao, K., Wada, O. and Yano, Y., *Clin. Chim. Acta*, **19**, 319 (1968).

77 Iwanow, E. D., *Folia Haematol.* (Leipzig), **89**, 233 (1968).
78a Granick, S. and Mauzerall, D., *J. Biol. Chem.*, **232**, 1101 (1958).
78b Granick, S. and Mauzerall, D., *J. Biol. Chem.*, **232**, 1119 (1958).
79 Burch, H. B. and Siegel, A. L., *Clin. Chem.*, **17**, 1038 (1971).
80a Shemin, D. and Wittenberg, J., *J. Biol. Chem.*, **192**, 315 (1951).
80b Dale, R. A., *Biochim. Biophys. Acta*, **261**, 310 (1972).
81 Aoki, Y., Wada, O., Urata, G., Takaku, F. and Nakao, K., *Biochem. Biophys. Res. Comm.*, **42**, 568 (1971).
82 Bottomley, S. S. and Smithee, G. A., *Biochim. Biophys. Acta*, **159**, 27 (1968).
83 Takaku, F. and Nakao, K., *Life Sciences*, **10**, 721 (1971).
84 Feldman, F. and Lichtman, H. C., *Biochim. Biophys. Acta*, **141**, 653 (1967).
85 Müller, M., Rosenthal, S. and Botscherowa, E., unpublished data (1970).
86 Izak, G., Wilner, T., Mager, J. and Karshai, A., *J. Clin. Invest.*, **39**, 1763 (1960).
87 Haschen, R. J., *Hoppe Seyler Z. Physiol. Chem.*, **342**, 194 (1965).
88 Haschen, R. J., Farr, W. and Groh, F., *Acta Biol. Med. German.*, **14**, 205 (1965).
89 Kochakian, C. D., *J. Biol. Chem.*, **155**, 579 (1944). Conference Metabolism Aspects Convalescence Trans., 17th, 187 (1948).
90 Nikkila, E. A., Pitkanen, E., Viropio, P. and Forsell, O., *Ann. Med. Intern. Fenn.*, **49**, 187 (1960).
91 Nishibe, H. and Makino, H., *Anal. Biochem.*, **43**, 357 (1971).
92 Pelikan, V., Kalab, M. and Tichy, J., *Clin. Chim. Acta*, **9**, 141 (1964).
93 Azizi, E., Dror, Y. and Wallis, K., *Clin. Chim. Acta*, **28**, 391 (1970).
94 Cabello, J., Basilio, C. and Prajoux, V., *Biochim. Biophys. Acta*, **48**, 148 (1961).
95 Nishibe, H. and Makino, H., *Clin. Chim. Acta*, **34**, 409 (1971).
96 Cabello, J., Prajoux, V. and Placa, M., *Biochim. Biophys. Acta*, **105**, 583 (1965).
97 Vetrella, M. and Barthelmai, W., *Monatschr. Kinderheilk.*, **119**, 265 (1971).
98 Caffrey, R. W., Tremblay, R., Gabrio, B. W. and Huennekens, F. M., *J. Biol. Chem.*, **223**, 1 (1956).
99 Sabater, J. and Puliol, M., *Enzyme*, **12**, 382 (1971).
100 Scheuch, D., *Acta Biol. Med. German.*, **11**, 941 (1963).
101 Smith, L., Jr., Sullivan, M. and Huguley, C. M., Jr., *J. Clin. Invest.*, **40**, 656 (1961).
102 Smith, L. H., Jr. and Baker, F. A., *J. Clin. Invest.*, **38**, 798 (1959).
103 Tashian, R. E., Riggs, S. K. and Yu, Y.-S. L., *Arch. Biochem. Biophys.*, **117**, 320 (1966).
104 Tanis, R. J., Tashian, R. E. and Yu, Y.-S. L., *J. Biol. Chem.*, **245**,

6003 (1970).
105 Reynaud, J., Luccioni, F., Bouthier, M., Savary, J. and Derrien, Y., *Biochemie*, **53**, 1095 (1971).
106 Tashian, R. E., *Proc. Soc. Exp. Biol. Med.*, **108**, 364 (1961).
107 Shinagawa, Y. and Ogura, M., *Kagaku* (Tokyo), **31**, 554 (1961).
108a Funakoshi, S. and Deutsch, H. F., *J. Biol. Chem.*, **246**, 1088 (1971).
108b Funakoshi, S. and Deutsch H. F., *J. Biol. Chem.*, **245**, 4913 (1970).
109 Rapoport, S. and Hofmann, E. C. G., *Biochem. Z.*, **326**, 493 (1955).
110 Moore, M. J., Funakoshi, S. and Deutsch, H. F., *Biochem. Genet.*, **5**, 497 (1971).
111 Rieder, R. F. and Weatherall, D. J., *Nature*, **203**, 1364 (1964).
112 Eng., L.-I. L. and Tarail, R., *Nature*, **211**, 47 (1966).
113 Wittels, B. and Hochstein, P., *J. Biol. Chem.*, **242**, 126 (1967).
114 Higashi, T., Yogi, M. and Hirai, H., *J. Biochem.*, **49**, 707 (1961).
115 Balcerzak, S. P., Vester, J. W. and Doyle, A. P., *J. Lab. Clin. Med.*, **67**, 742 (1967).
116 Paniker, N. V. and Iyer, G. Y. N., *Canad. J. Biochem.*, **43**, 1029 (1965).
117a Feinstein, R. N., Sacher, G. A., Howard, J. B. and Braun, J. T., *Arch. Biochem. Biophys.*, **122**, 338 (1967).
117b Feinstein, R. N., *Biochem. Genet.*, **4**, 135 (1970).
118a Aebi, H., Heiniger, J. P. and Lauber, E., *Helv. Chim. Acta*, **47**, 1428 (1964).
118b Aebi, H., Bossi, E., Cantz, M., Matsubara, Sh. and Suter, H., *in*: Beutler, E.: Hereditary Disorders of Erythrocyte Metabolism (New York, London: Grune & Stratton, 1968), p. 41.
119 Rapoport, S., Nieradt-Hiebsch, Ch. and Thamm, R., *Acta Biol. Med. German.*, **21**, 291 (1968).
120a Syllm-Rapoport, I., Reichelt, E., Remitschka, M.-E., Gerber, G., Nieradt-Hiebsch, Ch., Thamm, R. and Rapoport, S., VI. Internationales Symposium über Struktur und Funktion der Erythrozyten. Berlin (1970), *in*: Abhandlungen der Deutschen Akademie der Wissenschaften zu Berlin (Berlin: Akademie-Verlag, 1971), p. 487.
120b Syllm-Rapoport, I., Reichelt, E., Remitschka, M. E., Gerber, G., Nieradt-Hiebsch, Ch., Thamm, R. and Rapoport, S., unpublished data (1970).
121 Stansell, M. J. and Deutsch, H. F., *J. Biol. Chem.*, **240**, 4299 (1965).
122 Cantz, M., Mörikofer-Zwez, St., Bossi, E., Kaufmann, H., von Wartburg, J. P. and Aebi, H., *Experientia*, **24**, 119 (1968).
123 Sass, M. D., *Nature*, **197**, 503 (1963).
124 Thorup, O. A., Carpenter, J. T. and Howard, P., *Brit. J. Haematol.*, **10**, 542 (1964).
125 Guardamagna, C., Massari, N. and Santambrogio, C., *G. Gerontol.*, **8**, 161 (1960).

126 Granick, S. and Mauzerall, D., *Fed. Proc.*, **17**, Abstr. 919 (1958), p. 233.

127 Langelaan, D. E., Losowsky, M. S. and Toothill, C., *Clin. Chim. Acta*, **27**, 453 (1970).

128 Arakawa, T., Fujii, M. and Hirono, H., *Tohoku J. Exp. Med.*, **88**, 305 (1966).

129 Altenbrunn, H. J., Rapoport, S. and Hahn, Ch., *Acta Biol. Med. German.*, **2**, 599 (1959).

130 Wiley, J. S. and Whittam, R., *Biochim. Biophys. Acta*, **115**, 235 (1966).

131 Hokin, L. E. and Hokin, M. R., *Nature*, **189**, 836 (1961).

132 Wilmanns, W. and Jaenicke, L., *Klin. Wochenschr.*, **41**, 1077 (1963).

133 Wilmanns, W., *Folia Haematol.* (Leipzig), **89**, 216 (1968).

134 Wilmanns, W., *Z. Ges. Exp. Med.*, **147**, 154 (1968).

135 Smith, L. H., Jr. and Baker, F. A., *J. Clin. Invest.*, **38**, 798 (1959).

136 Rose, Z. B., *Adv. Exp. Med. Biol.*, **6**, 137 (1970).

137 Schröter, W. and Kalinowsky, W., *Clin. Chim. Acta*, **25**, 283 (1969).

138 Rose, Z. B., *J. Biol. Chem.*, **243**, 4810 (1968).

139 Chen, Shi-Han, Anderson, J. A. and Giblett, E. R., *Biochem. Genet.*, **5**, 481 (1971).

140 Roigas, H., Inaugural Dissertation Humboldt-Universität (Berlin, 1962).

141 Rose, Z. B. and Liebowitz, J., *J. Biol. Chem.*, **245**, 3232 (1970).

142 De Verdier, C.-H., *Biochem. J.*, **92**, 389 (1964).

143 Rose, Z. B., *Eed. Proc.*, **28**, 727 (1969).

144 Harkness, D. R. and Roth, S., *Biochem. Biophys. Res. Comm.*, **34**, 849 (1969).

145 Sauer, G., Jentsch, G. and Rapoport, S., *Folia Haematol.* (Leipzig), **90**, 210 (1968).

146 Srivastava, S. K. and Beutler, E., *Biochem. Med.*, **5**, 317 (1971).

147 Rapoport, S. M., Leva, E. and Guest, G. M., *J. Comp. Physiol.*, **19**, 103 (1942).

148 Rosenthal, S., Ruprecht, A. and Zank, W., *Folia Haematol.* (Leipzig), **90**, 142 (1968).

149 Lindigkeit, R., *Folia Haematol.* (Leipzig), **74**, 3 (1956).

150 Prehn, S. and Belkner, J., *Acta Biol. Med. German.* (in press).

151 Oski, F. A., Brigandi, E. and Noble, L., *Pediatrics*, **44**, 84 (1969).

152 Kraus, A. P., Langston, M. F. and Lynch, B. L., *Biochim. Biophys. Res. Comm.*, **30**, 173 (1968).

153 Arakawa, T., Tamura, T., Higashi, O., Ohara, K., Tanno, K., Honda, Y., Narisawa, K., Konno, T., Wada, Y., Sato, Y. and Mizuno, T., *Tohoku J. Exp. Med.*, **94**, 3 (1968).

154 Rubinstein, D., Ph. D. Thesis, McGill University, Montreal, Canada (1952–1953), cited *in*: Bishop, Ch. and Surgenor, D. M.: The Red

Blood Cell (New York, London: Academic Press, 1964), p. 35.
155 Kesselring, K., Diplomarbeit, Humboldt-Universität zu Berlin (Berlin, 1956).
156 Beutler, E., Paniker, N. and Trinidad, F., *Biochem. Med.*, **5**, 325 (1971).
157 Isselbacher, K. J., Anderson, E. P., Kurahashi, K. and Kalckar, H. M., *Science*, **123**, 635 (1956).
158 Ng, W. G., *Exp. Eye Res.*, **11**, 402 (1971).
159a Ng, W. G., Donnell, G. N. and Bergren, W. R., *J. Lab. Clin. Med.*, **66**, 115 (1965).
159b Gesche, M. and Menne, F., *Z. Klin. Chem. Klin. Biochem.*, **10**, 430 (1972).
160 Mathai, C. K. and Beutler, E., *Enzymologia*, **33**, 224 (1967).
161 Blume, K. G. and Beutler, E., *J. Biol. Chem.*, **246**, 6507 (1971).
162 Vigneron, C., *Enzyme*, **12**, 426 (1971).
163 Beutler, E. and Mitchell, M., *J. Lab. Clin. Med.*, **72**, 527 (1968).
164 Colombo, J. P., *Klin. Wochenschr.*, **43**, 1074 (1965).
165 Beutler, E., Baluda, M. C. and Halasz, A., *J. Lab. Clin. Med.*, **67**, 947 (1966)
166 Tesoriere, G., Vento, R., Magistro, D. and Dones, F., *Ital. J. Biochem.*, **19**, 139 (1970).
167 Ababei, L. and Moisiu, M., *Blut (München) Z. Ges. Blutforsch.*, **20**, 363 (1970).
168 Glock, G. E. and McLean, P., *Biochem. J.*, **55**, 400 (1953).
169 Lepke, S. and Passow, M., *J. Gen. Physiol.*, **51**, 365 (1968).
170 Sass, M. D., Vorsanger, E. and Spear, P. W., *Clin. Chim. Acta*, **10**, 21 (1964).
171 Vetrella, M. and Barthelmai, W., *Z. Kinderheilk.*, **110**, 99 (1971).
172 Jacobasch, G., Helbig, W., Syllm-Rapoport, I., Pester, H., Heine, K.-M., Boese, Ch., Otto, F. M. and Blau, H.-J., *Deutsche. Gesundh.*, **24**, 1441 (1969).
173 Brewer, G. P. and Powell, R. D., *Nature*, **199**, 704 (1963).
174 Report of a WHO Scientific Group, WHO Technical Report Series No. 366 (1967).
175 Grieger, M. and Jacobasch, G., unpublished data (1971).
176 Bonsignore, A., Fornaini, G., Fantoni, A., Leonaini, G. and Segni, P., *J. Clin. Invest.*, **43**, 5 (1964).
177 Butenandt, O., *Acta Haematol.*, **43**, 348 (1970).
178 Kahrig, C. and Rapoport, S., *Acta Biol. Med. German.*, **6**, 238 (1961).
179 Horecker, B. L. and Smyrniotis, P. Z., *J. Biol. Chem.*, **193**, 371 (1951).
180 Koshland, D. E., Jr., Nemethy, G. and Fillmer, D., *Biochemistry*, **5**, 365 (1966).

181 Eaton, G. M., Brewer, G. J. and Tashian, R. E., *Nature*, **212**, 944 (1966).
182 Eigen, M. and Hammes, G. G., *Adv. Enzymol.*, **25**, 1 (1963).
183 Hutton, J., *Biochem. Genet.*, **5**, 315 (1971).
184 Herz, F., Kaplan, E. and Gleiman, E. J., *Proc. Soc. Exp. Biol. Med.*, **124**, 1185 (1967).
185 Smith, J. E., McCants, M. and Parks, P., *Comp. Biochem. Physiol.*, **26**, 137 (1968).
186a Kirkman, H. N., Kidson, Ch. and Kennedy, M., *in*; ed. by Beutler, E.: Hereditary Disorders of Erythrocyte Metabolism (New York, London: Grune & Stratton, 1968), p. 126.
186b Beutler, E., *in*; ed. by Beutler, E.: Hereditary Disorders of Erythrocyte Metabolism (New York, London: Grune & Stratton, 1968), p. 126.
187 Trandafirescu, M., Rener, C. and Ababei, L., Abstracts: VI. Internationales Symposium über Struktur und Funktion der Erythrozyten (Berlin, 1970).
188 Kornfeld, R. and Noll, C., *Biochim. Biophys. Acta*, **170**, 77 (1968).
189 Bishop, Ch. and Surgenor, D. M., The Red Blood Cell (New York, London: Academic Press, 1964).
190 Nappi, L., Guidone, M., Branca, F. and Bordi, B., *Rass. Med. Sper.* (Napoli), **11**, Fasc. 6 (1964).
191 Hamfelt, A., *Clin. Chim. Acta*, **16**, 19 (1967).
192 Levy, L. M., Walter, H. and Sass, M. D., *Nature*, **184**, 643 (1959).
193 Fischer, I. and Walter, H., *Biochim. Biophys. Acta*, **184**, 660 (1969).
194 Bishop, Ch. and Van Gastel, C., *Haematologia*, **3**, 29 (1969).
195a Nisselbaum, J. S., *Fed. Proc.*, **24**, 356, Abstr., 1253 (1965).
195b Nisselbaum, J. S. and Bodansky, O., *Science*, **149**, 195 (1965).
196 Sandring, K.-H., Rohde, A. and Rost, J., *Folia Haematol.* (Leipzig), **89**, 209 (1968).
197 Chen, S.-H. and Giblett, E. R., *Amer. J. Hum. Genet.*, **23**, 419 (1971).
198 Buhler, H., Götze, T. and Götze, E., *Acta Biol. Med. German.*, **10**, 199 (1963).
199 Chen, S.-H. and Giblett, E. R., *Science*, **173**, 148 (1971).
200 Mohler, D. N., Majerus, P. W., Minnich, V., Hess, Ch. and Garrick, M. D., *New Eng. J. Med.*, **283**, 1253 (1970).
201 Majerus, P. W., Brauner, M. J., Smith, M. B. and Minnich, V., *J. Clin. Invest.*, **50**, 1637 (1971).
202 Jackson, R. C., *Biochem. J.*, **111**, 309 (1969).
203 Mills, G. C., *J. Biol. Chem.*, **229**, 189 (1957).
204 Mills, G. C., *J. Biol. Chem.*, **234**, 502 (1959).
205 Vetrella, M., Barthelmai, W. and Rietkötter, J., *Klin. Wochenschr.*, **29**, 481 (1967).
206 Boguslawska-Jaworska, J. and Kaplan, J. P., *Clin. Chim. Acta*, **26**,

459 (1969).
207 Necheles, T. F., Steinberg, M. H. and Cameron, D., *Brit. J. Haematol.*, **19**, 605 (1970).
208 Flatz, G., *Humangenetik*, **11**, 221 (1971).
209a Flohe, L., Eisele, B. and Wendel, A., *Hoppe Seyler Z. Physiol. Chem.*, **352**, 151 (1971).
209b Flohe, L., Loschen, G., Günzler, W. A. and Eichele, E., *Z. Physiol. Chem.*, **353**, 987 (1972).
209c Günzler, W. A., Vergin, H., Müller, J. and Flohe, L., *Z. Physiol. Chem.*, **353**, 1001 (1972).
209d Flohe, L., Günzler, W. A. and Schock, H. H., *FEBS Letters*, **32**, 132 (1973).
210 Jocelyn, P. C., *Biochem. J.*, **77**, 363 (1960).
211 Wagenknecht, Ch., Grützner, J., Prockat, U. and Wagenknecht, C., VI. Internationales Symposium über Struktur und Funktion der Erythrozyten Berlin 1970. *in*; Abhandlungen der Deutschen Akademie der Wissenschaften zu Berlin (Berlin: Akademie-Verlag, 1971).
212 Flatz, G., *Humangenetik*, **11**, 269 (1971).
213 Flatz, G., *Humangenetik*, **11**, 278 (1971).
214 Blume, K.-G., Rüdiger, H. W. and Löhr, G. W., *Biochim. Biophys. Acta*, **151**, 686 (1968).
215 Blume, K.-G., von Lingen, A., Löhr, G. W. and Rüdiger, H. W., *Humangenetik*, **6**, 266 (1968).
216 Eifler, R. and Wagenknecht, C., *Acta Biol. Med. German.*, **13**, 674 (1964).
217 Fornaini, G., Dacha, M., Fazi, A., Gargano, M. and Schiave, E., *Ital. J. Biochem.*, **19**, 345 (1970).
218 Scott, E. M., Duncan, I. W. and Ekstrand, V., *J. Biol. Chem.*, **238**, 3928 (1963).
219 Staal, G. E. J., Visser, J. and Veeger, C., *Biochim. Biophys. Acta*, **185**, 39 (1969).
220 Staal, G. E. J., Helleman, P. W., De Wael, J. and Veeger, C., *Biochim. Biophys. Acta*, **185**, 63 (1969).
221 Icen, A., *Scand. J. Clin. Lab. Invest.*, **20**, 96 (1967).
222 Beutler, E. and Ye, M. K. Y., *Blood*, **21**, 585 (1963).
223 Waller, H. D., *in*; ed. by Beutler, E.: Hereditary Disorders in Erythrocyte Metabolism (New York, London: Grune & Stratton, 1968), p. 185.
224 Hochberg, A., Rigbi, M. and Dimant, E., *Biochim. Biophys. Acta*, **90**, 464 (1964).
225 Grignani, F. and Löhr, G. W., *Klin. Wochenschr.*, **38**, 796 (1960).
226 Powell, R. D. and Brewer, G. J., *Klin. Wochenschr.*, **41**, 200 (1963).
227 Pescarmona, G. P., Bosia, A. and Arese, P., *Experientia*, **26**, 719 (1970).

228 Mills, G. C., *Fed. Proc.*, **30**, Part II, 1059, Abstr. 37 (1971).
229 Tanner, M. J. A. and Gray, W. R., *Biochem. J.*, **125**, 1109 (1971).
230 Fuhrmann, M., Inaugural Dissertation, Humboldt-Universität Berlin, Medizinische Fakultät Berlin (1962).
231 Schrier, S. L., Doak, L. S. and Carr, B., *Amer. J. Physiol.*, **210**, 139 (1966).
232 Schrier, S. L., *Biochim. Biophys. Acta*, **135**, 591 (1967).
233 Ronquist, G., *Acta Chem. Scand.*, **21**, 1484 (1967).
234 Oguchi, M., Hashimoto, T., Minakami, S. and Yoshikawa, H., *J. Biochem.*, **60**, 99 (1966).
235 Oguchi, M., *J. Biochem.*, **68**, 427 (1970).
236 Wolny, M., Wolny, E. and Baranowski, T., *Bull. Acad. Pol. Sci.*, **16**, 18 (1968).
237a Maretzki, D. and Rapoport, S., *Acta Biol. Med. German.*, **29**, 207 (1972).
237b Maretzki, D. and Rapoport, S., unpublished data (1971).
238a Eylar, E. H., Madoff, M., Brody, O. and Oncley, J. L., *J. Biol. Chem.*, **237**, 1992 (1962).
238b Eylar, E. H. and Matioli, G. T., *Science*, **147**, 869 (1965).
239 Cornblath, M., Levin, E. Y., Marquetti, E. and Hause, E. Y., *Fed. Proc.*, **19**, 68, Abstr. 37 (1960).
240 Haschen, R. J., *Biochem. Z.*, **334**, 560 (1961).
241 Haschen, R. J., *Acta Biol. Med. German.*, **9**, 15 (1962).
242 Valentine, W. M. and Tanaka, K. R., *Acta Haematol.*, **26**, 303 (1961).
243 Cohen, P. P. and Sober, E. K., *Cancer Res.*, **5**, 631 (1945).
244 Herschko, A., Wind, E. and Mager, J., *Bull. Res. Counc. Isr., Sec. A*, **11**, No. 1, 64 (1962).
245 Langelaan, D. E., Losowsky, M. S. and Toothill, C., *Clin. Chim. Acta*, **26**, 245 (1969).
246 Yoneyama, Y., Ohyama, H., Sugita, Y. and Yoshikawa, H., *Biochim. Biophys. Acta*, **62**, 261 (1962).
247 Yoneyama, Y., Ohyama, H., Sugita, Y. and Yoshikawa, H., *Biochim. Biophys. Acta*, **74**, 635 (1963).
248 Kübler, W., Schneider, W. and Gross, R., *Arch. Klin. Med.*, **215**, 67 (1968).
249 Syllm-Rapoport, I., *Folia Haematol.*, **83**, 244 (1964).
250 Jacobasch, G., Raderecht, H.-J., *Acta Biol. Med. German.*, **17**, 275 (1966).
251 Åkerblom, O., De Verdier, C.-H., Eriksson, Å., Garby, L. and Högmann, C., *Folia Haematol.* (Leipzig), **91**, 142 (1968).
252 Christensen, W. R., Plimton, C. H., Ball, E. G. and Hughes, D., *J. Biol. Chem.*, **180**, 791 (1949).
253 Rapoport, S., *in*: Campbell, P. N. and Greville, G. W., *Essays*

Biochem., **4**, 69 (1968).
254 Hinterberger, U., Ockel, E., Gerischer-Mothes, W. and Rapoport, S., *Acta Biol. Med. German.*, **7**, 50 (1961).
255 Gerber, G. K. G., Schultze, M. and Rapoport, S. M., *Europ. J. Biochem.*, **17**, 445 (1970).
256 Kaplan, J.-C. and Beutler, E., *Science*, **159**, 215 (1968).
257 Holmes, E. W. and Malone, J. J., *Science*, **156**, 646 (1967).
258 Malone, J. I., Winegrad, I., Oski, F. A. and Holmes, E. W., *New Eng. J. Med.*, **279**, 1071 (1968).
259 Schröter, W. and Tillmann, W., *Biochem. Biophys. Res. Comm.*, **31**, 92 (1968).
260 Tillmann, W. and Schröter, W., *Klin. Wochenschr.*, **47**, 762 (1969).
261 Kalckar, H. M., Anderson, E. P. and Isselbacher, K. J., *Biochim. Biophys. Acta*, **20**, 262 (1956).
262 Schwarz, V., Golberg, L., Komrower, G. M. and Holzel, A., *Biochem. J.*, **62**, 34 (1956).
263 Riabov, S., Inouye, T., Parker, D. and Hsia, D. Y.-Y., *Biochim. Biophys. Acta*, **99**, 175 (1965).
264a Portius, H. J. and Repke, K., *Naturwissenschaften*, **47**, 43 (1960).
264b Portius, H. J. and Repke, K., *Naunyn Schmiedeberg Arch. Pharmakol. Exptl. Pathol.*, **239**, 284, 299 (1960).
265 Brown, B. T., Golder, W. S. and Wright, S. E., *Aust. J. Exp. Biol. Med. Sci.*, **39**, 545 (1961).
266 Axelrod, L. R. and Werthessen, N. T., *Arch. Biochem. Biophys.*, **83**, 567 (1959).
267 Hershko, A., Hershko, C. and Mager, J., *Isr. J. Med. Sci.*, **4**, 939 (1968).
268 Kelley, W. N., Greene, M. L., Rosenbloom, F. M., Henderson, J. F. and Seegmiller, J. E., *Ann. Intern. Med.*, **70**, 155 (1969).
269 Kelley, W. N., Rosenbloom, F. M., Henderson, J. F. and Seegmiller, J. E., *Biochem. Biophys. Res. Comm.*, **28**, 340 (1967).
270 Henderson, J. F., Brox, L. W., Kelley, W. N., Rosenbloom, F. M. and Seegmiller, J. E., *J. Biol. Chem.*, **243**, 2514 (1968).
271 McDonald, J. A. and Kelley, W. N., *Fed. Proc.*, **30**, Part II, 1207, Abstr. 905 (1971).
272 Adams, E., Davis, N. C. and Smith, E. L., *J. Biol. Chem.*, **199**, 845 (1952).
273 Panadopoulus, K., Kovatsis, A. and Karavouas, G., Chromica, Spec. ed. **83** (1957) cited *in*: Bishop, Ch. and Surgenor, D. M., The Red Blood Cell (New York, London: Academic Press, 1964), p. 35.
274 Banaschak, H., *Acta Biol. Med. German.*, **18**, 581 (1957).
275 Vanderheiden, B. S., *Biochim. Biophys. Acta*, **215**, 555 (1970).
276 Vanderheiden, B. S., *Biochem. Genet.*, **3**, 289 (1969).

277 Liakopoulou, A. and Alivisatos, S. G. A., *Biochim. Biophys. Acta*, **89**, 158 (1964).
278 Chern, Ch. J., Macdonald, A. B. and Morris, A. J., *J. Biol. Chem.*, **244**, 5489 (1969).
279 Altman, K. J., *Arch. Biochem. Biophys.*, **42**, 478 (1953).
280 Heller, P., Weinstein, H. G., West, M. and Zimmermann, H. J., *J. Lab. Clin. Med.*, **55**, 425 (1960).
281 Belfiore, F., Calcara, G. and Bonaventura, S., *Boll. Soc. Ital. Biol. Sper.*, **34**, 1577 (1963).
282 Rapoport, S. and Sarkar, S. R., *Acta Biol. Med. German.*, **11**, 335 (1963).
283 Sarkar, S. R. and Rapoport, S., *Acta Biol. Med. German.*, **11**, 323 (1963).
284 Priem, F., Diplomarbeit, Humboldt-Universität zu Berlin (Berlin, 1967).
285 Bruns, F. H., Dünnwald, E. and Noltmann, E., *Biochem. Z.*, **330**, 497 (1958).
286 Henkel, H.-D., Inaugural Dissertation Humboldt-Universität zu Berlin (Berlin, 1962).
287 Rosa, J. and Schapira, F., *Nature*, **204**, 883 (1964).
288 Dioguardi, N., Agostoni, A., Fiorelli, G. and Manucci, P. M., *Enzym. Biol. Clin.* (Basel), **4**, 31 (1964).
289 Starkeweather, W. H., Cousineau, L., Schoch, H. K. and Zarafonetis, C. J., *Blood*, **26**, 63 (1965).
290 Haschen, R. J., *Biochem. Z.*, **334**, 569 (1961).
291 Warrendorf, E. M. and Rubinstein, D., *Canad. J. Biochem.*, **49**, 919 (1971).
292 Altman, K. J., Whatman, R. N. and Salomon, K., *Arch. Biochem. Biophys.*, **33**, 168 (1952).
293 James, A. T., Lowelock, J. E. and Webb, J., *Biochem. J.*, **73**, 106 (1959).
294 Rowe, C. E., *Biochem. J.*, **73**, 438 (1959).
295 Rowe, C. E., Allison, A. C. and Lowelock, J. E., *Biochim. Biophys. Acta*, **41**, 310 (1960).
296 O'Donnell, V. J., Ottolenghi, P., Malkin, A., Denstedt, O. F. and Heard, R. D. H., *Canad. J. Biochem.*, **36**, 1125 (1958).
297 Sloviter, H. A. and Bose, R. K., *Biochim. Biophys. Acta*, **116**, 156 (1966).
298 Sloviter, H. A. and Tanaka, S., *Biochim. Biophys. Acta*, **137**, 70 (1967).
299 Sloviter, H. A., Janic, V. and Cirkovic, T., *J. Lipid Res.*, **11**, 82 (1970).
300 Marks, P. A., Gellhorn, A. and Kidson, Ch., *J. Biol. Chem.*, **235**, 2579 (1960).

301 Raderecht, H. J., Binnewies, S. and Schölzel, E., *Acta Biol. Med. German.*, **8**, 199 (1962).
302 Snyder, M. and Reddy, W. J., *J. Lab. Clin. Med.*, **77**, 459 (1971).
303 Sarkar, S. R., *Acta Biol. Med. German.*, **11**, 597 (1963).
304 Sarkar, S. R., *Acta Biol. Med. German.*, **12**, 67 (1964).
305 Shrago, E. and Falcone, A. B., *Biochim. Biophys. Acta*, **73**, 7 (1963).
306 Shrago, E., *Arch. Biochem. Biophys.*, **109**, 57 (1965).
307 Davidson, R. G. and Cortner, J. A., *Nature*, **215**, 761 (1967).
308 Bertino, J. R., Simmons, B. and Dono Hue, D. M., *J. Biol. Chem.*, **237**, 1314 (1962).
309 Shrago, E. and Falcone, A. B., *Biochim. Biophys. Acta*, **67**, 147 (1963).
310 Rapoport, S. and Wagenknecht, C., *Hoppe Seyler Z. Physiol. Chem.*, **309**, 196 (1957).
311 Zamudio, I. and Canessa, M., *Biochim. Biophys. Acta*, **120**, 165 (1966).
312 Zamudio, I., Cellino, M. and Canessa-Fischer, M., *Arch. Biochem. Biophys.*, **129**, 336 (1969).
313 Kiese, M., Schneider, C. and Waller, H. D., *Naunyn Schmiedeberg Arch. Phamakol. Exptl. Pathol.*, **231**, 158 (1957).
314a Kuma, F., Ishizawa, S., Hirayama, K. and Nakajima, H., *J. Biol. Chem.*, **247**, 550 (1972).
314b Kuma, F. and Inomata, H., *J. Biol. Chem.*, **247**, 556 (1972).
315 Sugita, Y., Nomura, S. and Yoneyama, Y., *J. Biol. Chem.*, **246**, 6072 (1971).
316 Shimizu, Ch. and Matsuura, F., *Agr. Biol., Chem.*, **32**, 587 (1968).
317a Hegesh, E. and Avron, M., *Biochim. Biophys. Acta*, **146**, 91 (1967).
317b Hegesh, E. and Avron, M., *Biochim. Biophys. Acta*, **146**, 397 (1967).
317c Hegesh, E., Calmanovici, N. and Avron, M., *J. Lab. Clin. Med.*, **72**, 339 (1968).
317d Hegesh, E., Calmanovici, N., Lupo, M. and Bochkowsky, R., *J. Lab. Clin. Med.*, **77**, 859 (1971).
318a Scott, E. M., *J. Clin. Invest.*, **39**, 1176 (1960).
318b Scott, E. M. and Griffith, J. V., *Biochim. Biophys. Acta*, **34**, 584 (1959).
318c Scott, E. M., *Biochem. Biophys. Res. Comm.*, **9**, 59 (1962).
318d Scott, E. M., *in*; Beutler, E. (Ed.): Hereditary Disorders of Erythrocyte Metabolism (New York, Grune and Stratton, 1968), p. 102.
319 Scott, E. M. and McGraw, J. C., *J. Biol. Chem.*, **237**, 249 (1962).
320 Hsieh, H.-S. and Jaffé, E. R., *J. Clin. Invest.*, **50**, 196 (1971).
321 Wagenknecht, C., Zinsmeyer, J. and Nack, B., *Folia Haematol.* (Leipzig), **89**, 158 (1968).
322 McDonald, Ch. D. and Huisman, T. H. J., *Clin. Chim. Acta*, **7**, 555 (1962).
323 Huennekens, F. M., Caffrey, R. W., Basford, R. E. and Gabrio, B. W., *J. Biol. Chem.*, **227**, 261 (1957).

324 Huennekens, F. M., Kerwar, G. K. and Kajita, A., *in*: ed. by Beutler, E.: Hereditary Disorders of Erythrocyte Metabolism (New York, London: Grune & Stratton, 1968), p. 87.

325 Kajita, A., Kerwar, G. K. and Huennekens, F. M., *Arch. Biochem. Biophys.*, **130**, 662 (1969).

326 Hultquist, D. E. and Passon, P. G., *Nat. New Biol.*, **229**, 252 (1971).

327 Scott, E. M., Duncan, I. W. and Ekstrand, V., *J. Biol. Chem.*, **240**, 481 (1965).

328a Hopkinson, D. A., Corney, G., Cook, P. J. L. and Robson, E. B., *Ann. Hum. Genet.*, **34**, 1 (1970).

328b Schwartz, J. M., Paress, P. S., Fagelman, K. and Fogel, L., *in*; Ramot, B. (Ed.): Red cell Structure and Metabolism (Academic Press, New York, 1971), p. 135.

329a Brewer, G. J., Eaton, J. W., Knutsen, C. S. and Beck, G. C., *Biochem. Biophys. Res. Comm.*, **29**, 198 (1967).

329b Kaplan, J.-C. and Beutler, E., *Biochem. Biophys. Res. Comm.*, **29**, 605 (1967).

329c Bloom, G. E. and Zarkowsky, H. S., *New Engl. J. Med.*, **281**, 919 (1969).

330a Adachi, K. and Okuyama, T., *J. Biochem.*, **70**, 365 (1971).

330b Adachi, K. and Okuyama, T., *Biochim. Biophys. Acta.*, **268**, 629 (1972).

331 Hofmann, E. and Noll, F., *Acta Biol. Med. German.*, **6**, 1 (1961).

332 Ng, W. G., Donnel, G. N. and Bergren, W. R., *Nature*, **217**, 64 (1968).

333 Alivasatos, S. G. A., Kashket, S. and Denstedt, O. F., *Canad. J. Bio-Chem. Physiol.*, **34**, 46 (1956).

334 Hofmann, E. C. G., Karadschova, M. and Klecker, J., *Folia Haematol.* (Leipzig), **76**, 372 (1959).

335a Preiss, J. and Handler, P., *J. Biol. Chem.*, **225**, 259 (1957).

335b Preiss, J. and Handler, P., *J. Biol. Chem.*, **233**, 493 (1958).

336 Haberman, V. and Habermanova, S., *Folia Haematol.* (Leipzig), **78**, 690 (1962).

337 Parks, R. E., Cheng, Y.-C. and Agarwal, R. P., *Fed. Proc.*, **30**, No 3, Abstr. 693 (1971).

338 Del Bauffe, D., Paysant, M. and Polonovski, J., *Bull. Soc. Chem. Biol.* **50**, 1431, 1439 (1968).

339 Schneider, R. P. and Kirschner, L. B., *Biochim. Biophys. Acta*, **202**, 283 (1970).

340 Layzer, R. B., Rowland, L. P. and Bank, W. J., *J. Biol. Chem.*, **244**, 3823 (1969).

341 Layzer, R. B. and Conway, M. M., *Biochim. Biophys. Res. Comm.*, **40**, 1259 (1970).

342 Raderecht, H.-J., *Folia Haematol.* (Leipzig), **91**, 132 (1968).

343 I. International Symposion of the Biochem. Soc. GDR and the All-Union Biochem. Soc. Acad. Sci. USSR, Reinhardsbrunn, 1971, Reaction Mechanism and Control Properties of Phosphotransferases (Akademie Verlag, Berlin, 1973).

344a Kühn, B., Jacobasch, G. and Rapoport, S., *Acta Biol. Med. German.*, **23**, 1 (1969).

344b Kühn, B., Kinetische Charakterisierung der Phosphofructokinase an Erythrocyten, Inaugural-Dissertation, Biowissenschaftliche Fakultät der Humboldt-Universität zu Berlin, 1973.

345 Wenzel, K.-W., Kuhfahl, E., Liebe, St., Zimmermann, G. and Gauer, J., VI. Internationales Symposium über Struktur und Funktion der Erythrocyten, Berlin (1970), *in*: Abhandlungen der Deutschen Akademie der Wissenschaften. (Berlin: Akademie-Verlag, 1971), p. 307.

346 Wenzel, K.-W., Gauer, J., Zimmermann, G. and Hofmann, E., *FEBS Letters*, **19**, 281 (1972).

347 Wenzel, K.-W., Zimmermann, G., Gauer, J., Diezel, W., Liebe, St. and Hofmann, E., *FEBS Letters*, **19**, 285 (1972).

348 Noltmann, E. and Bruns, F. H., *Hoppe Seyler Z. Physiol. Chem.*, **313**, 194 (1958).

349 Santachiara, A. S. B. and Modiano, G., *Nature*, **223**, 625 (1969).

350 Spencer, N., Hopkinson, D. A. and Harris, H., *Nature*, **204**, 742 (1964).

351 Hopkinson, D. A. and Harris, H., *Nature*, **208**, 410 (1965).

352 Renninger, W. and Spielmann, W., *Humangenetik*, **8**, 64 (1969).

353 Marks, P. A., *Science*, **127**, 1338 (1958).

354 Glock, G. E. and McLean, P., *Biochem. J.*, **56**, 173 (1954).

355 Haut, A., Tudhope, G. R., Cartwright, G. E. and Wintrobe, M. M., *J. Clin. Invest.*, **41**, 579 (1962).

356 Temkine, H., *Bull. Soc. Chim. Biol.*, **48**, 771 (1966).

357 Tsuboi, K. and Fukunaga, K., *J. Biol. Chem.*, **246**, 7586 (1971).

358 Bruns, F. M. and Vahlhaus, E., *Naturwissenschaften*, **43**, 180 (1956).

359 Carter, N. D. and Parr, C. W., *Nature* (London), **216**, 511 (1967).

360a Watanabe, S. and Yoshida, A., *Fed. Proc.*, **30**, Part II, 1207, Abstr. 903 (1971).

360b Yoshida, A. and Watanabe, S., *J. Biol. Chem.*, **247**, 440 (1972).

360c Yoshida, A., Watanabe, S., Chen, S.-H., Giblett, E. R. and Malcolm, L. A., *J. Biol. Chem.*, **247**, 446 (1972).

360d Maretzki, D., Tsamaloukas, A. G., Küttner, G., Krüger, S., Groth, J. and Rapoport, S., Comperative Studies of Glyceraldehyde-3-phosphate Dehydrogenase from Man and Rabbit VII. International Symposium on Structure and Function of Erythrocytes, Berlin, 1973, Akademie-Verlag, Berlin, 1974.

361 Hashimoto, T. and Yoshikawa, H., *J. Biochem.*, **56**, 279 (1964).

362 Chen, S.-H., Malcolm, L. A., Yoshida, A. and Giblett, E. R., *Amer. J. Hum. Genet.*, **23**, 87 (1971).

363 Weser, C., Inaugural Dissertation Humboldt-Universität zu Berlin (Berlin, 1962).

364 Guarino, A. J. and Sable, H. Z., *J. Biol. Chem.*, **215**, 515 (1955).

365 Bruns, F. H., Noltmann, E. and Vahlhaus, E., *Biochem. Z.*, **330**, 483 (1958).

366 Urivetzky, M. and Tsuboi, K. K., *Arch. Biochem. Biophys.*, **103**, 1 (1963).

367 Fontanelle, L. J. and Henderson, J. F., *Biochim. Biophys. Acta*, **177**, 177 (1969).

368 Meyskens, F. L. and Williams, H. E., *Metabolism*, **20**, 737 (1971).

369 Hershko, A., Razin, A. and Mager, J., *Biochim. Biophys. Acta.*, **184**, 64 (1969).

370 Hershko, A. and Mager, J., *Isr. J. Chem.*, **6**, 100 (1968).

371 Hershko, A., Razin, A., Shoshani, T. and Mager, J., *Biochim. Biophys. Acta.*, **149**, 59 (1967).

372 Fox, I. H. and Kelley, W. N., *J. Biol. Chem.*, **246**, 5739 (1971).

373 Fortier, N. L., Galland, L. and Lionetti, F. J., *Arch. Biochem. Biophys.*, **119**, 69 (1967).

374 Morrison, W. L. and Neurath, H., *J. Biol. Chem.*, **200**, 39 (1953).

375 Künzel, W., Wagenknecht, C. and Rapoport, S., *Acta. Biol. Med. German.*, **7**, 609 (1961).

376 Götze, E. and Rapoport, S., *Biochem. Z.*, **326**, 53 (1954).

377 Götze, E., Lindigkeit, R. and Rapoport, S., *Biochem. Z.*, **326**, 48 (1954).

378 Götze, E. and Rapoport, S., *Biochem. Z.*, **327**, 305 (1955).

379 Reichelt, D., Jacobsohn, E. and Haschen, R. J., VI. Internationales Symposium über Struktur und Funktion der Erythrocyten, Berlin (1970). *in*: Abhandlungen der Deutschen Akademie der Wissenschaften zu Berlin (Berlin: Akademie-Verlag, 1971), p. 505.

380 Tsuboi, K. K. and Hudson, P. B., *J. Biol. Chem.*, **224**, 879 (1957).

381 Tsuboi, K. K. and Hudson, P. B., *J. Biol. Chem.*, **224**, 889 (1957).

382 Turner, B. M., Fisher, R. A. and Harris, H., *Europ. J. Biochem.*, **24**, 288 (1971).

383 Edwards, Y. E., Hopkinson, D. A. and Harris, H., *Ann. Hum. Genet.*, **34**, 395 (1971).

384 Kim, B. K., Cha, S. and Parks, R. E., Jr., *J. Biol. Chem.*, **243**, 1763 (1968).

385 Kim, B. K., Cha, S. and Parks, R. E., Jr., *J. Biol. Chem.*, **243**, 1771 (1968).

386 De Verdier, C.-H. and Gould, B. J., *Biochim. Biophys. Acta*, **68**, 333 (1963).

387 De Verdier, C.-H., VI. Internationales Symposium über Struktur

und Funktion der Erythrocyten, Berlin (1970) *in*: Abhandlungen der Deutschen Akademie der Wissenschaften zu Berlin (Berlin: Akademie Verlag, 1971).

388 Lionetti, F. J. and Fortier, N. L., *Biochim. Biophys. Acta*, **119**, 462 (1966).

389 Agarwal, R. P. and Parks, R. E., *J. Biol. Chem.*, **244**, 644 (1969).

390 Hamfelt, A., *Clin. Chim. Acta*, **16**, 7 (1967).

391 Malkin, A. and Denstedt, O. F., *Canad. J. Biochem. Physiol.*, **34**, 121 (1956).

392 Scheuch, D. and Rapoport, S., *Acta Biol. Med. German.*, **6**, 23 (1961).

393 Scheuch, D. and Rapoport, S., *Folia Haematol.* (Leipzig), **78**, 148 (1962).

394 Buruiana, L. M. and Hadarag, E. L., *Naturwissenschaften*, **52**, 520 (1965).

395 Pynes, G. and Younathan, E. S., *J. Biol. Chem.*, **242**, 2119 (1967).

296 Herx, F., Herold, F. S. and Kaplan, E., *Proc. Soc. Exptl. Biol. Med.*, **121**, 536 (1966).

397 Paglia, D. E. and Valentine, W. N., *J. Lab. Clin. Med.*, **76**, 202 (1970).

398 Jacobasch, G., Grieger, M., Piersig, A., Minkwitz, H. G., Redmann, M., Lachmann, P., Lange, U. and Friedrich, U., VI. Internationales Symposium über Struktur und Funktion der Erythrocyten Berlin (1970), (Berlin: Akademie-Verlag, 1971), p. 349.

399 Tanaka, K. R., Valentine, W. N. and Miwa, S., *Blood*, **19**, 267 (1962).

400 Tanaka, K. R. and Valentine, W. N., *in*: ed. by Beutler, E., Hereditary Disorders of Erythrocyte Metabolism (New York, London: Grune & Stratton, 1968), p. 229.

401 Koler, R. D., Bigley, R. H. and Stenzel, P., *in*: ed. by Beutler, E.: Hereditary Disorders of Erythrocyte Metabolism (New York, London: Grune & Statton, 1968), p. 249.

402 Blume, K. G., Hoffbauer, R. W., Busch, D., Arnold, H. and Löhr, G. W., *Biochim. Biophys. Acta*, **227**, 364 (1971).

403 Koster, J. F., Staal, G. E. J. and Van Milligen-Boersma, L., *Biochim. Biophys. Acta*, **226**, 362 (1971).

404 Solvonuk, P. F. and Collier, H. B., *Canad. J. Biochem. Physiol.*, **33**, 38 (1955).

405 Jagemann, K. and Rosenthal, S., *Folia Haematol.* (Leipzig), **83** (1965).

406 Williamson, R. and Mathias, A. P., *Biochem. J.*, **89**, 139 (1963).

407 Stavy, L., Feldman, M. and Elson, D., *Biochim. Biophys. Acta*, **91**, 606 (1964).

408 Adachi, K., Nagano, K., Nakao, T. and Nakao, M., *Biochim. Biophys., Acta*, **92**, 59 (1964).

409 Rosenthal, S., Prehn, S. and Rapoport, S., *Acta Biol. Med. German.*,

17, 667 (1966).
410 Rosenthal, S., Jagemann, K., Prehn, S. and Heinemann, G., *Acta Biol. Med. German.*, **18**, 329 (1967).
411 Rosenthal, S., Rapoport, S. and Heinemann, G., *Acta Biol. Med. German.*, **13**, 946 (1964).
412 Prehn, S. and Rosenthal, S., *Folia Haematol.* (Leipzig), **90**, 156 (1968).
413 Kinzel, D. and Rosenthal, S., *Folia Haematol.* (Leipzig), **90**, 167 (1968).
414 Rowley, P. T. and Barnes, F., *Fed. Proc.*, **25**, 645, Abstr. 2570 (1966).
415 Rowley, P. T. and Morris, J. A., *J. Biol. Chem.*, **242**, 1533 (1967).
416 Farkas, W. and Marks, P. A., *J. Biol. Chem.*, **243**, 6464 (1968).
417 Burka, E. R., *Science*, **162**, 1287 (1968).
418 Burka, E. R., *J. Clin. Invest.*, **48**, 1724 (1969).
419 Burka, E. R., *J. Clin. Invest.*, **50**, 60 (1971).
420 Sierralta, W. and Minguell, J., *Bioch. Biophys. Res. Comm.*, **41**, 50 (1970).
421 Goto, S. and Mizuno, D., *Arch. Biochem. Biophys.*, **145**, 64 (1971).
422 Goto, S. and Mizuno, D., *Arch. Biochem. Biophys.*, **145**, 71 (1971).
423 Dickens, F. and Williamson, D. H., *Biochem. J.*, **64**, 567 (1956).
424 Ballou, D., Palmer, G. and Massey, V., *Biochem. Biophys. Res. Comm.*, **36**, 898 (1969).
425a McCord, J. M. and Fridovich, J., *J. Biol. Chem.*, **244**, 6049 (1969).
425b Bannister, J., Bannister, W. and Wood, E., *Europ. J. Biochem.*, **18**, 178 (1971).
425c Wood, E., Dalgleish and Bannister, W., *Europ. J. Biochem.*, **18**, 187 (1971).
425d Carrico, R. J. and Deutsch, H. F., *J. Biol. Chem.*, **245**, 723 (1970).
426 Wilmanns, W., Sauer, M. and Gelingsky, P., *Blut.* (München) *Z. Ges. Blutforsch.*, **19**, 457 (1969).
427 Farina, M. V., Polli, E. E. and Bianchi, P. A., *Biochim. Biophys. Acta*, **103**, 512 (1965).
428 Brownstone, Y. S. and Denstedt, O. F., *Canad. J. Biochem. Physiol.*, **39**, 533 (1961). cited *in*: Bishop, C., The Red Blood Cell (New York, London: Academic Press, 1964), p. 35.
429 Konttinen, A. and Viherroski, M., *Clin. Chim. Acta.*, **22**, 145 (1968).
430 Massod, M.F., McGuire, S. L. and Werner, K. R., *Amer. J. Clin. Path.*, **55**, 465 (1971).
431 Schouten, H., Van Eps, L. W. S. and Boudier, A. M. S., *Clin. Chim. Acta*, **10**, 474 (1964).
432 Markkanen, T., Heikinheimo, R., Dahl, M., *Acta Haematol.*, **42**, 148 (1969).
433 Markkanen, T., Peltola, O. and Koskelo, P., *Acta Haematol.*, **46**, 142 (1971).

434 Markkanen, T., Peltola, O. and Dahl, M., *Biol. Neonat.*, **18**, 468 (1971).

435a Knapp, A., *Dtsch. Ges. Wesen.*, **25**, 372 (1970).

435b Hoffmann, J., Knapp, A., Rietz, K. and Milner, Ch., *Clin. Chim. Acta*, **33**, 415 (1971).

436 Chong, Y. H., *Amer. J. Clin. Nutr.*, **23**, 261 (1970).

437a Brin, M., Dibble, M. V., Peel, A., McMullen, E., Borquin, A. and Chen, N., *Amer. J. Clin. Nutr.*, **17**, 240 (1965).

437b Heinrich, P. C. and Wiss, O., *Helv. Chim. Acta*, **54**, 2658 (1971).

438 Bruns, F. H., Dünwald, E. and Noltmann, E., *Biochem. Z.*, **330**, 497 (1958).

439 Schneider, A. S., Valentine, W. N., Baughan, M. A., Paglia, D. E., Shore, N. A. and Heins, H. L., *in*: ed. by Beutler, E.: Hereditary Disorders of Erythrocyte Metabolism (New York, London: Grune & Stratton, 1968), p. 265.

440 Schneider, A. S., Dunn, J., Ibsen, K. H. and Weinstein, J. M., *in*: ed. by Beutler, E., Hereditary Disorders of Erythrocyte Metabolism. (New York, London: Grune & Stratton, 1968), p. 273.

441 Tsuboi, K. K., Penefsky, Z. J. and Hudson, P. B., *Arch. Biochem. Biophys.*, **68**, 54 (1957).

442 Ng, W. G., Donnell, G. N., Hodgman, J. E. and Bergren, W. R., *Nature*, **214**, 283 (1967).

443 Cornblath, M., Steiner, D. F., Bryan, P. and King, J., *Clin. Chim. Acta*, **12**, 27 (1965).

444 Kalckar, H. M. and Maxwell, E. S., *Physiol. Rev.*, **38**, 77 (1958).

445 Tsuboi, K. K., Fukunaga, K. and Petricciani, J. C., *J. Biol. Chem.*, **244**, 1008 (1969).

446 Granick, S. and Mauzerall, D., *J. Biol. Chem.*, **232**, 1141 (1958).

447 Niethammer, D. and Huennekens, F. M., *Arch. Biochem. Biophys.*, **146**, 564 (1971).

448 Horst, W. D., Gattanell, P., Unbano, S. and Sheppard, H., *Life Science*, **8**, 473 (1969).

449a Assicot, M. and Bohuon, C., *Biochimie*, **53**, 871 (1971).

449b Männl, H. F. H., Hempel, K. and Kübler, W., Naunyn Schmiedebergs, *Arch. Pharm.*, **266**, 398 (1970).

449c Axelrod, J. and Cohn, C. K., *J. Pharmakol. Exp. Ther.*, **176**, 650 (1971).

449d Gugler, R., Hengstmann, J. H. and Dengler, H. J., *Arch. Int. Pharmadynamic Ther.*, **201**, 353 (1973).

450a Bonsignore, D., Calissano, P. and Cartasegna, C., *Med. Lavoro*, **56**, 199 (1965).

450b Bonsignore, D., Calissano, P. and Cartasegna, C., *Med. Lavoro*, **56**, 727 (1965).

451 Bonsignore, D., *Med. Lavoro*, **57**, 654 (1966).

452 De Bruin, A. and Jong-Heisterkamp, G. T., *Ann. Biol. Clin.*, **26**, 717 (1968).
453a Hernberg, S. and Nikkanen, J., *Lancet*, **1**, 63 (1970).
453b Hernberg, S., Nikkanen, J. and Mellin, G., *Arch. Environ. Health*, **21**, 140 (1970).
454a Hager-Aronsen, B., Abdulla, M. and Fristedt, B. J., *Arch. Environ. Health*, **23**, 440 (1971).
454b Valloton, M. N., Guillemin, M. and Lob, M., *Schweiz. Med. Wschr.*, **103**, 547 (1973).
454c Coller, H. B., *Clin. Biochem.*, **4**, 222 (1971).
454d Weißberg, J. B., Lipschutz, F. and Oski, F. A., *New Engl. J. Med.*, **284**, 565 (1971).
455 Jaffe, E. R. and Hsieh, H.-S., *Seminars Hematol.*, **8**, 417 (1971).
456 Paniker, N. V. and Beutler, E., *J. Animal Sci.*, **34**, 75 (1972).
457 Sheppard, H. and Burghardt, Ch. R., *Biochem. Pharmakol.*, **22**, 427 (1973).
458 Moses, S. W., Chayoth, R., Levin, S., Lazarovitz, E. and Rubinstein, D., *J. Clin. Invest.*, **47**, 1343 (1968).
459 Arnold, W. J. and Kelley, W. N., *J. Biol. Chem.*, **246**, 7398 (1971).
460 Wehinger, H., *Klin. Wochenschr.*, **50**, 339 (1972).
461 Wehinger, H. and Peikert, B., *Helv. Paediat. Acta.*, **28**, 117 (1973).
462 Passon, P. G. and Hultquist, D. E., *Biochim. Biophys. Acta*, **275**, 62 (1972).
463 Sudo, T., Kikuno, M. and Kurihara, T., *Biochim. Biophys. Acta*, **255** 640 (1972).
464 Smith, J. E., Kiefer, S. and Lee, M., *Comp. Biochem. Physiol.*, **43 B**, 113 (1973).
465 Gupta, J. D., Irvine, S. and Harley, J. D., *Aust. J. Exp. Biol. Med. Sci.* **50**, 511 (1972).
466 Partsch, G. and Altmann, H., *Experimentia*, **26**, 267 (1973).
467 Hilgertova, J., Strakova, M., Vrbova, H., Gregorova, J., Sonka, J. and Josifko, M., *Clin. Chim. Acta*, **36**, 511 (1972).
468 Emerson, P. M., Mason, D. Y. and Cuthbert, J. E., *Brit. J. Haematol.*, **22**, 667 (1972).
469a Wendel, A., Schaich, E., Weber, U. and Flohe, L., *Hoppe Seylers Z. Physiol. Chem.*, **353**, 514 (1972).
469b Wendel, A. and Flohe, L., *Hoppe Seylers Z. Physiol. Chem.*, **353**, 523 (1972).
470a Spencer-Peet, J., *Clin. Chim. Acta*, **10**, 481 (1964).
470b Cornblath, M., Steiner, D. F., Bryan, P. and King, J., *Clin. Chim. Acta*, **12**, 27 (1965).
471a Moses, S. W. and Bashan, N., *Isr. J. Med. Sci.*, **7**, 1213 (1971).
471b Moses, S. W., Bashan, N. and Gutman, A., *Europ. J. Biochem.*, **30**,

205 (1972).
471c *Ibid.*, *Blood*, **40**, 836 (1972).
472a Mannervik, B., Lindström, L. and Bartfai, T., *Europ. J. Biochem.*, **29**, 276 (1972).
472b Mannervik, B., Gorna-Hall, B. and Bartfai, T., *Europ. J. Biochem.*, **37**, 270 (1973).
473a Müller, M. M., Dobrovits, H. and Stemberger, A., *Z. Klin. Chem. Klin. Biochem.*, **10**, 535 (1972).
473b Müller, M. M. and Dobrovits, H., *Preparative Biochem.*, **2**, 375 (1972).
474 Bloos, J. and Sauer, H.-J., *Klin. Wochenschr.*, **50**, 991 (1972).
475 Yoneyama, Y. and Sugita, Y., Methemoglobin Réduction in Human Erythrocytes: 7. International Berlin Symposium on Structure and Function of Erythrocytes, 22.-25. 8. 73 Berlin (Akademie-Verlag Berlin, 1974).
476 Niedel, J. and Dietrich, L. S., *J. Biol. Chem.*, **248**, 3500 (1973).
477 Rogers, L. E., *Amer. J. Clin. Pathol.*, **59**, 31 (1973).
478 Lewis, W. H. P. and Harris, H., *Nature*, **215**, 351 (1967).
479 Witheller, J. and Wilson, D. B., *J. Biol. Chem.*, **247**, 2217 (1972).
480 Tarui, S., Kono, N. and Uyeda, K., *J. Biol. Chem.*, **247**, 1138 (1972).
481a Staal, G. E. J., Koster, J. F., Bänziger, J. M. and van Milligen-Boerma, L., *Biochim. Biophys. Acta*, **276**, 113 (1972).
481b Staal, G. E. J. and Koster, J. F., *FEBS Letters*, **23**, 29 (1972).
481c Staal, G. E. J., *Int. J. Biochem.*, **4**, 74 (1973).
482 Lee, L. M. Y., *Arch. Biochem. Biophys.*, **148**, 607 (1972).
483 Tsai, M. Y. and Kemp, R., *J. Biol. Chem.*, **248**, 785 (1973).
484 Kühn, B., Jacobasch, G., Gerth, Ch. and Rapoport, S., manuscript submitted.
485 Ropers, H. and Op'thof, J., *Vox Sang.*, **18**, 244 (1970).
486 Fox, I. H. and Kelley, W. N., *J. Biol. Chem.*, **247**, 2126 (1972).
487a Cornblath, M., Levin, E. Y., Marquetti, E. and House, E. Y., *Fed. Proc.*, **19**, 68, Abstr. 37/1 (1960).
487b Moses, S. W., Chayoth, R., Levin, S., Lazarovitz, E. and Rubinstein, D., *J. Clin. Invest.*, **47**, 1343 (1968).
488 Chern, Ch. J., Rittenberg, M. B. and Black, J. A., *J. Biol. Chem.*, **247**, 7173 (1972).
489a Boivin, P., Galand, C. and Demartial, M.-C., *Path. Biol.*, **20**, 583 (1972).
489b Garreau, H. and Buc-Temkine, H., *Biochemie*, **54**, 1103 (1972).
489c Koster, J. F., Slee, R. G., Staal, G. E. J. and van Berkel, J. C., *Biochim. Biophys. Acta*, **258**, 763 (1972).
490 Imamura, K. and Tanaka, T., *J. Biochem.*, **71**, 1073 (1972).
491 De Jimenez, E. S., Ma. de la Paz, De Miles L. and Roman, P. R., *Europ. J. Biochem.*, **28**, 538 (1972).

492a Fee, J. A. and Gaber, B. P., *J. Biol. Chem.*, **247**, 60 (1972).
492b Fee, J. A., Natter, R. and Baker, G. S., *Biochim. Biophys. Acta*, **29**, 96 (1973).
493 Beutler, E. and Guinto, E., *Blood*, **41**, 559 (1973).
494 Romeo, G. and Levin, E. Y., *Proc. Nat. Acad. Sci.*, **63**, 856 (1969).

The Primary Structures of Hemoglobin Molecules and Their Phylogenetic Implications

G. MATSUDA, H. TAKEI and T. MAITA

Department of Biochemistry, Nagasaki University, School of Medicine, Nagasaki, Japan

The primary structures of hemoglobins derived from various kinds of living organisms, including human hemoglobin are generally already determined, or have been studied. The present authors compared the primary structures of these hemoglobins, and calculated mutual minimum mutation distances from the differences. According to the results, the more distant the divergence point in the evolution of these animals becomes, the larger the minimum mutation distances become. This suggests a relationship between the evolution of living organisms and the mutation of the primary structures of proteins. On the basis of these minimum mutation distances, phylogenetic trees of the α and β polypeptide chains of various hemoglobins have been already made. On the other hand, the primary structure of an ancestral hemoglobin chain has been assumed on the basis of various methods. The authors assumed human γ polypeptide chain to be the closest to the β polypeptide chain of an ancestral homeothermal animal. Furthermore, a consideration of the relationship between phylogeny and function was made.

INTRODUCTION

Since the original living organisms appeared on the earth about 3 billion years ago, evolution has occurred continuously and has produced a nearly infinite variety. In order to classify this complicated animate world, a classification based upon the form and habit of these living organisms was initiated, and gradually the conception of the evolution of living organisms was born. Darwin gave natural selection as a factor in evolution. On the other hand, in the latter half of the twentieth century, there has been a strong tendency to study various vital phenomena at the molecular level. This tendency extended to the study of the evolution of living organisms. For instance, Anfinsen[1)] tried to investigate the process of evolution of living organisms by comparing the primary structures of homologous proteins. Ingram[2] compared the primary structures of α, β, γ and δ polypeptide chains of human hemoglobin, and suggested that 4 kinds of structure genes corresponding to these 4 polypeptide chains, which were originally a single kind, were created by gradual evolution and separation, and further, the rate of evolution of these structure genes was different. Pauling and Zuckerkandl[3] calculated that 10×10^6 years were needed for the mutation of one amino acid, from differences in the amino acid sequences between the primary structures of α polypeptide chains of human hemoglobin and horse hemoglobin. This was the first report to show the rate of evolution of protein molecules as a numerical value. Fitch and Margoliash[4] prepared a phylogenetic tree showing the evolution of cytochrome c derived from various living organisms, and further suggested the primary structure of ancestral cytochrome c. Goodman *et al.*[5] made phylogenetic trees showing the evolution of hemoglobin and fibrinopeptide, and further calculated the percentages of mutational divergence from an assumed ancestral mammalian hemoglobin to various present mammalian hemoglobins. From the results of these studies using 3 computer programs, it was recognized that the rate of evolution of hemoglobin molecules was not always constant, but changed considerably, and in particular, the rate of evolution in higher primates gradually decreased. Comparative studies on the primary structures of protein are also carried from the viewpoint of population genetics, and reports on mechanism, rate, and so forth of the evolution of protein molecules have been published. Kimura[6] and King and Jukes[7] proposed a theory that exchanges of amino acid sequences in proteins occur mainly by neutral mutation regardless of natural selection.

The study of molecular evolution based upon comparison of the primary structures of protein is still in the initial stages, and many problems remain. Some concrete results have been obtained, however.

THE PRIMARY STRUCTURES OF HEMOGLOBIN MOLECULES

Since hemoglobin is widely distributed in nature, its isolation and purification is comparatively easy, and in addition its primary and tertiary structure are studied in detail, it is considered to be one of the most sutiable proteins for the study of molecular evolution. Mammalian hemoglobins are tetramers, consisting of 2 kinds of polypeptide chains, generally designated as $\alpha_2\beta_2$. In 1961, Braunitzer *et al.*[8]

and Konigsberg *et al.*[9] determined the primary structure of the α and β polypeptide chains of human adult hemoglobin. This α chain consists of 141 amino acid residues, and the β chain 146 amino acid residues. Human fetal hemoglobin, which is present as the main component in human fetus, possesses a γ polypeptide chain in place of the β polypeptide chain of human adult hemoglobin, and it is designated as $\alpha_2\gamma_2$. The primary structure of this γ chain was determined by Schroeder *et al.*[10] It consists of 146 amino acid residues, like the β chain of human adult hemoglobin. It is known that there are 2 kinds of γ polypeptide chain, having glycine or alanine residue at the 136th position from the N-terminus.[11] Furthermore, AII component, which is a minor component of human adult hemoglobin possesses a δ polypeptide chain[12,13] in place of the β polypeptide chain, and is designated as $\alpha_2\delta_2$. This δ chain consists of 146 amino acid residues like the β and γ chains.

While studying the primary structure of human hemoglobin, studies on the primary structure of horse hemoglobin were carried out. This is considered to be very important, particularly in relation to the tertiary structure of horse hemoglobin. Horse hemoglobin contains 2 main components, which are designated as fast component and slow component respectively. This difference depends upon the presence of 2 kinds of α polypeptide chain. First of all, the primary structure of the α polypeptide chain of slow component was determined by Matsuda *et al.*[14] Subsequently, the primary structure of the β polypeptide chain was determined by Smith *et al.*,[15] and then the α polypeptide chain of the fast component was determined by Kilmartin *et al.*[16] These α polypeptide chains and the β polypeptide chain consist of 141 amino acid residues, and 146 amino acid residues, respectively, like human hemoglobin, and between the 2 α polypeptide chains, amino acid exchanges were recognized at 2 positions. On the other hand, Perutz *et al.*[17–20] carried out detailed studies on the tertiary structures of horse hemoglobin and human hemoglobin, and the conformations of these hemoglobins became clear.

An interest is taken in the primary structure of nonhuman primate hemoglobins because of their direct connection with human hemoglobin from the viewpoint of molecular evolution. Amino acid compositions of tryptic peptides of the α and β polypeptide chains from chimpanzee hemoglobin[21] were analyzed. The results are recognized to be quite similar to those from human hemoglobin. Further, the primary structures of α and β polypeptide chains of hemoglobins from gorilla,[22]

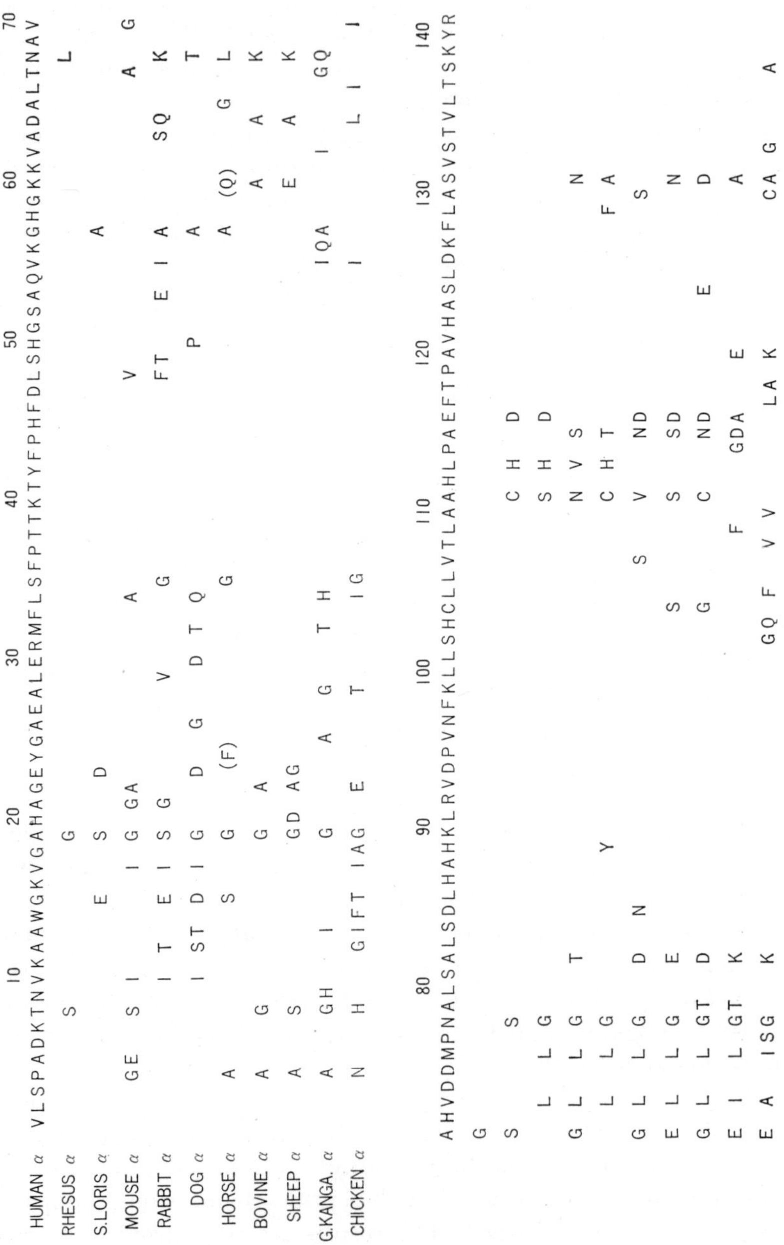
10 20 30 40 50 60 70
HUMAN α VLSPADKTNVKAAWGKVGAHAGEYGAEALERMFLSFPTTKTYFPHFDLSHGSAQVKGHGKKVADALTNAV
RHESUS α S G L
S.LORIS α E S D A
MOUSE α GE S I I G GA A V A G
RABBIT α I T E I S G V G FT E I A SQ K
DOG α I ST D I G D G D T Q P A T
HORSE α A S G (F) G A (Q) G L
BOVINE α A G G A A A K
SHEEP α A S GD AG E A K
G.KANGA. α A GH I G A G T H IQA I GQ
CHICKEN α N H GIFT IAG E T IG I L I I
80 90 100 110 120 130 140
AHVDDMPNALSALSDLHAHKLRVDPVNFKLLSHCLLVTLAAHLPAEFTPAVHASLDKFLASVSTVLTSKYR
G
S S C H D
L L G S H D
G L L G T N V S N
L L G Y C H T F A
G L L G D N S V ND S
E L L G E S S SD N
G L L GT D G C ND E D
E I L GT K F GDA E A
E A ISG K GQ F V V LA K CA G A

Fig. 1

rhesus monkey,[23] Japanese monkey,[24] crab-eating monkey,[25] slow loris,[26] and β and δ polypeptide chains of spider monkey hemoglobin[27] are already determined or have almost been determined.

As for other hemoglobins, studies on the primary structures of the α and β polypeptide chains of mouse hemoglobin,[28,29] α and β polypeptide chains of rabbit hemoglobin,[30,31] α and β polypeptide chains of dog hemoglobin,[32] β polypeptide chain of camel hemoglobin,[33] α and β polypeptide chains of 11ama hemoglobin,[34] α and β polypeptide chains of pig hemoglobin,[35,36] α and β polypeptide chains of bovine hemoglobin,[37] β polypeptide chain of bovine fetal hemoglobin,[38] α and β (A, B, C) polypeptide chains of sheep hemoglobin,[39–43] β polypeptide chain of sheep fetal hemoglobin,[43] α and β (A, C) polypeptide chains of goat hemoglobin,[44–46] β (C) polypeptide chain of barbary sheep hemoglobin,[47] α and β polypeptide chains of gray kangaroo hemoglobin,[48] α and β polypeptide chains of chicken hemoglobin,[49,50] β polypeptide chain of frog hemoglobin,[51] α polypeptide chain of carp hemoglobin,[52] and so forth have been carried out.

Figure 1 shows a comparison of the primary structures of α polypeptide chains of hemoglobins from human, rhesus monkey, slow loris, mouse, rabbit, dog, horse, cow, sheep, gray kangaroo and chicken. The α polypeptide chains of the hemoglobins shown all consist of 141 amino acid residues. Figure 2 shows a comparison of the primary structures of β polypeptide chains of human, rhesus monkey, slow loris, mouse, rabbit, dog, horse, cow, gray kangaroo and chicken, and the γ polypeptide chain of human hemoglobin. The β and γ polypeptide chains shown consist of 146 amino acid residues except for the β polypeptide chain of bovine hemoglobin which consists of 145 amino acid residues.

Fig. 1. Comparison of the primary structures of 11 kinds of α polypetide chains. In this figure, HUMANα, RHESUSα, S. LORISα, MOUSEα, RABBITα, DOGα, HORSEα, BOVINEα, SHEEPα, G. KANGA.α and CHICKENα refer to the α polypeptide chains of hemoglobins from human, rhesus monkey, slow loris, mouse, rabbit, dog, horse (slow and fast components), bovine, sheep, gray kangaroo and chicken (AII component), respectively. In the polypeptide chains other than the α polypeptide chain of human hemoglobin, amino acid sequences are shown only when differences occur as compared with human α chain. One letter amino acid abbreviations are used as follows; A: Ala, C: CysH, D: Asp, E: Glu, F: Phe, G: Gly, H: His, I: Ile, K: Lys, L: Leu, M: Met, N: Asn, P: Pro, Q: Gln, R: Arg, S: Ser, T: Thr, V: Val, W: Trp, Y: Tyr.

```
                   10        20        30        40        50        60        70
HUMAN β    VHLTPEEKSAVTALWGKVNVDEVGGEALGRLLVVYPWTQRFFESFGDLSTPDAVMGNPKVKAHGKKVLGA
RHESUS β           N   T                   L                S
S.LORIS β      G                D                           S S                S
MOUSE β        DA  A  SG      A                   Y S      SA  I   A         IT
RABBIT β      SS               E                            SAN   N          A
DOG β          A    L SG                   I         D           S A         NS
HORSE β     Q SG   A  L   D   EE                     D      N G              HS
BOVINE β   -M  A   A    F S  H                               A    D          DS
G.KANGA. β     A   N I S     AIEQT         I     S   DH     NAK   A    L   A   V
CHICKEN β    W A   QLI G       A C A   A   I         A   N  S T IL   M R     TS
HUMAN γ    G F E D ATI S       EDA   T               D   N  SAS I            TS

         80        90       100       110       120       130       140   146
FSDGLAHLDNLKGTFATLSELHCDKLHVDPENFRLLGNVLVCVLAHHFGKEFTPPVQAAYQKVVAGVANALAHKYH
     N          Q                K                   Q
     N          K                         V        D   Q  S
     N          S                      MI I  G  L  D   AA   F        A
  E  S          K                         I  S         Q
     KN         K                K                     Q
 GE VH          A                        AL V R    D   EL  S
    MK   D      A                K        V   RN  N    VL  DF                R
 G AIKN         K                K    II IC  E        IDT V W  L
 G AVKN     IN  SQ                   DI II   A  S D   EC   W  L RV  H    R
LG AIK   D      Q                K        T   I        E   SW  M T(A)S  SSR
```

Fig. 2

↓

The hemoglobins described above all exist as tetramers. It is known, however, that different characteristics are seen in the hemoglobins of some lower animals. For instance, hemoglobin of cyclostomata, regarded as the lowest form of vertebrate, is a monomer. It is known to dimerize under conditions of deoxygenation. Regarding such hemoglobins, the primary structures of hemoglobins of lampetra fluviatilis[53)] and petromyzon marinus[54)] are already determined. Further, erythrocruorin[55)] of chironomus thummi, a much lower animal, has been investigated. This erythrocruorin contains more than 10 components. Of these 4 components are monomers and 6 are dimers. A component which is a tetramer was found, though it is present in very small amounts. The primary structures of CTTIII component[56)] and CTTI component[57)] of chironomus thummi thummi are already determined. Further, a leghemoglobin provides a very interesting case for study. This is obtained from bean plant and bacteria of the rhizobium genus in symbiosis with it. The primary structure of this leghemoglobin[58)] has been determined.

PHYLOGENY OF THE α AND β POLYPEPTIDE CHAINS OF HEMOGLOBIN MOLECULES

It is assumed that the α and β polypeptide chains of hemoglobin from chimpanzee, which is an anthropoid, possess exactly the same primary structure as human hemoglobin. It is also assumed that the α and β polypeptide chains of hemoglobin from gorilla, which is also an anthropoid, has 1 amino acid exchange as compared with the α and β polypeptide chains of human hemoglobin, based on analysis of amino acid compositions of the tryptic peptides. Furthermore, it is recognized that there are, respectively, 4 and 8 amino acid exchanges between the α and β polypeptide chains from hemoglobin of rhesus

Fig. 2. Comparison of the primary structures of 11 kinds of β and γ polypeptide chains. In this figure, HUMANβ, RHESUSβ, S. LORISβ, MOUSEβ, RABBITβ, DOGβ, HORSEβ, BOVINEβ, G. KANGA.β, CHICKENβ and HUMANγ refer to the β polypeptide chains of hemoglobins from man, rhesus monkey, slow loris, mouse, rabbit, dog, horse, bovine, gray kangaroo and chicken (AII component) and the γ polypeptide chain of human fetal hemoglobin, respectively. In the polypeptide chains other than the β polypeptide chain of human hemoglobin, amino acid sequences are shown only when differences occur as compared with the human β chain. One letter amino acid abbreviations are used as in Fig. 1.

monkey,[23] which belongs to macaca genus, and those of human hemoglobin. Comparing the α and β polypeptide chains of hemoglobin from slow loris,[26] which belongs to prosimiae, with those of human hemoglobin, 9 and 11 amino acid exchanges are recognized, respectively.

Comparing the primary structures of α and β polypeptide chains of horse hemoglobin[14–16] with those of human hemoglobin, 18 amino acid exchanges are recognized in the α chain of slow component, 20 amino acid exchanges in the α chain of fast component, and 26 amino acid exchanges in the β chain. As to gray kangaroo hemoglobin,[48] 27 amino acid exchanges are recognized in the α chain, and 38 amino acid exchanges in the β chain as compared with human hemoglobin. Further, between chicken hemoglobin (AII component)[49,50] and human hemoglobin, 35 amino acid exchanges are recognized in the α chain, and 45 amino acid exchanges in the β chain. The number of amino acid exchanges thus gradually increases as the divergence in the evolution of living organisms becomes more distant. This suggests that protein molecules have evolved with the evolution of living organisms.

Table I shows differences among the amino acid sequences of 11 kinds of α polypeptide chains as minimum mutation distances. Table II shows differences among the amino acid sequences of 10 kinds of β polypeptide chains and 1 kind of γ polypeptide chain as

TABLE I. Minimum mutation distances of the α polypeptide chains of chicken and mammalian hemoglobins.

	Human	Rhesus	S. Loris	Mouse	Rabbit	Dog	Horse	Bovine	Sheep	G. Kang	Chicken
Human		5	10	21	28	25	22	21	27	34	45
Rhesus	5		13	22	28	26	19	18	25	31	46
S. Loris	10	13		22	27	21	23	23	26	36	51
Mouse	21	22	22		31	27	29	21	28	38	51
Rabbit	28	28	27	31		32	31	29	36	42	55
Dog	25	26	21	27	32		31	30	31	39	54
Horse	22	19	23	29	31	31		20	23	36	49
Bovine	21	18	23	21	29	30	20		14	32	49
Sheep	27	25	26	28	36	31	23	14		36	56
G. Kang	34	31	36	38	42	39	36	32	36		54
Chicken	45	46	51	51	55	54	49	49	56	54	

minimum mutation distances. Minimum mutation distances in these tables show the differences between the amino acid sequences of 2 kinds of hemoglobins (shown in Figs. 1 and 2) considering the number of mutations of the genetic codes. In the case of deletion, it was calculated as 2. In the case of α polypeptide chain of horse hemoglobin, only slow component is shown.

TABLE II. Minimum mutation distances of the β and γ polypeptide chains of chicken and mammalian hemoglobins.

	Human	Rhesus	S. Loris	Mouse	Rabbit	Dog	Horse	Bovine	G. Kang	Chicken	Human γ
Human		10	15	31	16	18	32	32	53	59	50
Rhesus	10		15	35	15	18	35	34	50	55	46
S. Loris	15	15		31	13	21	29	36	52	55	42
Mouse	31	35	31		33	35	42	44	60	60	53
Rabbit	16	15	13	33		25	32	36	49	58	47
Dog	18	18	21	35	25		35	36	51	51	47
Horse	32	35	29	42	32	35		37	60	61	50
Bovine	32	34	36	44	36	36	37		58	67	48
G. Kang	53	50	52	60	49	51	60	58		59	57
Chicken	59	55	55	60	58	51	61	67	59		52
Human γ	50	46	42	53	47	47	50	48	57	52	

Then, taking the α polypeptide chain of human hemoglobin as a standard in Table I, minimum mutation distances between this human α polypeptide chain and those of other animals are enlarged as points of divergence in the evolution of living organisms gradually goes far off. However, if the α polypeptide chain of chicken hemoglobin is taken as a standard, no remarkable difference is recognized concerning minimum mutation distances between chicken and mammal hemoglobins. This may suggest that the molecular evolution of this hemoglobin is divergent.

Minimum mutation distances between the β polypeptide chain of mouse hemoglobin and the β polypeptide chain of hemoglobin of other mammals are shown to be comparatively high in Table II. This is considered to be because the β polypeptide chain of mouse hemoglobin is strongly influenced by the rate of alternation of generations. The authors are especially interested in the γ polypeptide chain of human fetal hemoglobin. They consider that this possesses the primary structure closest to the ancestral β polypeptide chain of homeothermal animals. Minimum mutation distances between human γ polypeptide chain and β polypeptide chains of other homeothermal animals are similar, as shown in Table II. This may suggest that the rate of molecular evolution of γ polypeptide chain is extremely slow. Also among many abnormal human hemoglobins, there are fewer hemoglobins containing anomalies of the γ polypeptide chain than of the α and β polypeptide chains. In 1866, a recapitulation theory was proposed by Haeckel. The authors wish to reconsider this theory. Protein that existed at a early period of phylogeny of living organisms may appear subsequently at a period of ontogenesis

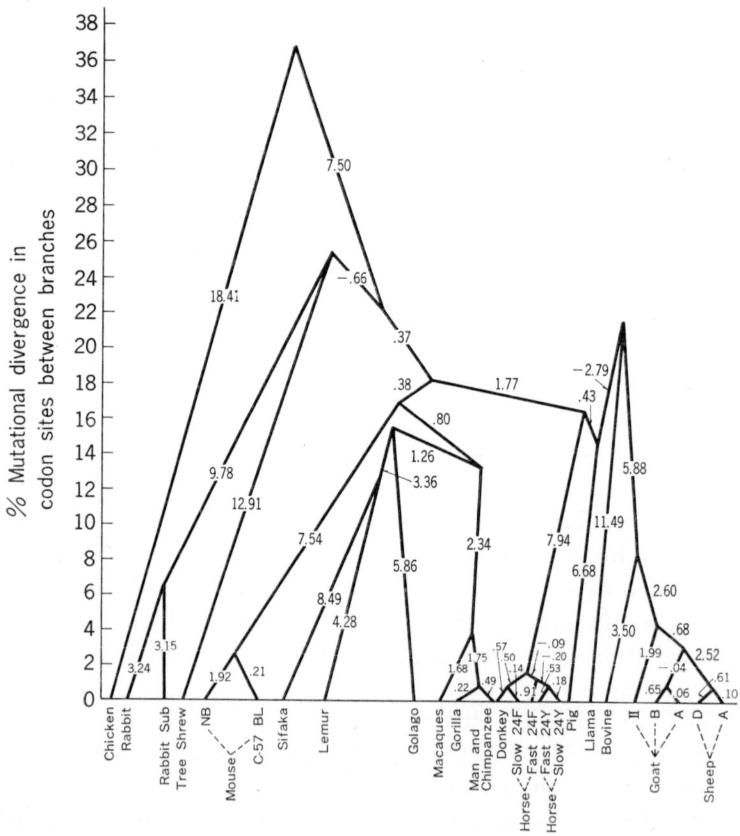

Fig. 3. Phylogenetic tree of the α polypeptide chains of chicken and mammalian hemoglobins (Goodman *et al.*,[5] 1971).

of individual organisms exhibiting little evolution.

Goodman *et al.*[5] compared the primary structures of α and β polypeptide chains of hemoglobins from various kinds of animals, and then prepared their phylogenetic trees. Figure 3 is a phylogenetic tree of α polypeptide chains of mammalian and chicken hemoglobins, and Fig. 4 is a phylogenetic tree of β-like polypeptide chains of mammalian hemoglobins.

Braunitzer *et al.*[59] arranged α and β polypeptide chains of human hemoglobin in 2 lines, making gaps at suitable places in their amino acid sequences. Then, between these 2 polypeptide chains, a high homology was recognized. Common amino acid residues in these 2 polypeptide chains were seen at 66 positions. The gaps in these amino acid sequences were called sequence gaps. These α and β polypeptide

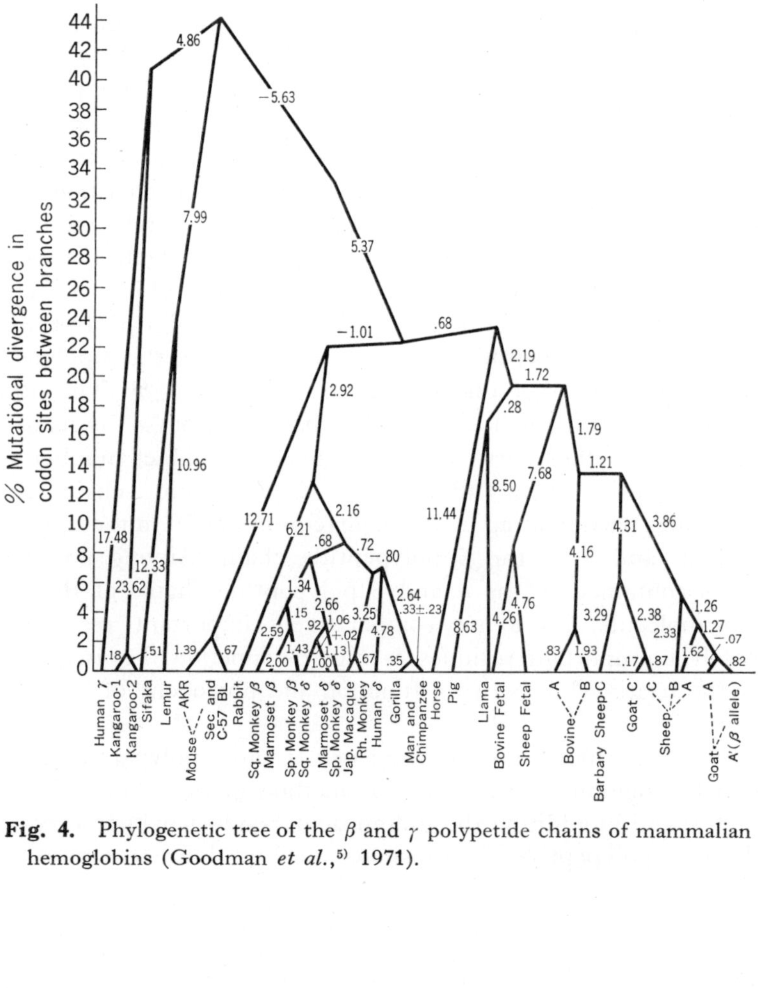

Fig. 4. Phylogenetic tree of the β and γ polypetide chains of mammalian hemoglobins (Goodman *et al.*,[5] 1971).

chains possess proximal His at α 87 and β 92, respectively, and distal His at α 58 and β 63, respectively. Proximal His residues and distal His residues can be arranged in exactly opposite positions by making these sequence gaps. On the other hand, in the study of the tertiary structure of hemoglobin, a high homology is recognized between the conformations of α and β polypeptide chains. This is very similar to the homology of these primary structures. Furthermore, in the tertiary structures of α and β polypeptide chains, the positions where differences are recognized seem to correspond to the sequence gaps in these primary structures.

A CORRELATION OF PHYLOGENY AND FUNCTION OF HEMOGLOBIN MOLECULES

The 2 α polypeptide chains and 2 β polypeptide chains composing hemoglobin molecules possess 1 heme each. Amino acid residues participating in the combination with this heme number 19 in the α polypeptide chain and 21 in the β polypeptide chain. These 40 amino acid residues are considered to be highly important in relation to the function of hemoglobin. It is said that amino acid residues participating in contacts between polypeptide chains are significant in relation to heme-heme interactions and Bohr's effect. There are contacts between the same kind of polypeptide chain, such as $\alpha^1\alpha^2$ and $\beta^1\beta^2$, and between different kinds of polypeptide chain, such as $\alpha^1\beta^1$ and $\alpha^1\beta^2$. In the latter case, taking 1 α polypeptide chain as a standard, α^1, the β polypeptide chain which is a larger distance from α^1 is named β^1. The other β polypeptide chain, which is a smaller distance from α^1 is named β^2. Amino acid residues participating in this $\alpha^1\beta^1$ contact number 16 in the α polypeptide chain and 18 in the β polypeptide chain. Amino acid residues participating in $\alpha^1\beta^2$ contact number 10 in the α polypeptide chain and 9 in the β polypeptide chain. Among amino acid residues contained in the α and β polypeptide chains of the hemoglobin molecule, there are comparatively important residues and relatively unimportant residues as regards function. Figures 5 and 6 show the relationship between function and phylogeny of hemoglobin molecules.

In Fig. 5, the amino acid sequence of the α polypeptide chain of human hemoglobin is drawn by the method of Schroeder and Huisman,[60,61] and in addition the amino acid residues which vary in 11 kinds of α polypeptide chains shown in Fig. 1 are compared with

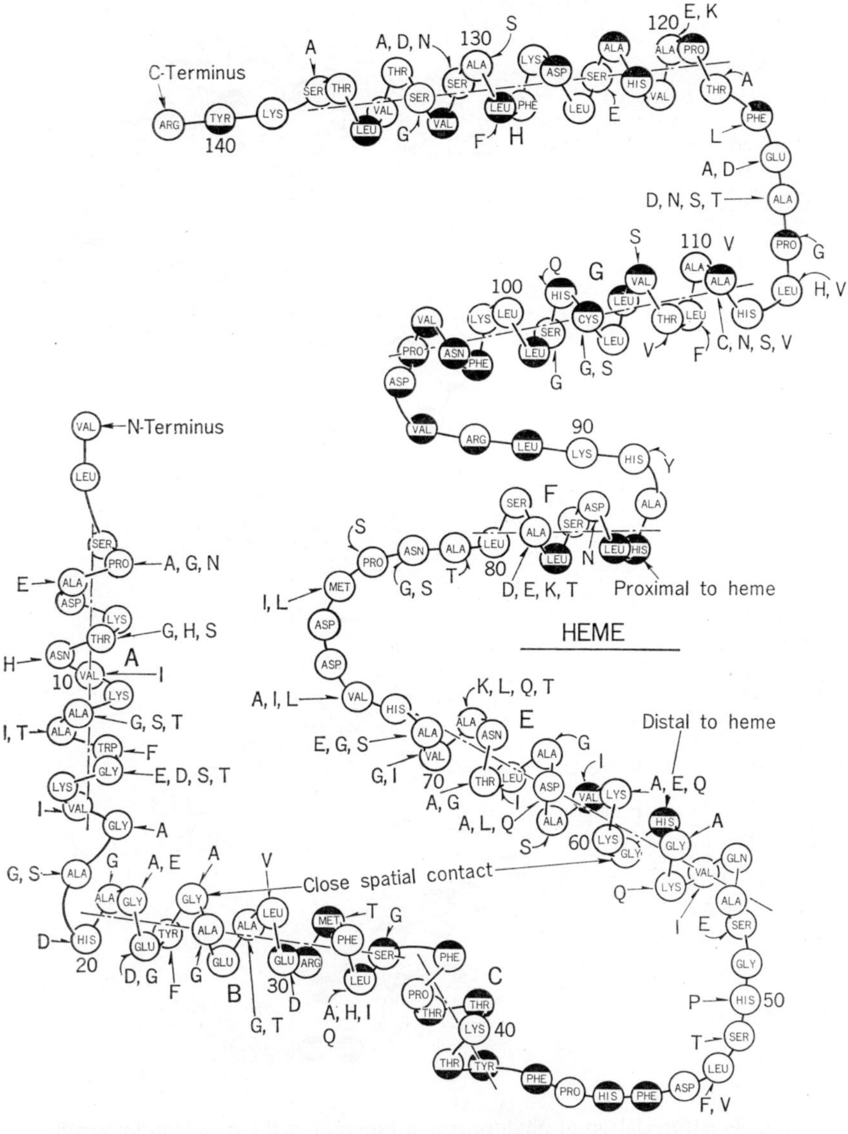

Fig. 5. Correlation of phylogeny and function of the α polypeptide chains of chicken and mammalian hemoglobins. In this figure, amino acid sequences of the α polypeptide chain of human hemoglobin are drawn by the method of Schroeder and Huisman[60,61] and in addition, amino acid residues which vary in 11 kinds of α polypeptide chains shown in Fig. 1, are compared with the human α polypeptide chain. ⊖: heme contact, ◓: $\alpha^1\beta^1$ contact, ◒: $\alpha^1\beta^2$ contact.

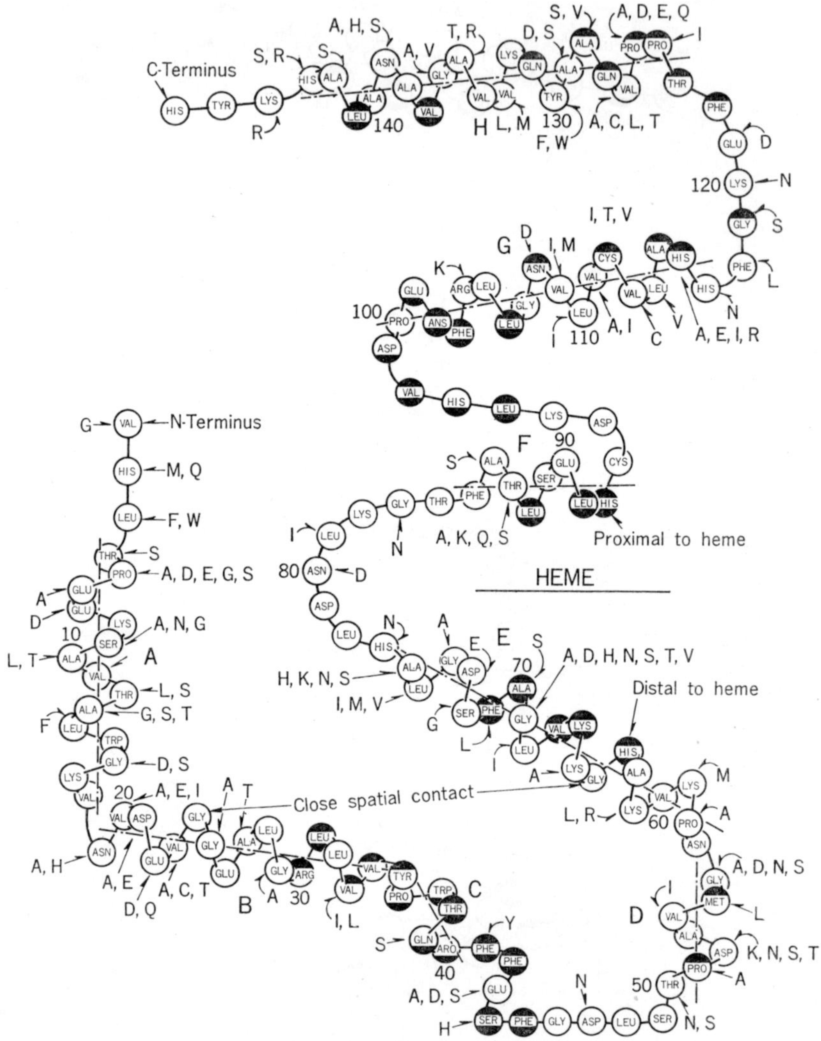

Fig. 6. Correlation of phylogeny and function of the β and γ polypeptide chains of chicken and mammalian hemoglobins. In this figure, amino acid sequences of the β polypetide chain of human hemoglobin are drawn by the method of Schroeder and Huisman[60,61] and in addition amino acid residues which vary in 11 kinds of β and γ polypeptide chains shown in Fig. 2, are compared with human β polypeptide chain. ⊖: heme contact, ◓: $\alpha^1\beta^1$ contact, ◒: $\alpha^1\beta^2$ contact.

human α polypeptide chain. Also, amino acid residues participating in contact with heme, and in $\alpha^1\beta^1$ and $\alpha^1\beta^2$ contacts are shown. In Fig. 6, the amino acid sequence of the β polypeptide chain of human hemoglobin is drawn by the method of Schroeder and Huisman,[60,61] as in the case of Fig. 5, and the amino acid residues which vary in 11 kinds of β and γ polypeptide chains shown in Fig. 2 are compared with human β polypeptide chain.

As shown above, in amino acid residues which are considered to be comparatively important for the function of hemoglobin, there are relatively few amino acid exchanges in comparison with other locations. For instance, in the α polypeptide chain, α32, α39, α42, α43, α45, α46, α58, α62, α83, α86, α87, α91, α93, α97, α98, α101, α129, α132, and α136 are known to participate in contact with heme; α30, α31, α34, α35, α36, α103, α104, α106, α107, α111, α114, α117, α119, α122, α123, and α126 participate in $\alpha^1\beta^1$ contact; α38, α41, α42, α91, α92, α93, α94, α95, α96, and α140 participate in $\alpha^1\beta^2$ contact. However, α42, α91 and α93, have 2 roles. Of the 42 amino acid residues which are considered to be comparatively important for the function of hemoglobin in this α polypeptide chain, amino acid exchanges at 12 amino acid residues are shown in Fig. 5, and this is approximately 29%. Of the 99 amino acid residues other than the above residues, amino acid exchanges at 58 amino acid residues are shown in Fig. 5, and this is approximately 59%. In the β polypeptide chain, β31, β38, β41, β42, β44, β45, β63, β66, β67, β70, β71, β88, β91, β92, β96, β98, β102, β103, β106, β137, and β141 participate in contact with heme; β30, β33, β34, β35, β51, β55, β108, β112, β115, β116, β119, β122, β123, β124, β125, β127, β128 and β131 participate in $\alpha^1\beta^1$ contact; β36, β37, β39, β40, β97, β98, β99, β101, and β102 participate in $\alpha^1\beta^2$ contact. However, β98 and β102 have 2 roles. Of the 42 amino acid residues which are considered to be comparatively important for the function of hemoglobin in this β polypeptide chain, amino acid exchanges at 16 amino acid residues are shown in Fig. 6, and this is approximately 35%. Of the 100 amino acid residues other than the above residues, amino acid exchanges at 65 amino acid residues are shown in Fig. 6, and this is approximately 65%.

From the above observations, the molecular evolution of the α and β polypeptide chains of hemoglobin molecules is restricted in relation to the function of hemoglobin. It may be assumed that this is due to natural selection.

REFERENCES

1 Anfinsen, C. B., Molecular Basis of Evolution (John Wiley & Sons Inc., New York, 1959).

2 Ingram, V. M., *Nature*, **189**, 704 (1961).

3 Pauling, L. and Zuckerkandl, E., *Acta Chem. Scand.*, **17**, 9 (1963).

4 Fitch, W. M. and Margoliash, E., *Science*, **155**, 279 (1967).

5 Goodman, M., Barnabas, J., Matsuda, G. and Moore, G. W., *Nature*, **233**, 604 (1971).

6 Kimura, M., *Nature*, **271**, 624 (1968).

7 King, J. L. and Jukes, T. H., *Science*, **164**, 788 (1969).

8 Braunitzer, G., Gehring-Müller, R., Hilschmann, H., Hilse, K., Hobom, G., Rudloff, V. and Wittmann-Liebole, B., *Z. Physiol. Chem.*, **325**, 283 (1961).

9 Konigsberg, W., Guidotti, G. and Hill, R. J., *J. Biol. Chem.*, **236**, PC 55 (1961).

10 Schroeder, W. A., Shelton, J. R., Shelton, J. B., Cormick, J. and Jones, R. T., *Biochemistry*, **2**, 992 (1963).

11 Schroeder, W. A., Huisman, T. H. J., Shelton, J. R., Shelton, J. B., Kleihauer, E. F., Dozy, A. M. and Robberson, B., *Proc. Natl. Acad. Sci. U.S.*, **60**, 537 (1968).

12 Ingram, V. M. and Stretton, A. O. W., *Biochim. Biophys. Acta*, **63**, 20 (1962).

13 Jones, R. T., *Cold Spring Harbor Symp. Quant. Biol.*, **29**, 297 (1964).

14 Matsuda, G., Gehring-Müller, R. and Braunitzer, G., *Biochem. Z.*, **338**, 669 (1963).

15 Smith, D. B. and Chung, W. P., *Canad. J. Biochem.*, **48**, 1160 (1970).

16 Kilmartin, J. V. and Clegg, J. B., *Nature*, **213**, 269 (1967).

17 Perutz, M. F., Rossmann, M. G., Cullis, A. F., Muirhead, H., Will, G. and North, A. C. T., *Nature*, **185**, 416 (1960).

18 Perutz, M. F., Muirhead, H., Cox, J. M. and Goaman, L. C. G., *Nature*, **219**, 131 (1968).

19 Perutz, M. F., *Proc. Roy. Soc.*, **173**B, 113 (1969).

20 Perutz, M. F. and Lehman, H., *Nature*, **219**, 902 (1968).

21 Rifkin, D. B. and Konigsberg, W., *Biochim. Biophys. Acta*, **104**, 457 (1965).

22 Zuckerkandl, E. and Schroeder, W. A., *Nature*, **192**, 984 (1961).

23 Matsuda, G., Maita, T., Takei, H., Ota, H., Yamaguchi, M., Miyauchi, T. and Migita, M., *J. Biochem.*, **64**, 279 (1968).

24 Matsuda, G., Maita, T., Ota, H., Araya, A., Nakashima, Y., Ishii, U. and Nakashima, M., *Int. J. Protein Res.*, in press.

25 Wade, P. T., Barnicot, N. A. and Huehns, E. R., *Biochim. Biophys. Acta*, **221**, 450 (1970).

26 Matsuda, G., Maita, T., Watanabe, B., Ota, H., Araya, A., Goodman, M. and Prychodko, W., *Int. J. Protein Res.*, in press.

27 Boyer, S. H., Crosby, E. F., Fuller, G. L., Noyes, A. N. and Adams, J. G., *Biochem. Genet.*, **5**, 405 (1971).

28 Popp, R. A., *J. Mol. Biol.*, **27**, 9 (1967).

29 Rifkin, D. B., Rifkin, M. R. and Konigsberg, W., *Proc. Natl. Acad. Sci.*, **55**, 586 (1966).

30 Brunitzer, G., Flamm, U., Best, J. S. and Schrank, B., *Z. Physiol. Chem.*, **347**, 207 (1966).

31 Braunitzer, G., Best, J. S., Flamm, U. and Schrank, B., *Z. Physiol. Chem.*, **349**, 1073 (1968).

32 Jones, R. T., Atlas of Protein Sequence and Structure, Vol. 5 (National Biomedical Research Foundation, Washington, D. C., 1972) P.D–58 and D–70.

33 Banerjee, S. and Bhown, A. S., *Biochim. Biophys. Acta*, **100**, 503 (1965).

34 Braunitzer, G., Hilse, K., Rudloff, V. and Nilschmann, N., *Advances in Protein Chemistry*, Vol. 19 (Academic Press, New York, 1964), p. 34.

35 Yamaguchi, Y., Horie, H., Matsuo, A., Sasakawa, S. and Satake, K., *J. Biochem.*, **58**, 186 (1965).

36 Braunitzer, G. and Kohler, H., *Z. Physiol. Chem.*, **343**, 290 (1966).

37 Schroeder, W. A., Shelton, J. R., Shelton, J. B., Robberson, B. and Babin, D. R., *Arch. Biochem. Biophys.*, **120**, 124 (1967).

38 Babin, D. R., Schroeder, W. A., Shelton, J. R., Shelton, J. B. and Robberson, B., *Biochemistry*, **5**, 1297 (1966).

39 Beale, D., *Biochem. J.*, **103**, 129 (1967).

40 Wilson, J. B., Brandt, G. and Huisman, T. H. J., *J. Biol. Chem.*, **243**, 3687 (1968).

41 Huisman, T. H. J., Dozy, A. M., Wilson, J. B., Efremov, G. D. and Vaskov, B., *Biochim. Biophys. Acta*, **160**, 467 (1968).

42 Boyer, S. H., Hathaway, P., Pascasio, F., Bordley, J., Orton, C. and Naughton, M. A., *J. Biol. Chem.*, **242**, 2211 (1967).

43 Wilson, J. B., Edwards, W. C., McDaniel, M., Dobbs, M. M. and Huisman, T. H. J., *Arch. Biochem. Biophys.*, **115**, 385 (1966).

44 Huisman, T. H. J., Adams, H. R., Dimmock, M. O., Edwards, W. E., and Wilson, J. B., *J. Biol. Chem.*, **242**, 2534 (1967).

45 Huisman, T. H. J., Brandt, G. and Wilson, J. B., *J. Biol. Chem.*, **243**, 3675 (1968).

46 Adams, H. R., Boyd, E. M., Wilson, J. B., Miller, A., Huisman, T. H. J., *Arch. Biochem. Biophys.*, **127**, 398 (1968).

47 Huisman, T. H. J., Dasher, G. A., Moretz, W. H., Dozy, A. W., Wilson, J. B. and Vilet, G. V., *Biochem. J.*, **107**, 745 (1968).

48 Air, G. M., Thompson, E. O. P., Richardson, B. J. and Sharman, G. B., *Nature*, **229**, 391 (1971).

49 Matsuda, G., Takei, H., Wu, K. C. and Shiozawa, T., *Int. J. Protein Res.*, **3**, 173 (1971).
50 Matsuda, G., Maita, T., Mizuno, K. and Ota, H., *Nature*, in press.
51 Chauvet, J. P. and Acher, R., *FEBS Letters*, **10**, 136 (1970).
52 Hilse, K. and Braunitzer, G., *Z. Physiol. Chem.*, **349**, 433 (1968).
53 Braunitzer, G. and Fujiki, H., *Naturwissenschaften*, **56**, 322 (1969).
54 Li, S. L. and Riggs, A., *J. Biol. Chem.*, **245**, 6149 (1970).
55 Braun, V., Crichton, R. R. and Braunitzer, G., *Z. Physiol. Chem.*, **349**, 197 (1968).
56 Buse, G., Braig, S. and Braunitzer, G., *Z. Physiol. Chem.*, **350**, 1686 (1969).
57 Braunitzer, G., personal communication.
58 Ellfolk, N. and Sievers, G., Atlas of Protein Sequence and Structure, Vol. 5 (National Biomedical Research Foundation, Washington, D. C., 1972) P. D-81.
59 Braunitzer, G., Hilschmann, N. and Wittmann-Liebold, B., *Z. Physiol. Chem.*, **325**, 94 (1961).
60 Schroeder, W. A., *Ann. Rev. Biochem.*, **32**, 301 (1963).
61 Huisman, T. H. J. and Schroeder, W. A., CRC Critical Reviews in Clinical Laboratory Science (July, 1970), p. 471.

Gas Transport

I. Tyuma

Department of Physicochemical Physiology, Medical School,
Osaka University, Osaka, Japan

One of the central functions of the blood is to transfer oxygen from the lungs to the tissues and carbon dioxide from the tissues to the lungs. Of the total amount of oxygen and carbon dioxide carried by the blood, less than 5% is found to be in simple physical solution (Table I). The remainder of the transport of the 2 gases involves complex reversible chemical reactions, in which hemoglobin, the pigment protein of erythrocytes, plays a key role. This chapter outlines present knowledge of the reversible chemical reactions occurring in human blood or hemoglobin solutions.

TRANSPORT OF OXYGEN

As indicated in Table I, 100 ml of standard human arterial blood contains 20.3 ml oxygen (oxygen content), of which only 0.3 ml is physically dissolved. The remainder, 20 ml, is reversibly bound to ferrous heme iron in hemoglobin. Since the combination of the heme iron with oxygen is stoichiometric, the oxygen-combining capacity (oxygen capacity) of 1 gram of hemoglobin is 1.38 ml, the oxygen

TABLE I. Standard values for blood gases.

	Arterial blood	Mixed venous blood
Oxygen		
pO_2 (mmHg)	100	40
O_2 content (vol %)	20.3	15.5
Dissolved O_2 (vol %)	0.3	0.12
Carbon dioxide		
pCO_2 (mmHg)	40	46.5
Total CO_2 (vol %)	49.0	53.1
Dissolved CO_2 (vol %)	2.6	2.9
Plasma pH	7.40	7.376

capacity of 100 ml normal blood containing 15 grams hemoglobin being 20.7 ml.

1) Oxygen Equilibrium Curve

The combination of hemoglobin with oxygen can conveniently be described in terms of an oxygen equilibrium curve; a plot of oxygen saturation, Y, or its percentage, y, against oxygen pressure, p, or log p. Some representative oxygen equilibrium curves are illustrated in Fig. 1, which includes the best available data for human adult whole blood, obtained by Roughton *et al.*[1)]

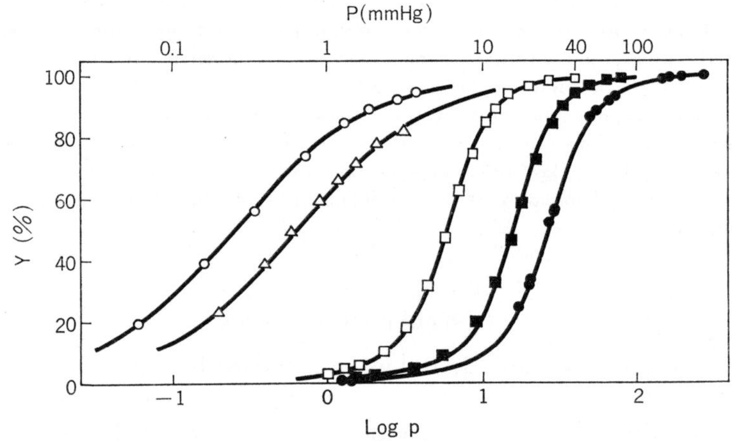

Fig. 1. Oxygen equilibrium curve of human blood, hemoglobin, and hemoglobin subunits. 1, β chains. 2, α chains. 3, stripped Hb A in 0.1 *M* NaCl. 4, stripped Hb A in 0.1 *M* NaCl+2 m*M* 2,3-DPG. 5, Adult whole blood, plotted from the data of Roughton *et al.*[1)] Other experimental conditions are as shown in Table II. Symbols refer to experimental points and solid lines are the simulated curves constructed from Eqs. (8) or (1) using the estimates of k's or K and *n* listed in Table II.

As seen in the figure, the curve for whole blood and hemoglobin displays a characteristic sigmoid shape. This is physiologically important for oxygen transport. At pO_2 of 100 mmHg (a standard value for alveolar pO_2) the blood equilibrium curve (curve 5) indicates about 97% oxygen saturation, and the saturation changes only slightly with minor alterations of the alveolar pO_2. On the other hand, the curve becomes very steep near pO_2=40 mmHg, *i.e.*, a normal value for mixed venous blood, facilitating the unloading of oxygen at the tissues. This remarkable feature is a characteristic of native hemoglobin, a tetramer composed of 2 different kinds of subunits. The α and β chains isolated from human adult hemoglobin (Hb A, $\alpha_2\beta_2$) show flat equilibrium curves with very high oxygen affinity (curves 1 and 2), although the latter chains exist in the tetrameric form, β_4.[2)]

The oxygen affinity of hemoglobin is conventionally expressed in terms of P_{50}, the oxygen pressure at y=50%. The P_{50} for human adult blood under physiological conditions is between 26 and 27 mmHg. The oxygen equilibrium curves for other animals are summarized in the handbook "Respiration and Circulation",[3)] and experimental methods for the determination of the equilibrium curves are reviewed in the recent monograph of Antonini and Brunori.[4)]

Hill's equation: An empirical but very simple way of describing the oxygen equilibrium curve is the Hill equation,[5)]

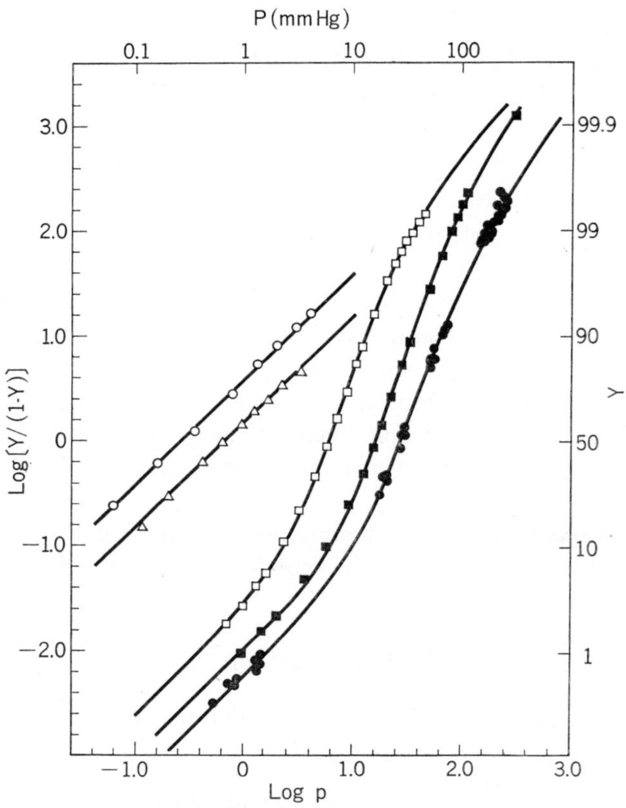

Fig. 2. Hill plots of the data shown in Fig. 1.

$$Y = \frac{y}{100} = \frac{Kp^n}{1+Kp^n} \tag{1}$$

where $K=1/(P_{50})^n$ and n is a constant which determines the sigmoidicity of the equilibrium curve. On rearrangement, and taking logarithms, Eq. (1) gives

$$\log [Y/(1-Y)] = \log K + n \log p\,. \tag{2}$$

Thus, a plot of log [Y/(1—Y)] against log p, the Hill plot, should yield a straight line making an angle with the log p axis having a tangent equal to n, and an intercept on the log [Y/(1—Y)] axis equal to log K. The plots for the isolated chains shown in Fig. 2 conform to Eq. (2), the value of n being unity. The plots for hemoglobin and whole blood also roughly fit the Hill equation at values of y between 20 and 90% with n=2.7 to 2.8. They deviate, however, from the equation at both ends, the slope approaching unity.

Although the Hill equation itself has no direct physical meaning, Wyman[6] has shown that the value of n defined by

$$n = \frac{d \ln [Y/(1-Y)]}{d \ln p} \tag{3}$$

is related to the overall free energy of interaction among the oxygen combining sites (homotropic interactions), ΔF_I, and that the Hill plot will tend toward an asymptote of unit slope at the ends unless ΔF_I is infinite. For this reason and for simplicity (only 2 parameters), the Hill plot is still in general use for the presentation of binding data in the reactions of hemoglobin, and the value of n is considered to represent the magnitude of the "heme-heme" interaction. In a strict sense, however, the value of n itself is not proportional to ΔF_I (Table II).[6]

Adair's equation: Since 1 hemoglobin molecule contains 4 hemes, it is reasonable to assume that the reaction of the hemoglobin molecule with oxygen takes place in 4 stages[7];

$$Hb(O_2)_{i-1}+O_2 \rightleftharpoons Hb(O_2)_i\,, \quad i=1 \text{ to } 4. \tag{4}$$

The corresponding oxygen saturation function, Adair's equation, can be described in a general form;

$$Y = \frac{A_1p+2A_2p^2+3A_3p^3+4A_4p^4}{4(1+A_1p+A_2p^2+A_3p^3+A_4p^4)} \tag{5}$$

where A's are composite constants including the appropriate equilibrium constants. However, if one assumes that the 4 hemes in the hemoglobin molecule are all equivalent in their reaction with oxygen, A's are related to the equilibrium (association) constants, K's, for the reactions (4) in the following simple way;

$$A_i = \prod_{j=1}^{i} K_j . \quad (6)$$

Since the intrinsic association constants (corrected for statistical factors), k's, for the reactions (4) are given by

$$k_i = K_i[i/(5-i)], \quad (7)$$

the Adair equation can be written as,

$$Y = \frac{k_1p + 3k_1k_2p^2 + 3k_1k_2k_3p^3 + k_1k_2k_3k_4p^4}{1 + 4k_1p + 6k_1k_2p^2 + 4k_1k_2k_3p^3 + k_1k_2k_3k_4p^4} . \quad (8)$$

TABLE II. Intrinsic association constants (k's, $mmHg^{-1}$), P_{50} (mmHg), n_{max}, and ΔF_1 (cal/site) for the equilibrium of oxygen with human hemoglobins. Temperature: 25°C for hemoglobins, 37°C for whole blood. Hemoglobin concentration: 1.5×10^{-5} *M* (tetramer).

Conditions	k_1	k_2	k_3	k_4	P_{50}	n_{max}	ΔF_I	Ref.
Adult whole blood*	0.00545	0.0279	0.00617	2.63	26.6	2.76	3790	1
Hb A at pH 7.4†								
stripped	0.114	0.165	1.17	4.04	1.9	2.51	2080	10
in 0.1 *M* NaCl	0.0240	0.0743	0.0858	7.37	5.8	2.98	3390	11
in 2 m*M* 2,3-DPG	0.0135	0.00894	0.0431	4.23	15.3	3.09	3350	10
in 1.7 m*M* IHP	0.00450	0.00801	0.00372	0.415	70.8	2.38	2680	11
in 0.1 *M* NaCl +2 m*M* DPG	0.0103	0.0231	0.00838	11.2	15.5	3.05	4140	11
Hb A at pH 9.1**								
stripped	0.199	0.554	1.03	4.63	1.2	2.11	1860	12
in 2 m*M* DPG	0.141	0.279	0.920	4.85	1.6	2.38	2090	12
Hb F at pH 7.4†								
stripped	0.0739	0.227	0.297	4.65	2.7	2.44	2450	11
in 2 m*M* 2,3-DPG	0.0251	0.0198	0.0905	4.91	8.9	2.98	3120	11
α chains††		K=1.58			0.63	1.0	0	14
β chains††		K=4.0			0.25	1.0	0	14

* at pCO_2=40 mmHg and pH 7.4.
† 0.05 *M* bis-Tris-HCl.
** 0.05 *M* glycine-NaOH.
†† 0.1 *M* phosphate (pH 7.5), K is defined in Eq. (1).

The value of the 4 k's can be estimated on accurately determined oxygen equilibrium curves either by the least-squares method[1,8–12] or by trial-and-error curve fitting on the Scatchard[13] and Hill plots.[14,15] Once estimates of k's are obtained, the overall free energy of interaction can be simply evaluated by the following relationship;[14]

$$\Delta F_I = RT \ln (k_4/k_1). \qquad (9)$$

Table II lists the estimates of k's for human blood and hemoglobins under various conditions, as obtained by the least-squares method. It also includes P_{50} and the maximum value of the slope of the Hill plot, n_{max}, determined on simulated curves constructed from Eq. (8) and ΔF_I obtained by means of Eq. (9) from the estimates of k's. As seen in Figs. 1 to 4 the fit of the simulated curves to the experimental points is satisfactory, indicating the validity of the Adair equation, at least as a first approximation, in describing the oxygen equilibrium function of hemoglobin.

2) *Factors Affecting on the Oxygen Equilibrium Curve*

It is now well-established that protons, carbon dioxide, and 2,3-diphosphoglycerate (2,3-DPG) also combine with hemoglobin reversibly. Although the binding sites of these 3 ligands are remote from the heme iron atoms, the bindings are related to the oxygenation of the iron atoms, *i.e.*, oxygenation-linked binding;[6,16] there are interactions between the oxygen-binding sites and the sites for the 3 ligands (heterotropic interactions). Moreover, the bindings of the 3 ligands are mutually related, as will be described below.

Carbon dioxide: In 1904 Bohr, Hasselbalch, and Krogh[17] showed that increased pCO_2 shifts the oxygen equilibrium curve to the right (classical Bohr effect). There was much discussion at that time as to whether the shift due to CO_2 could be explained entirely by the concomitant change in pH, or whether CO_2 has, in addition, a specific effect. It has now been shown that CO_2 does exert a specific effect due to its direct combination with uncharged N-terminal α-amino groups of the α and β chains to form carbamino compounds;[18]

$$\text{Hb-NH}_2 + CO_2 \rightleftharpoons \text{Hb-NHCOOH} \rightleftharpoons \text{Hb-NHCOO}^- + H^+. \qquad (10)$$

The oxygenation of hemes favors the equilibrium to the left, promoting the unloading of carbon dioxide in the lungs. Conversely, increased pCO_2 aids the release of oxygen at the tissues. Since increased

pCO_2 inevitably makes the blood more acid, the classical Bohr effect is a composite of the specific effects of CO_2 and pH; the latter effect has conventionally been referred to as the Bohr effect.

pH: As shown in Fig. 3, the change of pH from 7.4 to 9.1 shifts the oxygen equilibrium curve to the left (alkaline Bohr effect), in-

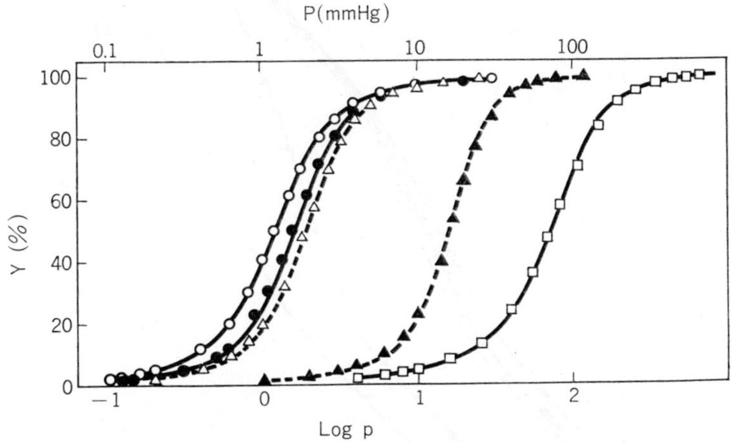

Fig. 3. Effect of pH and organic phosphates on the oxygen equilibrium curve of Hb A. Circles, in 0.05 *M* glycine-NaOH (pH 9.1); triangles and squares, in 0.05 *M* bis-Tris-HCl (pH 7.4); open circles and triangles, stripped; filled circles and triangles, in 2 m*M* 2,3-DPG; open squares, in 1.7 m*M* IHP. Other experimental conditions are shown in Table II. Solid and broken lines are the simulated curves constructed from Eq. (8) using the estimates of k's listed in Table II.

creasing the oxygen affinity of hemoglobin. Below pH 6, on the other hand, the oxygen affinity increases with decreasing pH (acid Bohr effect) (Figs. 5 and 6). However, titration experiments show that oxygenation of the hemoglobin molecule increases its acid strength (depresses the pK) in the pH range 6 to 9, while it increases the pK of certain groups of the protein below pH 6. This led to Wyman[16)] to postulate that there are 2 kinds of acidic groups in hemoglobin, the dissociation of which is linked to the oxygenation of the hemes in the molecule; the pK of one kind of group decreases and that of the other increases on oxygenation. The oxygenation-linked acidic groups involved in the alkaline Bohr effect have now been identified as the α-amino group of valine NA1(1)α and imidazole groups of histidines H5(122)α and HC3(146)β.[19)] The oxygenation of hemes dissociates a proton from

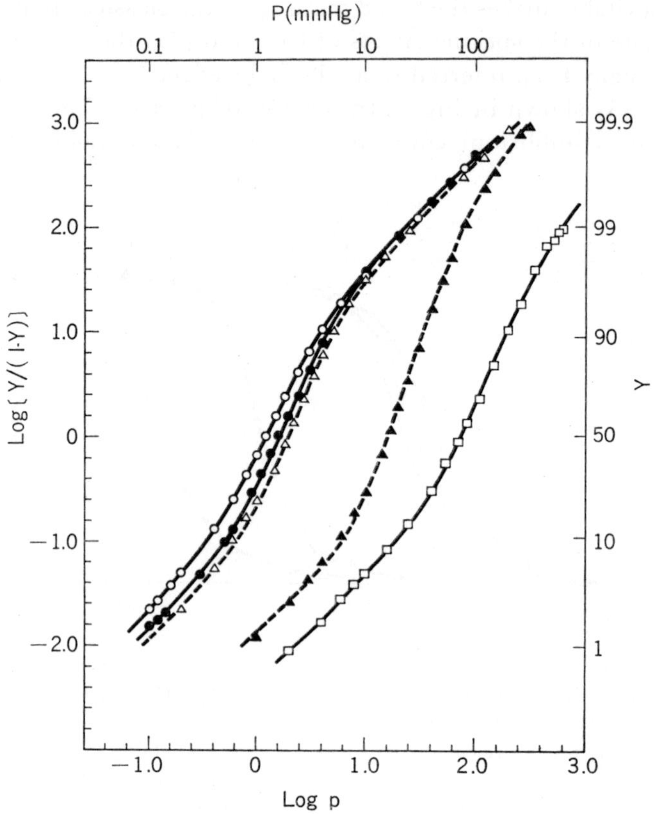

Fig. 4. Hill plots of the data shown in Fig. 3.

these groups, and protonation of the groups releases oxygen from the hemes. The relation is best described by the following equation theoretically derived by Wyman[6,16]:

$$\left(\frac{\partial \log \mathrm{p}}{\partial \,\mathrm{pH}}\right)_{\mathrm{Y}} = \left(\frac{\partial \mathrm{H}^+}{\partial \mathrm{Y}}\right)_{\mathrm{pH}}. \tag{11}$$

If the oxygen equilibrium curve is symmetrical, Eq. (11) can be written in the simplified form:

$$\left(\frac{\partial \log \mathrm{P}_{50}}{\partial \,\mathrm{pH}}\right) = \mathrm{H}^+_{\mathrm{HbO_2}} - \mathrm{H}^+_{\mathrm{Hb}} = \Delta\mathrm{H}^+, \tag{12}$$

where $\mathrm{H}^+_{\mathrm{HbO_2}}$ and $\mathrm{Hb}^+_{\mathrm{Hb}}$ indicate the number of protons per heme bound by oxy- and deoxyhemoglobin, respectively. The relation is

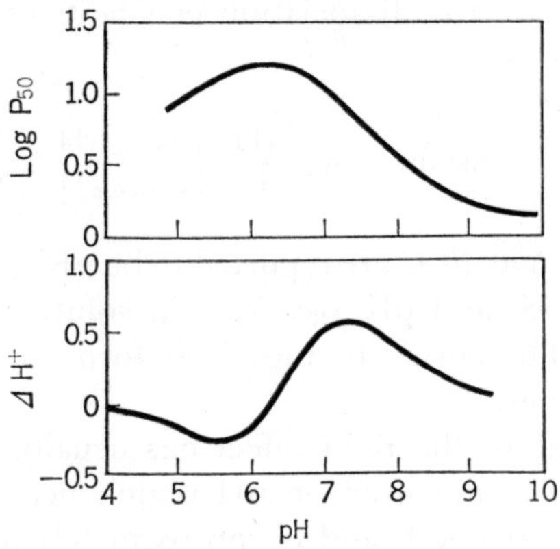

Fig. 5. The Bohr effect for Hb A at 20°C. Dependence of log P_{50} (upper panel) and ΔH^+ (lower panel) upon pH. Ionic strength 0.2 to 0.4 *M*; protein concentration about 5 mg/ml. From Antonini and Brunori.[4]

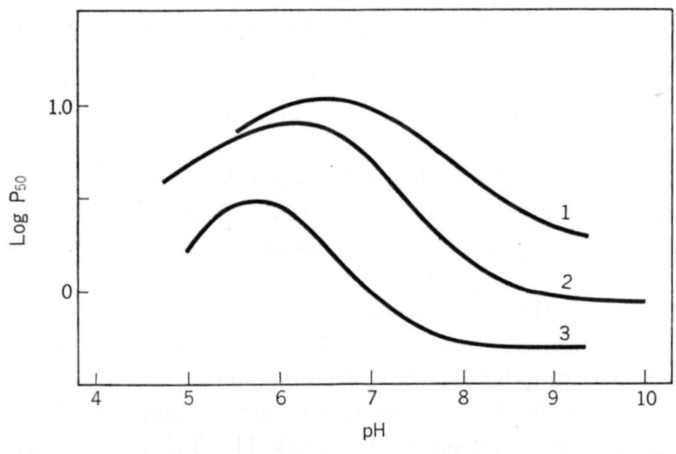

Fig. 6. Dependence of log P_{50} on pH in Hb A at different NaCl concentrations and 20°C. 1, in 2 *M*; 2, in 0.3 *M*; 3, in 10^{-6} to 10^{-3} *M*. From the data of Antonini *et al.*[20]

graphically represented in Fig. 5.

The pK of the 2 oxygenation-linked acidic groups can be calculated from measurements of ΔH^+ or log P_{50} at different pH values. The equations involved in the calculation are the following[16]:

$$-\Delta H^+ = \frac{K'_{HbO_2}}{H^+ + K'_{HbO_2}} - \frac{K'_{Hb}}{H^+ + K'_{Hb}} + \frac{K''_{HbO_2}}{H^+ + K''_{HbO_2}} - \frac{K''_{Hb}}{H^+ + K''_{Hb}} \qquad (13)$$

where K′ and K″ are the dissociation constants of the 2 groups and H^+ is the proton activity.

$$\log P_{50} = \text{constant} + \log \frac{(H^+ + K'_{Hb})(H^+ + K''_{Hb})}{(H^+ + K'_{HbO_2})(H^+ + K''_{HbO_2})} \tag{14}$$

The values for Hb A at 20°C are reported to be $pK'_{HbO_2}=6.26$, $pK'_{Hb}=5.46$, $pK''_{HbO_2}=6.45$, and $pK''_{Hb}=7.85$ in solutions of 0.1 to 0.4 *M* ionic strength.[21] The curves in Fig. 5 conform to Eqs. (13) and (14) with the above values.

The magnitude of the Bohr effect has usually been expressed as $\Delta H^+ = \Delta \log P_{50}/\Delta pH$ measured at pH region near 7 where the log P_{50} vs. pH curve is steepest, and is approximately linear (Fig. 5). The magnitude for Hb A in the absence of CO_2 is about −0.6,[16] while that for human adult whole blood under physiological conditions (pH 7.4, $pCO_2=40$ mmHg, and 37°C) is reported to be −0.48,[22] and it decreases with increasing pCO_2. The binding of CO_2 to the uncharged α-amino group of valine NA1(1)α releases protons (Eq. (10)) and this causes the equilibrium,

$$\text{Hb-NH}_3^+ \rightleftharpoons \text{Hb-NH}_2 + H^+ , \tag{15}$$

to be shifted to the right with the further release of protons. The released protons compensate for the uptake of protons by the other Bohr groups on deoxygenation, decreasing the magnitude of the Bohr effect.

Although the pH independence of the shape of the oxygen equilibrium curve has generally been accepted,[6] recent accurate measurements show that this is not the case.[9,12,23] Our results, shown in Figs. 3 and 4, clearly indicate the dependence of the shape upon pH, the value of n_{max} decreasing with increasing pH (Table II). The dependence of k's upon pH is also not uniform, k_4 being insensitive to pH change. Therefore, the magnitude of the Bohr effect considerably decreases above y=90% with increasing y (Fig. 4).

The isolated α and β chains show no Bohr effect at all.[2]

Temperature: Increase in temperature shifts the oxygen equlibrium curve to the right, facilitating the unloading of oxygen at the active tissues. The temperature coefficient for the shift was determined as $\Delta \log p = 0.024 \Delta T$ in human adult whole blood,[22] assuming a temperature-independent shape for the equilibrium curve. The heat of oxygenation of hemoglobin calculated from the temperature depen-

ınder various conditions ranges from −10.5 to −11.5 f O_2.[4] The magnitude of the Bohr effect decreases with ɔerature.[21] The heat of ionization of the groups re- ᵉe alkaline Bohr effect is 7 to 9 kcal per mole, whereas ı the acid Bohr effect appears to be very near to zero.[21]

ılts and organic phosphates: The profound influence of salts on ᵕ oxygen equilibrium function of hemoglobin has been recognized for a long time.[24] A comparison of curve 3 in Fig. 1 and the curve for stripped Hb A at the same pH in Fig. 3 (open triangles) clearly indicates that the presence of 0.1 *M* NaCl significantly shifts the equilibrium curve to the right. Below 1 *M*, increase in salt concentration decreases the oxygen affinity, although the effect markedly depends upon the type of ion.[25,26] The effect of salts in lowering the oxygen affinity undoubtedly reflects preferential binding of salts by the deoxy as opposed to the oxy form of hemoglobin.

As shown in Fig. 6, NaCl displaces the effective pH region for the Bohr effect toward higher pH values but scarcely affects the magnitude of the Bohr effect below 0.4 *M*.

Recently it has been established that 2,3-DPG, the major organic phosphate of human erythrocytes, tremendously decreases the oxygen affinity of hemoglobins.[27,28] As seen in Figs. 1 and 3, the effect is more marked in the absence of salts than in their presence, and disappears on the addition of 0.5 *M* NaCl.[29] Conversely, in 2 m*M* 2,3-DPG the oxygen equilibrium curve is essentially independent of the salt concentration. Therefore 2,3-DPG can be regarded as an especially effective case of the general salt effect on hemoglobin oxygenation. Benesch *et al.*[30,31] have shown that 2,3-DPG binds with an overwhelming preference for deoxyhemoglobin, not for fully oxygenated hemoglobin, and in a mole-for-mole ratio in 0.1 *M* NaCl at pH 7.3. The binding has been assumed to occur in the central cavity of β chains with salt bridges between the 4 negatively charged groups of 2,3-DPG and the positively charged groups of valine NA1(1), histidine H21(143), and lysine EF6(82).[19,32] The binding constant for fully deoxygenated Hb A under the above conditions was determined as $6.65 \times 10^4\ M^{-1}$ at 20°C by ultrafiltration.[31]

The affinity of 2,3-DPG for hemoglobin decreases with increasing pH[29] and at pH 9.1 the shift of P_{50} due to 2 m*M* DPG is only 0.4 mmHg as compared with the corresponding value of about 14 mmHg at pH 7.4 (Fig. 3 and Table II). The binding constant of 2,3-DPG for the deoxy form of Hb A decreases with increasing temperature and ΔH for the binding is reported to be -13.2 kcal per mole.[29] However, if the binding is assumed to occur when both the α-amino groups of valine NA1(1)β are protonated, the above value includes ΔH for the protonation reaction. The intrinsic binding constant corrected for the associated protonation reaction is found to be virtually temperature-independent.[33] Since CO_2 also combines with the N-terminal α-amino groups, but only when they are in the uncharged form (Eq. (10)), the gas inhibits the effect of 2,3-DPG competitively at pH's greater than 7.3, but not at lower pH.[34] Moreover, 2,3-DPG, especially in low concentrations, increases the magnitude of the Bohr effect,[29] shifting the ionization equilibria involving the N-terminal α-amino groups of the β chains in favor the protonation of deoxyhemoglobin (Eq. (15)): the protonation of these groups becomes linked to oxygenation in the presence of 2,3-DPG.[33] The interactions among the binding of O_2, 2,3-DPG, CO_2, and H^+ in hemoglobin are shown schematically in Fig. 7.

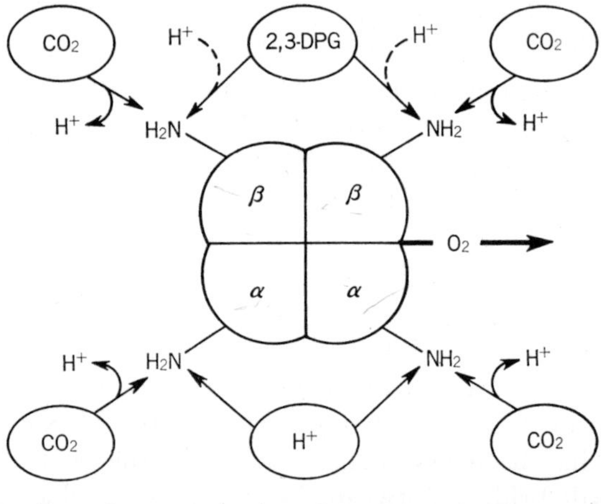

Fig. 7. A schematic representation of the interactions among the binding of O_2, 2,3-DPG, CO_2, and H^+ in hemoglobin. O_2 is released from hemoglobin when the processes proceed in the directions marked by arrows. On deoxygenation the direction of the processes is reversed.

2,3-DPG has no effect on the oxygen equilibrium curve of isolated α and β subunits.[35] Binding measurements, on the other hand, show that while α chains do not react with phosphate at all, the β chains bind 1 mole of 2,3-DPG per β_4 tetramer in both the oxy and deoxy forms.[35] The effect of ATP, which constitutes about a quarter of organic phosphates present in human red cells, on the oxygen equlibrium function of Hb A is very similar to that of 2,3-DPG.[15,27] As shown in Figs. 3 and 4, inositol hexaphosphate (IHP), the major organic phosphate of avian erythrocytes, is more effective than 2,3-DPG in lowering the oxygen affinity of Hb A.[15,30]

Since the concentration of 2,3-DPG and ATP in human erythrocytes is metabolically controlled, as described in other chapters of this book, organic phosphates can act as a prevailing regulator for oxygen transport. This has now been well-recognized under different and even pathological conditions, and its significance is discussed in detail in 2 recent symposium books.[36,37]

Carbon monoxide and methemoglobin: Carbon monoxide and nitric oxide combine with hemoglobin at the same site as does oxygen and in a similar way, but the affinity of the gases for hemoglobin is about 250 and 300,000 times, respectively, higher than that of oxygen.

Douglas *et al.*[38] have found that partial saturation of hemoglobin with CO not only destroys the oxygen-carrying function of the hemes combined with CO but also increases the oxygen affinity of the remaining hemes in this molecule and decreases the sigmoidicity of the oxygen equilibrium curve (Douglas-Haldane effect). Partial oxidation of the hemes in hemoglobin also has a very similar effect (Darling-Roughton effect[39]). Thus, partial carbonmonoxygenation or oxidation of hemoglobin in the circulating blood induces much more serious effects than loss of a similar amount of the circulating hemoglobin due to anemia.

3) *Fetal and Abnormal Hemoglobins*

Fetal hemoglobin: It has long been known that human fetal blood shows a higher oxygen affinity than adult blood[40,41] and this characteristic feature of the fetal blood has been ascribed to fetal hemoglobin (Hb F), $\alpha_2\gamma_2$, contained in it. We have shown, however, that the oxygen affinity of stripped Hb F is actually lower than that of Hb A, while the relationship is reversed in the presence of 2,3-DPG in concentrations roughly one-third of those of effective organic phosphates in the red cells (Fig. 8 and Table II).[42,43] This clearly indicates that the sensitivity of the fetal hemoglobin to 2,3-DPG is less than that of the adult one and that this is responsible for the fetal-maternal difference in the oxygen affinity of the blood, since the data on 2,3-DPG levels in these 2 kinds of blood show no significant difference.[44] The smaller effect of phosphate on Hb F can be ascribed to the loss of 2 of the 4 salt bridges

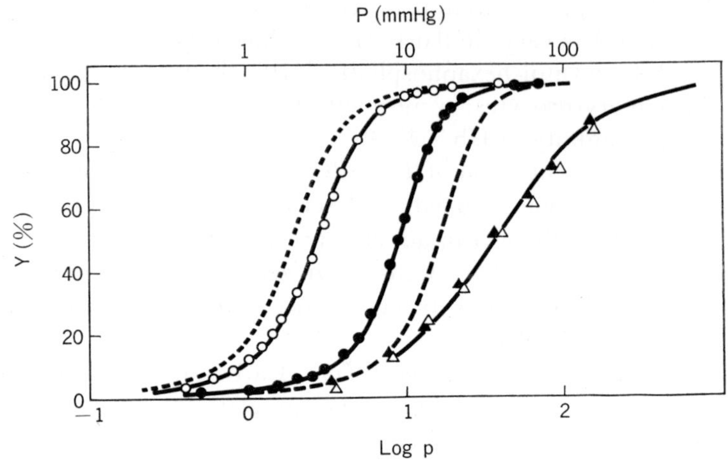

Fig. 8. Oxygen equilibrium curve of human fetal hemoglobin (25°C) and Hb M Boston (19.5°C). Curves for Hb A in the absence and presence of 2 m*M* 2,3-DPG at pH 7.4 indicated in Fig. 3 are shown for comparison (dotted and broken lines, respectively). Open circles, stripped Hb F; filled circles, Hb F in 2 m*M* 2,3-DPG; open triangles, Hb M Boston at pH 7.4; filled triangles, Hb M Boston at pH 6.5. Concentration of Hb M Boston, 6×10^{-4} *M* (tetramer) in 0.2 *M* phosphate. Other experimental conditions for Hb F are shown in Table II. Solid lines for Hb F are the simulated curves constructed from Eq. (8) by using the estimates of k's listed in Table II. The line for Hb M Boston is obtained from Eq. (1) with K= 0.0091 and $n=1.3$.

with 2,3-DPG in this hemoglobin, since histidine H21(143)β, assumed to be involved in the linkages, is replaced by uncharged serine in the γ chains (15).

Abnormal hemoglobins: More than 30 out of 150 abnormal hemoglobins reported to date show abnormal oxygen equilibrium functions. In general, the oxygen transport function of hemoglobin is insensitive to replacements of amino acid residues on its surface but extremely sensitive to replacements near the hemes and at the points of contact between α and β subunits.[45,46] The oxygen equilibrium curve of abnormal hemoglobin M Boston, in which the hemes of the α chains are permanently oxidized to the met form due to the replacement of the distal histidine E7(58)α by tyrosine, is shown in Fig. 7. Evidently the oxygen affinity of the β chains in the abnormal hemoglobin is very low, which is opposite to the result expected from the Darling-Roughton effect. Moreover Hb M Boston shows no Bohr effect and a markedly decreased *n* value.[47] In this case, therefore, the effect of amino acid replacement is not confined to the abnormal chains but extends to the partner chains, the primary structure of which is normal.

The oxygen equilibrium functions of other abnormal hemoglobins are fully discussed from the viewpoint of molecular pathology in 2 recent review articles.[45,46]

4) *Molecular Mechanism of Oxygen Binding in Hemoglobin*

The nature of the heme-heme interaction: As mentioned above, the isolated α and β chains show markedly higher oxygen affinities than Hb A, and no heme-heme interaction. Therefore the interaction among oxygen binding sites must be the result of constraints imposed on the deoxy form of hemoglobin, $\alpha_2\beta_2$. Figuratively speaking, "The first oxygen enters the molecule with more difficulty than the second owing to the necessity of breaking up a pre-existing partnership between the hemes."[16] X-ray crystallographic studies have shown that the distances between the heme iron atoms in the hemoglobin molecule are far too large (25 to 40 Å) for direct interactions to be effective.[48] The studies, however, also demonstrated significant differences in quaternary structure between the deoxy and oxy forms of hemoglobin, the heme separation between the β chains being about 7 Å larger in the former.[48] Moreover, it has been shown that deoxyhemoglobin tetramer is structurally constrained by the following salt bridges,[49]

$$\text{Arg HC3(141)}\alpha^1 \left\langle \begin{array}{l} \text{COO}^- \ldots\ldots\ldots\ldots\ldots\ldots\ldots {}^+\text{NH}_3\text{–Val NA1(1)}\alpha^2 \\ \text{guanidinium}^+ \ \ldots\ldots\ldots {}^-\text{OOC–Asp H9(126)}\alpha^2 \end{array} \right.$$

$$\text{His HC3(146)}\beta^1\text{–COO}^- \ldots\ldots\ldots\ldots\ldots\ldots\ldots\ldots {}^+\text{NH}_3\text{–Lys C6(40)}\alpha^2 ,$$

where the numbering of the subunits in tetrameric Hb A is according to Perutz,[50] the heme iron atom separation between α^1 and β^1 being larger than that between α^2 and β^1. In the presence of 2,3-DPG, the 4 salt bridges between the phosphate and the β chains will be an additional constraint.

The Perutz model: From these and other lines of X-ray crystallographic evidence, Perutz[19] has recently proposed a model for the sequence of cooperative oxygen binding in hemoglobin, in which the 6 salt bridges constraining the deoxyhemoglobin are broken stepwise during oxygenation. The outline of the model is as follows.

In deoxyhemoglobin, the α chains have enough room in the heme pocket for oxygen, but the β chains do not, so that the α chains are likely to react with oxygen first. Oxygenation of the heme of 1 of the α subunits, say α^1, triggers a change in the tertiary structure of the reacting subunit, which causes the links between arginine HC3(141)α^1 and the α^2 subunit to be broken, with the release of Bohr protons. Next, the α^2 chain reacts with oxygen followed by the rupture of the links between the C-terminal arginine and the α^1 subunit, with further release of Bohr protons. Since 4 of the 6 salt bridges constraining the deoxyhemoglobin will have been broken at this stage, the conformation of the tetramer becomes unstable and changes to the deoxy form, breaking the remainder of the salt bridges including those involved with 2,3-DPG. Thus, the reaction of the remaining β chains with oxygen, which also leads to the liberation of Bohr protons, will take place more easily than that of the α chains.

The similarity of the fourth oxygen association constant, k_4, for Hb A in the absence of NaCl to the corresponding constant for isolated β chains (Table II) may be taken to support the idea that the hemoglobin subunit which combines the last oxygen molecule comprises β chains. The model predicts that the total interaction energy among oxygen binding sites is between 6 and 12 kcal per mole of hemoglobin, since the bond energy per salt bridge may reasonably be assumed as 1 to 2 kcal per mole. As seen in Table II, the overall free energy of interaction, ΔF_I, for stripped Hb A and F in the absence of NaCl at pH 7.4 is 2080 and 2450 cal per site, *i.e.*, 8.3 and 9.8 kcal per mole, respectively, and within the predicted range. On the other hand, the proposal that each oxygenation step is accompanied by the release of Bohr protons seems unlikely, since k_4 is insensitive to pH changes (Table II).

The mechanism of action of DPG: The values of overall interaction energy shown in Table II are consistent with the salt-bridge formation between 2,3-DPG and deoxyhemoglobin proposed above. In the absence of NaCl, the increase in ΔF_I due to 2 m*M* 2,3-DPG is about 5.1 and 2.7 kcal per mole for Hb A and F, respectively, which are comparable to the bond energy for the assumed 4 and 2, respectively, salt bridges between phosphate and the non-α chains. The binding of phosphate to hemoglobin in an intermediate stage of oxygenation can be investigated in the following way.

If one assumes that 1 mole of the phosphate, A, combines with 1 mole of hemoglobin tetramer in any oxygenation stage, the equlibria can be described in terms of 5 reversible reactions,

$$Hb(O_2)_j + A \longleftrightarrow Hb(O_2)_j A\,, \quad j = 0 \text{ to } 4. \tag{16}$$

Let M_i be the binding constant for the *j*-th equilibrium, then the Adair constants, A's, in Eq. (5) are expressed as follows;

$$A_i = R_i \prod_{j=1}^{i} K_j \tag{17}$$

where

$$R_i = \frac{1+M_j[A]}{1+M_0[A]} \, . \tag{18}$$

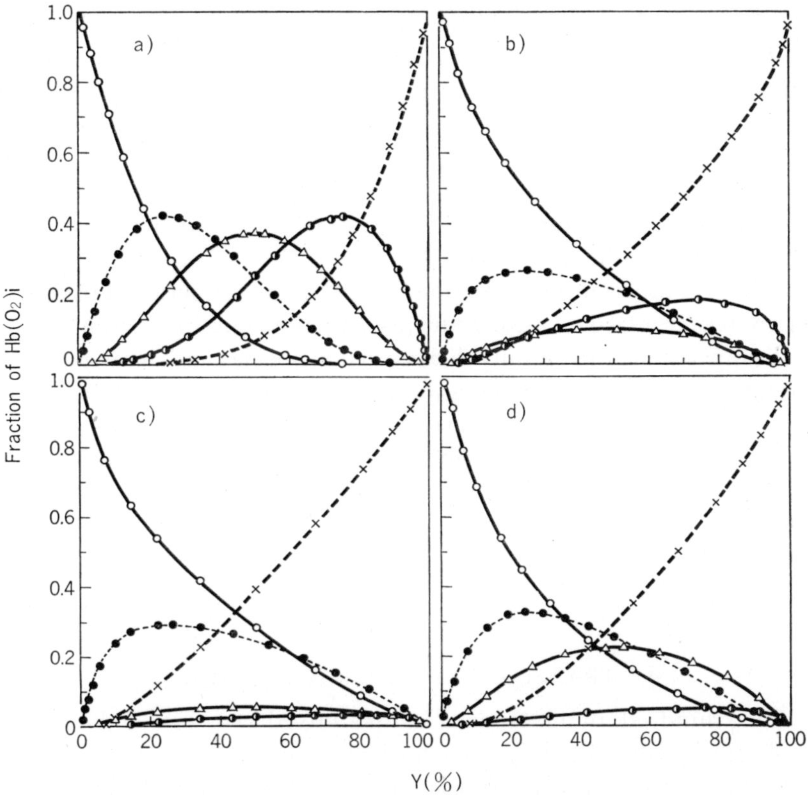

Fig. 9. Fractions of Hb A in various oxygenation stages, $Hb(O_2)_i$, in the absence of NaCl as a function of oxygen saturation, y, calculated from the estimates of k's shown in Table II. (a) no homotropic interaction, *i.e.*, $k_1=k_2=k_3=k_4$, (b) stripped, (c) in 2 m*M* 2,3-DPG, (d) in 1.7 m*M* IHP. Open circles, fully deoxygenated hemoglobin; filled circles, $Hb(O_2)_1$; open triangles, $Hb(O_2)_2$; half-filled circles, $Hb(O_2)_3$; crosses, $Hb(O_2)_4$.

Therefore, one can indirectly estimate the values of M's from analysis of the oxygen equilibrium curves on the basis of appropriate assumptions. The estimates for Hb A in the presence of 0.1 *M* NaCl at pH 7.4 and 25°C obtained by assuming $M_4=0$ are $M_0=3.10\times10^4\ M^{-1}$, $M_1=1.81\times10^4\ M^{-1}$, $M_2=2.58\times10^3\ M^{-1}$, and $M_3=0$,[11] the value for M_0, after correction for slight differences in pH and temperature, being very close to the corresponding value obtained by direct binding experiments.

These results clearly indicate that the links between phosphate and deoxyhemoglobin are also broken successively during oxygenation and DPG is expelled with the addition of the third oxygen molecule.

Fractions of hemoglobin in various oxygenation stages: The values of the 4 k's being defined, it is possible to calculate the fraction of $Hb(O_2)_i$ at a given oxygen saturation. It is also easily shown that the maximum fractions of $Hb(O_2)_1$, $Hb(O_2)_2$, and $Hb(O_2)_3$ are always obtained at y=25, 50, and 75%, and if there is no homotropic interaction the values are 27/64, 3/8, and 27/64, respectively, irrespective of the absolute value of k's (Fig. 9a).

Figure 9 illustrates the fraction of $Hb(O_2)_i$ as a function of oxygenation in representative cases. Evidently, homotropic interaction delays the disappearance of the fully deoxygenated species and accelerates the appearance of $Hb(O_2)_4$, reducing the maximum values of the fractions of other hemoglobin species in various intermediate oxygenation stages. In the presence of organic phosphates, the maximum fraction of $Hb(O_2)_3$ is below 5% and its presence can be neglected except in the region near y=100%. Thus, it can be said, as a first approximation, that the third and fourth oxygen molecules combine with hemoglobin simulataneously.

TRANSPORT OF CARBON DIOXIDE

One hundred ml of standard human mixed venous blood contains 53 ml CO_2 (Table I), only one-third of which is present in the red cells. The remaining two-thirds are found in the blood plasma. However, in the transport of carbon dioxide also, hemoglobin contained in the erythrocytes plays a dominant role. In contrast to the transport of oxygen, where only 1 type of chemical reaction, that with hemoglobin, is predominant the transport of carbon dioxide involves several different types of chemical reaction. Two enlightening reviews of the interrelations among these reactions and their historical buildup are given by Roughton.[51,52)]

1) Various Forms of Carbon Dioxide

When carbon dioxide dissolves in water, it is in the following equilibria at physiological pH:

$$CO_2+H_2O \rightleftharpoons H_2CO_3\,, \tag{19}$$

$$H_2CO_3 \rightleftharpoons H^++HCO_3^-\,. \tag{20}$$

In the absence of catalysts, the rate of reaction (19) is very slow, sufficiently to prevent attainment of equilibrium between the blood and its surroundings during passage through capillaries. However, in the presence of carbonic anhydrase, a zinc-containing enzyme present in red cells, the rate is enormously increased. The reaction (20) reaches equilibrium almost instantaneously. In blood plasma, total carbon dioxide exists in these 3 forms: dissolved CO_2, carbonic acid, and bicarbonate ions. Under physiological conditions, however, the amount of H_2CO_3 is less than 1/300 of that of dissolved CO_2 and can therefore be neglected. The overall process of (19) and (20) is conventionally described by the Henderson-Hasselbalch equation;

$$pH = pK'_1+\log\frac{[HCO_3^-]}{[CO_2]} = pK'_1+\log\frac{[HCO_3^-]}{a\cdot pCO_2}\,, \tag{21}$$

where K'_1 is the apparent first dissociation constant of carbonic acid and a is the solubility coefficient of CO_2 gas, the values for plasma being 8×10^{-7} *M* and 0.301 m*M* $mmHg^{-1}$, respectively, at 38°C. Since pH and pCO_2 can easily and accurately be determined by electrometric methods, the equation has widely been used for the estimation of bicarbonate (and total carbon dioxide) in blood plasma.

In the red cells, in addition to the above 3 forms, a significant fraction of CO_2 exists in the form of carbaminohemoglobin (Eq. (10)). Because CO_2 reacts only with uncharged amino groups, the fraction of hemoglobin combined with carbon dioxide, Z, is given by the following equation.

$$Z = \frac{K_CK_ZpCO_2}{K_CK_ZpCO_2+K_Z[H^+]+[H^+]^2} \tag{22}$$

where K_C is the equilibrium constant of the following reaction,

$$Hb\text{-}NH_2+CO_2 \rightleftharpoons Hb\text{-}NHCOO^-+H^+\,, \tag{10'}$$

and K_Z is the dissociation constant of reaction (15).

$$Hb\text{-}NH_3^+ \rightleftharpoons Hb\text{-}NH_2 + H^+ . \qquad (15)$$

The values of pK_C and pK_Z are reported to be 4.2–4.4 and 7.5–8.3, respectively, at 37°C.[53]

The presence of other forms of carbon dioxide in blood is still dubious.

2) Carbon Dioxide Equilibrium Curve

The carbon dioxide equilibrium curve, a plot of total carbon dioxide content against pCO_2 for deoxygenated and oxygenated whole blood is shown in Fig. 10. The 2 curves differ from the curve for a

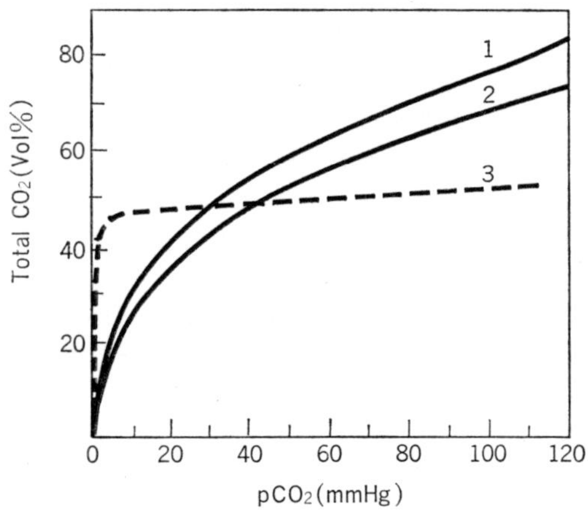

Fig. 10. Carbon dioxide equilibrium curve of human blood at 37°C. 1, deoxygenated blood. 2, oxygenated blood. 3, 24 m*M* $NaHCO_3$ solution.

simple solution of $NaHCO_3$ in the following 2 ways. Firstly, at $pCO_2 = 0$, the total CO_2 content of the blood is zero, whereas $NaHCO_3$ solution still contains an appreciable amount of HCO_3^-. Secondly, above $pCO_2 = 20$ mmHg, the total blood CO_2 content increases with increasing pCO_2, while the $NaHCO_3$ curve becomes flat. In view of the pCO_2 values of arterial and venous blood shown in Table I, this indicates that the simple bicarbonate solution is very poorly adapted for transporting CO_2 in the body.

The difference between the blood and $NaHCO_3$ curves is due to the presence of weak acids, especially hemoglobin, in the blood. The decrease of pCO_2 shifts both the equilibria (19) and (20) to the left.

In the blood, the shift is promoted by the dissociation of H^+ from the acidic groups of hemoglobin, *e.g.*, reaction (15). Normal blood contains ample hemoglobin for the neutralization of its total HCO_3^-. Conversely, an increase in pCO_2 shifts the equilibria to the right and the released protons are taken up by the dissociated groups of hemoglobin. Therefore the carbon dioxide-combining capacity of blood is directly proportional to its buffering capacity.

Figure 10 also shows that deoxygenated blood at any given pCO_2 binds much more carbon dioxide than does oxygenated blood, facilitating the loading of CO_2 at the tissues and the release of the gas at the lungs. The Bohr effect and oxygenation-linked carbaminohemoglobin formation are responsible for the higher carbon dioxide-combining capacity of deoxygenated blood. As described above, deoxyhemoglobin is a weaker acid than oxyhemoglobin and has a greater capacity for taking up hydrogen ions. Moreover, Ferguson[54)] showed that at pCO_2= 40 mmHg and 37°C oxyhemoglobin binds about 0.1 mole CO_2 per mole heme, whereas deoxyhemoglobin binds about 0.34 mole CO_2 per mole heme.

3) Role of Carbaminohemoglobin

On the basis of the above figures, Ferguson suggested that the role of carbaminohemoglobin in physiological CO_2 transport would amount to about 30%. It is clear from Eq. (22), however, that a decrease in H^+ concentration accompanied by the deoxygenation of hemoglobin (Bohr effect) at constant pCO_2 increases the fraction of carbaminohemoglobin. Wyman[16)] calculated the pH difference between oxy- and deoxyhemoglobin solutions in Ferguson's experiments as 0.096 assuming that the magnitude of the Bohr effect (ΔH^+) is 0.6 and that the buffer value of hemoglobin per heme is 2.9 Eq. per pH. He suggested that this pH difference might be sufficient to account for the extra CO_2 contained in the deoxyhemoglobin solutions without the need to suppose that the carbamino reactions of hemoglobin are oxygenation-linked. On this basis he thought that carbaminohemoglobin plays only a minor role in physiological CO_2 transport, the Bohr effect being capable of negotiating essentially all of the transport.

On the other hand, Rossi-Bernardi and Roughton[55)] have decisively demonstrated that even at the same pH and the same pCO_2 the total CO_2 content of deoxyhemoglobin solutions is always greater than that of oxyhemoglobin solutions and that the observed pH shifts on deoxygenation at pCO_2=40 mmHg are about half (ΔpH=0.048) of

Wyman's calculated shifts. They have also demonstrated that the presence of CO_2 evidently decreases the magnitude of the Bohr effect and increases the buffer capacity of both oxy- and deoxyhemoglobins, these 2 factors being responsible for the difference between the observed and calculated pH shifts. According to their calculations the difference in carbaminohemoglobin content between deoxy- and oxyhemoglobin solutions at $pCO_2=40$ mmHg, pH 7.2, and 37°C is 0.21 mole per mole heme, which is 87.5% of Ferguson's corresponding figure.

The above calculations, however, do not include the effect of 2,3-DPG, which is probably depleted in the hemoglobin solutions. An antagonism between carbamate formation and 2,3-DPG in hemoglobin solutions has been reported by Bauer[56] and Tomita and Riggs[34] probably because 2,3-DPG combines with 2 out of the 4 N-terminal α-amino groups in the hemoglobin molecule with which CO_2 is capable of forming carbamate. The role of carbaminohemoglobin in physiological CO_2 transport, therefore, seems to be still unsettled.[52,57]

4) Mechanism of Carbon Dioxide Transport

The chain of processes occurring when carbon dioxide passes from the tissues to the blood is shown schematically in Fig. 11, and its quantitative aspects are summarized in Table III. In the table, the figures for total CO_2, dissolved CO_2, Cl^-, net negative charges (amount of base electrochemically equivalent to the negatively charged protein ions), and volumes represent actual determinations. The amount of carbamino-CO_2 is calculated on the basis of the data of Rossi-Bernardi and Roughton[55] by assuming a linear decrease of the amount with oxygen saturation. HCO_3^- concentration is obtained by subtracting carbamino-CO_2 and dissolved CO_2 from total CO_2, and pH is calculated from Eq. (21). In view of the uncertainty of the role of carbaminohemoglobin, these indirectly obtained values should be taken as tentative.

Carbon dioxide produced by the tissues is released into the blood plasma in the form of dissolved CO_2. Some of the dissolved CO_2 stays in the plasma, but most of it diffuses into the red cells. In the plasma the hydration of CO_2 takes place very slowly due to the absence of carbonic anhydrase. The hydrogen ions produced by the ionization of carbonic acid are buffered by the plasma proteins (Pr) with a concomitant decrease in the net negative charges of the proteins from *a* to *b*.

In the red cells, the largest fraction of carbon dioxide is hydrated

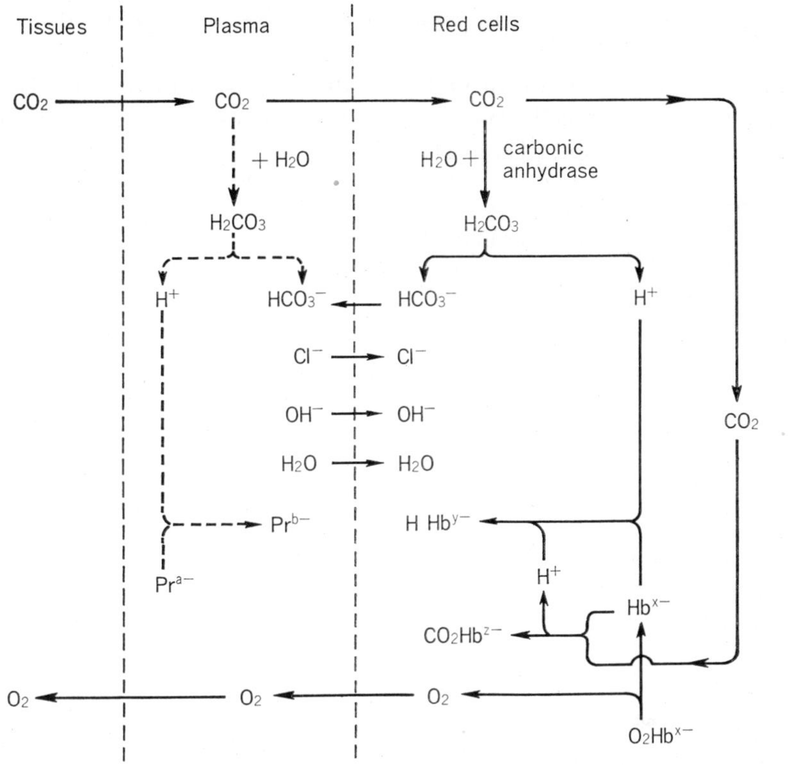

Fig. 11. A schematic representation of the processes occurring when carbon dioxide passes from the tissues to the blood. In the lungs CO_2 is liberated from the blood by a reversal of the direction of each process marked by arrows. For further details see text.

to form carbonic acid, which ionizes to give H^+ and HCO_3^-. These reactions are greatly accelerated by the presence of ample amounts of carbonic anhydrase on one hand and the immediate removal of the reaction products on the other. Hemoglobin, due to its Bohr effect on deoxygenation at the tissues as well as its protein buffer properties, mops up most of the hydrogen ions, and much of the bicarbonate diffuses into the plasma. The remaining CO_2 fraction combines with hemoglobin to form carbaminohemoglobin and H^+, the hydrogen ions being buffered by hemoglobin. The buffering of H^+ by hemoglobin decreases its negative charge from x to y, whereas the carbamino-CO_2 formation increases the charge to z.

The diffusion of HCO_3^- into the plasma is accompanied by the migration of Cl^- from the plasma into the red cells (chloride shift), since the membrane of the erythrocytes is practically impermeable to cations. A small amount of OH^- also diffuses inward from the plasma. Therefore, the red cell-plasma pH difference is slightly less in venous than in arterial blood (Table III).

TABLE III. Distribution of carbon dioxide between plasma and red cells. Adapted from Roughton[51] and Rossi-Bernardi and Roughton.[55]

	Arterial	Venous	(V-A)
Total CO_2 in whole blood	21.88	24.05	+2.17
Plasma			
Total CO_2	14.54	15.66	+1.12
Dissolved CO_2	0.71	0.81	+0.10
HCO_3^-	13.83	14.85	+1.02
Cl^-	57.71	56.84	−0.87
Net negative charges on plasma proteins	9.60	9.47	−0.13
pH	7.40	7.37	−0.03
Volume (ml per liter whole blood)	551.7	548.9	−2.8
Red Cells			
Oxyhemoglobin	8.7	6.0	−2.7
Total CO_2	7.34	8.39	+1.05
Dissolved CO_2	0.48	0.56	+0.08
HCO_3^-	6.05	6.44	+0.39
Carbamino-CO_2	0.81	1.39	+0.58
Cl^-	24.30	25.17	+0.87
Net negative charges on hemoglobin	18.58	16.61	−1.97
pH	7.19	7.17	−0.02
Volume (ml per liter whole blood)	448.3	451.1	+2.8

All quantities except pH and volume are expressed in milliequivalents (mEq) per liter of whole blood.

On the other hand, since the decreased negative charges on hemoglobin are mainly replaced by Cl^- and HCO_3^-, which are osmotically active, the total osmotic pressure of the interior of erythrocytes increases and water moves from the plasma into the cells. Consequently, the volume of the erythrocytes is a little larger in venous than in arterial blood (Table III).

Table III shows that of the total carbon dioxide transport by whole blood, 8.3% is due to changes in dissolved CO_2, 65% is due to changes in HCO_3^-, and 26.7% is due to changes in carbamino-CO_2. The table also indicates an almost equal contribution of the plasma and red cells to the transport. However, of the total HCO_3^- (1.02 mEq) carried in the plasma, about 85% (0.87 mEq=about 40% of the total CO_2 transported by whole blood) is due to the exchange of Cl^- from the plasma with HCO_3^- from the erythrocytes, the primary buffer capacity of the plasma proteins accounting for only 15%.

The contribution of hemoglobin to the transport of carbon dioxide can be evaluated from the decrease in its net negative charge (1.97 mEq), which is balanced by the increase in HCO_3^- (0.39 mEq), carbamino-CO_2 (0.58 mEq), and Cl^- (0.87 mEq). The ionic changes of hemoglobin thus account for about 85% (1.84 mEq) of the total CO_2 transport by whole blood. At the tissues 2.7 mEq of oxyhemoglobin is deoxygenated, which increases the negative charge on hemoglobin by 1.3 mEq if the magnitude of the Bohr effect (ΔH^+ per heme) is 0.48. Therefore, the Bohr effect and the ordinary buffering action of hemoglobin are responsible for about 60 and 25%, respectively, of the total carbon dioxide transport by whole blood.

REFERENCES

1 Roughton, F. J. W., DeLand, E. C., Kernohan, J. C. and Severinghaus, J. W., ed. by Rørth, M. and Astrup, P., Oxygen Affinity of Hemoglobin and Red-Cell Acid-Base Status (Munksgaard, Copenhagen, 1972), p. 73.

2 Tyuma, I., Benesch, R. E. and Benesch, R., *Biochemistry*, **5**, 2957 (1966).

3 Altman, P. L. and Dittmer, D. S., Respiration and Circulation, *Fed. Amer. Soc. Exptl. Biol.* (Bethesda, 1971).

4 Antonini, E. and Brunori, M., Hemoglobin and Myoglobin in Their Reactions with Ligands (North-Holland Publ. Co., Amsterdam, 1971).

5 Hill, A. V., *J. Physiol.*, **40**, p. iv (1910).

6 Wyman, J., *Adv. Protein Chem.*, **19**, 223 (1964).

7 Adair, G. S., *J. Biol. Chem.*, **63**, 529 (1925).

8 Roughton, F. J. W., Otis, A. B. and Lyster, R. L. J., *Proc. Roy. Soc. London Series B*, **144**, 29 (1955).

9 Roughton, F. J. W. and Lyster, R. L. J., *Hvalrådets Skrifter*, **48**, 185 (1965).

10 Imai, K., *Biochemistry*, **12**, 798 (1973).

11 Tyuma, I., Imai, K. and Shimizu, K., *Biochemistry*, **12**, 1491 (1973).

12 Tyuma, I., Kamigawara, Y. and Imai, K., *Biochim. Biophys. Acta*, **310**, 317 (1973).
13 Edsall, J. T., Felsenfeld, G., Goodman, D. S. and Gurd, F. R. N., *J. Amer. Chem. Soc.*, **76**, 3054 (1954).
14 Tyuma, I., Shimizu, K. and Imai, K., *Biochem. Biophys. Res. Comm.*, **43**, 423 (1971).
15 Tyuma, I., Imai, K. and Shimizu, K., *Biochem. Biophys. Res. Comm.*, **44**, 682 (1971).
16 Wyman, J., *Adv. Protein Chem.*, **4**, 410 (1948).
17 Bohr, C., Hasselbalch, K. and Krogh, A., *Scand. Arch. Physiol.*, **16**, 402 (1904).
18 Kilmartin, J. V. and Rossi-Bernardi, L., *Nature*, **222**, 1243 (1969).
19 Perutz, M. F., *Nature*, **228**, 726 (1970).
20 Antonini, E., Amiconi, G. and Brunori, M., ed. by Rørth, M. and Astrup, P., Oxygen Affinity of Hemoglobin and Red-Cell Acid-Base, Status, (Munksgaard, Copenhagen, 1972), p. 121.
21 Antonini, E., Wyman, J., Brunori, M., Fronticelli, C., Bucci, E. and Rossi-Fanelli, A., *J. Biol. Chem.*, **240**, 1096 (1965).
22 Severinghaus, J. W., *J. Appl. Physiol.*, **21**, 1108 (1966).
23 Glauser, S. C., *Fed. Proc.*, **22**, 516 (1963).
24 Barcroft, J. and Camis, M., *J. Physiol.*, **39**, 18 (1909).
25 Rossi-Fanelli, A., Antonini, E. and Caputo, A., *J. Biol. Chem.*, **236**, 397 (1961).
26 Enoki, Y. and Tyuma, I., *Jap. J. Physiol.*, **14**, 280 (1964).
27 Benesch, R. and Benesch, R. E., *Biochem. Biophys. Res. Comm.*, **26**, 162 (1967).
28 Chanutin, A. and Curnish, R. R., *Arch. Biochem. Biophys.*, **121**, 96 (1967).
29 Benesch, R. E., Benesch, R. and Yu, C. I., *Biochemistry*, **8**, 2567 (1969).
30 Benesch, R., Benesch, R. E. and Yu, C. I., *Proc. Nat. Acad. Sci. U.S.*, **59**, 526 (1968).
31 Benesch, R. E., Benesch, R., Renthal, R. and Gratzer, W. B., *Nature*, **234**, 174 (1971).
32 Bunn, H. F. and Briehl, R. W., *J. Clin. Invest.*, **49**, 1088 (1970).
33 Riggs, A., *Proc. Nat. Acad. Sci. U.S.*, **68**, 2062 (1971).
34 Tomita, S. and Riggs, A., *J. Biol. Chem.*, **246**, 547 (1971).
35 Benesch, R., Benesch, R. E. and Enoki, Y., *Proc. Nat. Acad. Sci. U.S.*, **61**, 1102 (1968).
36 Brewer, J., Red-Cell Metabolism and Function (Plenum Press, New York, 1970).
37 Rørth, M. and Astrup, P., Oxygen Affinity of Hemoglobin and Red-Cell Acid-Base Status (Munksgaard, Copenhagen, 1972).
38 Douglas, C. G., Haldane, J. S. and Haldane, J. B. S., *J. Physiol.*, **44**,

275 (1912).
39 Darling, R. C. and Roughton, F. J. W., *Amer. J. Physiol.*, **137**, 56 (1942).
40 Hasselhorst, G. and Stromberger, K., *Z. Geburtshilfe Gynäkol.*, **98**, 49 (1930).
41 Litarczek, C., Soloboziano, H., Aubert, H. and Cosmulesco, I., *Compt. Rend. Soc. Biol.*, **104**, 710 (1930).
42 Tyuma, I. and Shimizu, K., *Arch. Biochem. Biophys.*, **129**, 404 (1969).
43 Tyuma, I. and Shimizu, K., *Fed. Proc.*, **29**, 1112 (1970).
44 Schröter, W. and Winter, P., *Klin. Wochenschr.*, **45**, 255 (1967).
45 Perutz, M. F. and Lehman, H., *Nature*, **219**, 902 (1968).
46 Morimoto, H., Lehman, H. and Perutz, M. F., *Nature*, **232**, 408 (1971).
47 Suzuki, T., Hayashi, A., Yamamura, Y., Enoki, Y. and Tyuma, I., *Biochem. Biophys. Res. Comm.*, **19**, 691 (1965).
48 Muirhead, H. and Perutz, M. F., *Nature*, **199**, 633 (1963).
49 Perutz, M. F., Muirhead, H., Cox, J. M. and Goaman, L. C. G., *Nature*, **219**, 131 (1968).
50 Perutz, M. F., *J. Mol. Biol.*, **13**, 646 (1965).
51 Roughton, F. J. W., ed. by Fenn, W. O. and Rahn, H., Handbook of Physiology, Vol. 1 (American Physiological Society, Washington, 1964), p. 767.
52 Roughton, F. J. W., *Biochem. J.*, **117**, 801 (1970).
53 Siggaard-Andersen, O., *Scand. J. Clin. Lab. Invest.*, **27**, 351 (1971).
54 Ferguson, J. K. W., *J. Physiol.*, **88**, 40 (1936).
55 Rossi-Bernardi, L. and Roughton, F. J. W., *J. Physiol.*, **189**, 1 (1967).
56 Bauer, C., *Life Science*, **8**, 1041 (1969).
57 Rossi-Bernardi, L. and Roughton, F. J. W., *J. Physiol.*, **209**, 25 (1970).

The Role of Hemin in the Control of the Synthesis of Hemoglobin and of Other Proteins

I. M. LONDON and Y. BEUZARD*

Harvard-M. I. T. Program in Health Sciences and Technology
16–512 M. I. T., Cambridge, Massachusetts 02139, U.S.A.

Heme regulates the synthesis of hemoglobin by feedback inhibition of heme synthesis and by enhancement of the formation and coordinate assembly of the α and β chains of globin. Hemin is required for the maintenance of the initiation mechanism in globin synthesis. Current evidence suggests that hemin can inactivate or prevent the formation of an inhibitor which can compete with, or inactivate, M_3 and perhaps other initiation factors. A working hypothesis for the mechanism and site of action of hemin is presented.

The effect of hemin on protein synthesis is not restricted to heme proteins or to erythroid cells. Added hemin promotes the synthesis of carbonic anhydrase in rabbit reticulocytes, and of protein in intact and lysed Krebs II ascites tumor cells; it also promotes the translation of rabbit globin mRNA in the ascites tumor cell extract. A more general role for hemin in the synthesis of proteins in erythroid, and at least certain nonerythroid cells, has implications for an understanding of the consequences of iron deficiency and disorders of heme synthesis.

The role of heme in the synthesis of globin is the subject of very active investigation at present. Although iron deficiency anemia has been recognized for centuries, the mechanisms by which iron and heme affect the synthesis of hemoglobin have not been understood. In this discussion we shall be concerned primarily with the role of heme in the control of the synthesis of globin and of other proteins.

The synthesis of protein by reticulocytes[1–4] and by bone-marrow erythroid cells[4] is greatly enhanced by the addition of iron to the incubation medium. Iron also promotes the synthesis of heme[3,5] by serving as a substrate for combination with protoporphyrin and by

* Permanent address: INSERM Unit 91 Henri Mondor Hospital Creteil 9400 France.

serving as a cofactor in the formation of δ-aminolevulinic acid.[6] These findings gain added significance when one observes that the synthesis of heme and the synthesis of globin proceed in parallel (Fig. 1).[4] Although this parallelism may be disrupted by various

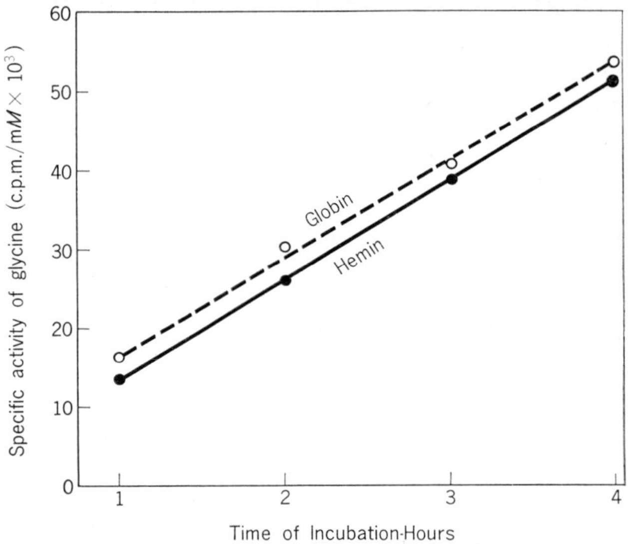

Fig. 1. The synthesis of heme and the incorporation of glycine into globin in rabbit bone marrow *in vitro* as a function of time of incubation.

changes in the conditions of incubation,[3] the evidence of parallel rates of synthesis raised the question of the existence of a mechanism for the coordination of the synthesis of heme and of globin.[1]

Some insight into this question was afforded by the findings that (a) hemin can control its own synthesis by inhibition of one or more steps prior to the formation of δ-aminolevulinic acid (ALA)[7] and (b) that hemin can promote the synthesis of globin in intact reticulocytes[8] (Fig. 2). The control of heme synthesis by heme has been reviewed recently[9] and will not be considered here beyond noting that hemin appears to serve both as an inhibitor of ALA formation, probably by inhibition of ALA synthetase activity, and also as a repressor of the synthesis of the enzyme, ALA synthetase.

The enhancement of globin synthesis following the addition of hemin to the incubation medium of intact reticulocytes is associated with an increase in the size and proportion of the polyribosomes.[10,11] Since added iron, as well as added hemin, serves to stimulate the syn-

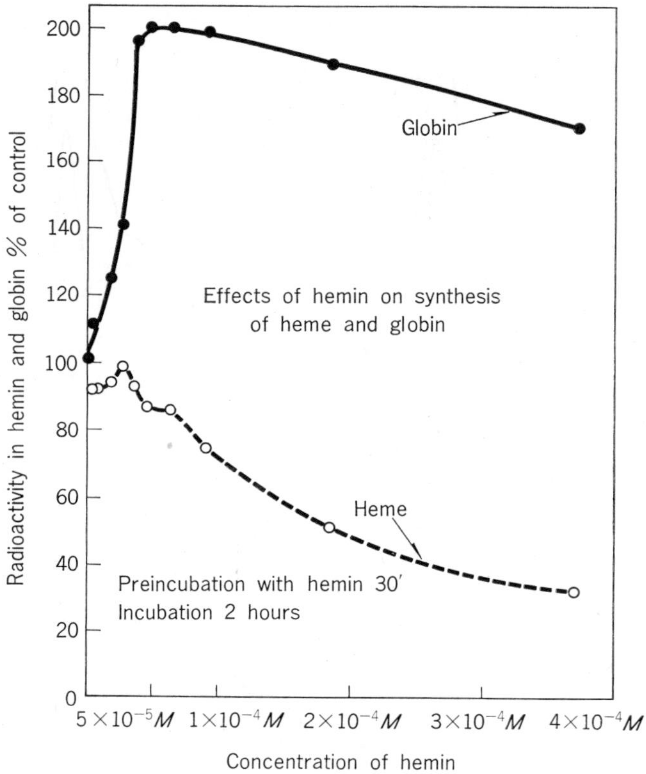

Fig. 2. The effects of various concentrations of added hemin on the utilization of [2-^{14}C]glycine for heme synthesis and of [1-^{14}C]valine for globin synthesis in rabbit reticulocytes.

thesis of globin, it was important to differentiate these effects. Accordingly, reticulocytes were incubated with added iron or added hemin in the presence of the iron-chelating agent, desferrioxamine methane sulfonate (Fig. 3). This agent inhibits globin synthesis and causes disaggregation of polyribosomes. These effects can be prevented by the simultaneous addition of hemin but not of iron. The results demonstrate that hemin acts directly to stimulate globin synthesis and does not serve merely as a source of iron.[10)]

Hemin enhances the synthesis of both α and β chains.[12)] In rabbit reticulocytes, incubation with added hemin serves also to promote the assembly of the hemoglobin tetramer. This effect on assembly is reflected in a disappearance of free β chains; a pool of free α chains persists, however. In rabbit bone-marrow cells, the addition of hemin

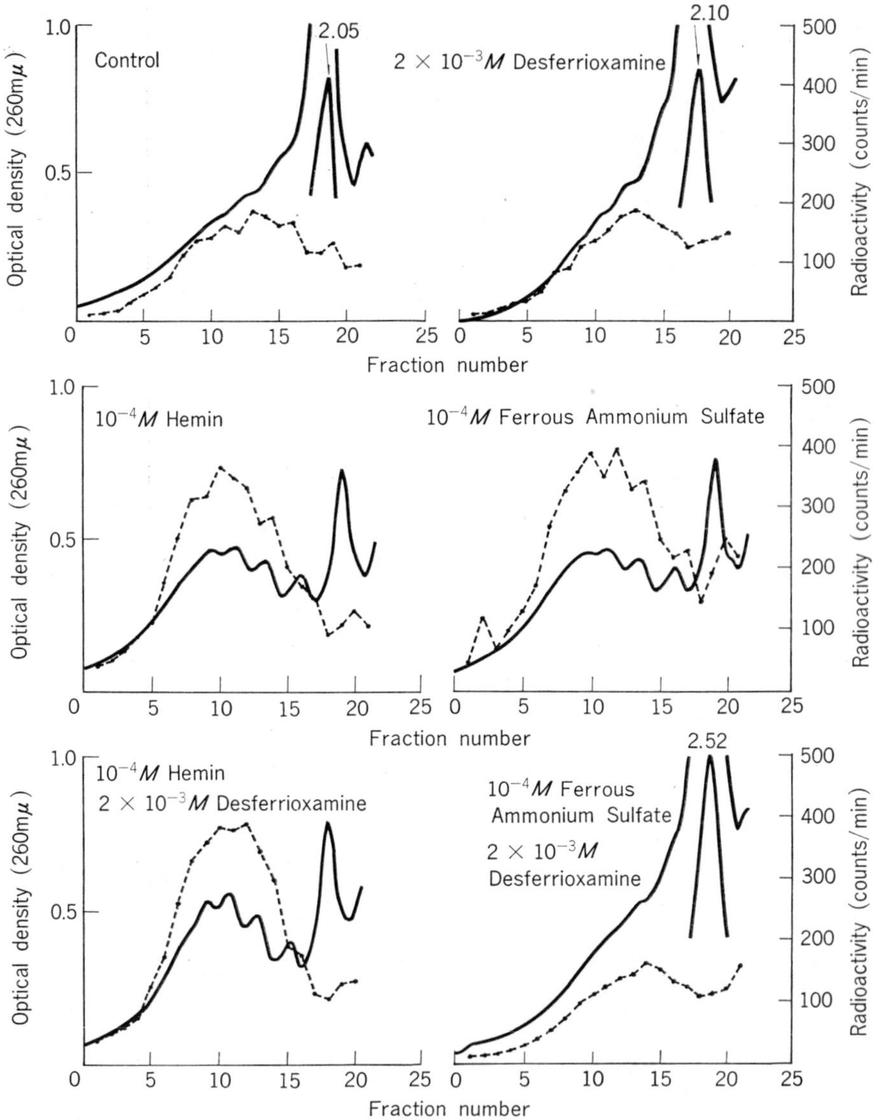

Fig. 3. Incubation for 30 min with no additions (control) or with the compounds indicated.
——, Optical density; ------, radioactivity.

results not only in enhanced synthesis of α and β chains but there is virtually complete disappearance of the pools of free α chains and of αb dimers.[13] These findings suggest that in addition to promoting the synthesis of α and β chains, hemin serves to promote the coordinate assembly of α and β chains in the formation of the hemoglobin tetramer.

The regulation of hemoglobin synthesis by heme is the first known example of control by the prosthetic group of the synthesis of both moieties of a complex protein. Disorders in the formation of heme will be reflected in disturbed synthesis and assembly of globin; disorders in the synthesis of globin will affect the synthesis of heme. This schema of regulation is helpful in understanding the induction and control of hemoglobin synthesis in developing erythroid cells, and it provides a framework for clarifying various disorders of hemoglobin metabolism in man.[14]

The mechanism by which hemin enhances the synthesis of globin has been studied for the most part in reticulocyte lysates. The effect of hemin on the size and proportion of polyribosomes focussed attention on the initiation of globin synthesis as a likely site for the action of hemin. Indeed, it was soon found that the addition of hemin resulted in increased *de novo* synthesis of both α and β chains, *i.e.*, increased initiation from the amino-terminal valine residues.[15]

Hemin is required for the prolonged maintenance of the initiating mechanism; in the absence of added hemin, several rounds of protein

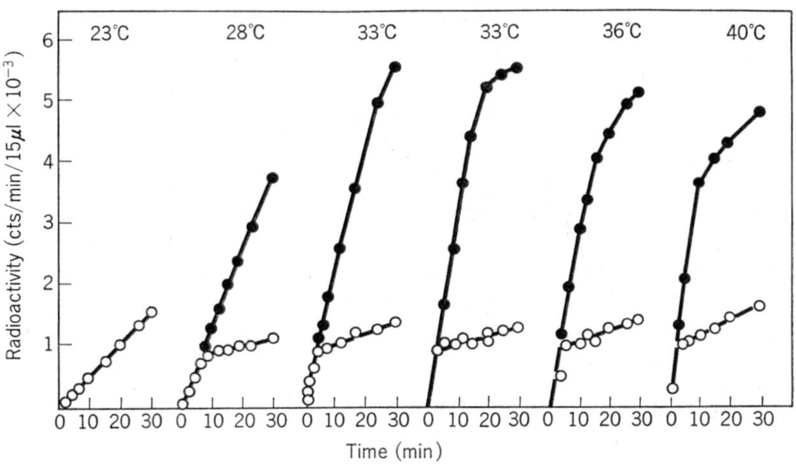

Fig. 4. The effect of temperature on protein synthesis by the lysate. —○—○—, Control; —●—●—, hemin, 3×10^{-5} *M*.

synthesis occur at the initial rate, but within 10 minutes after the start of incubation at temperatures above 25°C, "shut-off" occurs, *i.e.*, there is an abrupt decline in the rate (Fig. 4).[15–17]

Addition of hemin after the start of an incubation is often ineffective in prolonging protein synthesis by the lysate. On those occasions when hemin is effective, there is a distinct lag before synthesis resumes after the addition of hemin (Fig. 5).[16,18] A lysate that has "shut-off" because of lack of added hemin will make protein again at a higher rate if S-100 with hemin is added to it; hemin alone is generally ineffective under these conditions.[16,19] The factor present in S-100 has

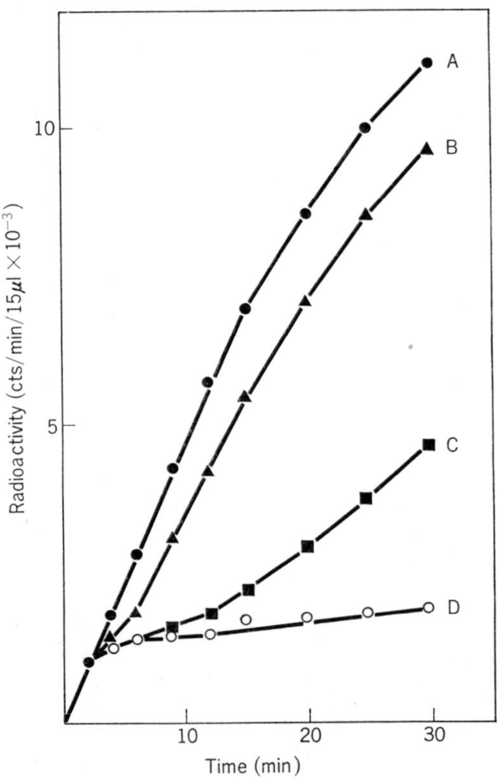

Fig. 5. The effect of adding hemin after the start of an incubation. 3×10^{-3} *M* hemin was added at zero time to 1 sample (curve A), and after 1 min and 5 min of incubation, respectively, at 35°C to 2 other samples (curves B and C) to give a final concentration of 3×10^{-5} *M*. Curve A, Hemin from 0 min; curve B, hemin from 1 min; curve C, hemin from 5 min; curve D, control.

been partially purified (Kosower, Vanderhoff, and London, unpublished data). As yet it is not clear what its relationship is to initiation factors in reticulocytes S-100, which may stimulate the translation of poly U[20,21] or natural mRNA[22] or to the initiation factors which can be extracted from ribosomes with 0.5 *M* KCl.[23–26]

The S-100 from an incubated lysate contains an inhibitor of protein synthesis,[27] and incubation of S-100 alone results in the formation of this inhibitor in the absence of ATP or protein synthesis. Formation of the inhibitor is prevented by hemin at concentrations which prolong synthesis by the lysate.[28] The inhibitor is effective in blocking initiation even when the lysate contains optimal concentrations of hemin, *i.e.*, the inhibitor is irreversible. These properties tended to make this inhibitor an attractive candidate for the role of preventing prolonged synthesis in the absence of added hemin. However, the rate of formation of this irreversible inhibitor seemed to be too slow to account for the rapid onset of shut-off, which usually occurs within 5 minutes at 35°C. Furthermore, inhibitor could not be demonstrated immediately after shut-off in lysates containing no added hemin.[19] To test the hypothesis of the irreversible inhibitor more directly, the following experiment was performed[16]: initially, standard incubation in the presence or absence of added hemin was performed. Shut-off in the absence of hemin occurred in 5 minutes. In the second part, the same lysate was incubated for 10 minutes without hemin or master mix (amino acids, ATP-generating system, ATP, GTP, KCl and $MgCl_2$) and then an identical incubation, as in the first part, was performed with and without added hemin. There was no significant decline in the capacity to synthesize protein due to this preincubation. If shut-off at 5 minutes had been due to the formation of an irreversible inhibitor, it should have accumulated in the 10-minute preincubation and should have inhibited synthesis. These results rendered unlikely the possibility that shut-off is caused by an irreversible inhibitor with the properties described above,[27] but they did not exclude the possibility of a reversible inhibitor which could be inactivated by hemin or of an inhibitor which could be formed quickly by protein synthesis.[16]

The existence of a reversible inhibitor which can be observed during the early period of incubation without hemin and which can be inactivated by hemin and by cooling has recently been reported.[29] This reversible inhibitor is distinct from the irreversible inhibitor described above, but the suggestion has been made that it may be an intermediate in the formation of the irreversible inhibitor. Since the reversible inhibitor can be inactivated by hemin, it may be part of the regulatory process by which hemin controls the synthesis of globin in the intact cell.

The relationships between hemin, the initiation fraction of Miller and Schweet, prepared by extraction of ribosomes with 0.5 *M* KCl, and an inhibitor in the S-100 have been the subject of further investigation.[30] These studies provide evidence that the initiation fraction can block and reverse the action of the inhibitor. The inhibitor acts on initiation, most likely through interference with reactions dependent on the initiation fraction. At low concentrations of initiation fraction, its stimulatory effect is greatly potentiated by hemin; at high concentrations of initiation fraction, the effect of hemin is much less marked. On incubation of intact reticulocytes in the absence of added iron, an inhibitor with properties similar to the S-100 inhibitor is demonstrable.

The site of action of hemin in the process of initiation is as yet uncertain. There is evidence, however, that in the absence of added hemin, the formation of the complex between the 40 S ribosomal subunit and the initiator methionyl-tRNA is impaired.[31] Other studies indicate that in the absence of added hemin there is loss of activity of an initiation factor which inhibits the association of 40 S and 60 S ribosomal subunits and which is required for the binding of globin mRNA to ribosomes.[32] This factor has properties very similar to the M_3 of Anderson *et al.*[26] and to the mRNA-binding activity of Heywood.[33] Studies in our own laboratory with preparations of M_3, generously provided by French-Anderson, indicate that (a) M_3 can promote the resumption of protein synthesis in a reticulocyte lysate in which shut-off has occurred in the absence of added hemin; (b) M_3 can overcome the inhibitory effect of double-stranded RNA (dsRNA) on protein synthesis, an inhibitory effect described previously (34); and (c) hemin can overcome partially the inhibitory effect of dsRNA.

It is important to note that, until the initiation factors have been more highly purified, one should reserve judgement on the site and mechanism of action of hemin and its relationship to 1 or more initiation factors. As a working hypothesis, however, we present the following schema.

Hemin prevents the formation of an inhibitor from a proinhibitor or reverses the formation of the inhibitor. The inhibitor and M_3 compete for the same site or sites in the initiation process, or alternatively, the inhibitor may inactivate M_3. In either case, the effect of M_3 is to promote the formation of active initiation complexes. The steps in this process appear to be as follows:

$$40\ S + \text{met-tRNA}_F + \text{mRNA} \longrightarrow 40\ S\text{-met-tRNA}_F\text{-mRNA} \quad (1)$$

$$40\ S - \text{met-tRNA}_F - \text{mRNA} + 60\ S \rightarrow 80\ S\text{-met-tRNA}_F\text{-mRNA} \quad (2)$$

There is evidence that the first step is divisible into the formation of a 40 S-met-tRNA$_F$ complex which then reacts with mRNA to form the 40 S-met-tRNA$_F$-mRNA complex.[35]

The inactivation of M_3, or competition with it, by inhibitor formed in the absence of hemin will result in diminished formation of the active initiation complex.

The elucidation of these mechanisms must await further purification of the initiation factors and of the reversible inhibitor and analysis of the sequence of steps in the formation of the initiation complex. It is then that the mechanism of action of hemin and the inhibitory effects of dsRNA and oxidized glutathione[36] may be better understood.

In addition to the question of the role of hemin in initiating globin synthesis, there is the closely related question of the specificity of the effect of hemin. Does hemin affect the initiation of nonheme proteins, and if so, does this occur not only in erythroid cells but in other cells in which hemoglobin synthesis does not occur? These questions have been considered in studies[37] which examine (1) the effect of added hemin on the synthesis of carbonic anhydrase as well as of globin in the rabbit reticulocyte; (2) the effect of added hemin on the synthesis of protein in intact Krebs II ascites tumor cells; and (3) the effect of

TABLE I. Effect of hemin on the synthesis of hemoglobin and of carbonic anhydrase in intact rabbit reticulocytes.

		Control cpm/mg	Hemin ($5 \times 10^{-4}\ M$) Added cpm/mg	Ratio of specific activity Plus Hemin/Control
Experiment I	Hemolysate	6,500	12,500	1.8
	Purified hemoglobin	6,400	12,300	1.8
	Purified carbonic anhydrase	86	159	1.8
Experiment II	Hemolysate	4,500	14,500	3.1
	Purified hemoglobin	4,500	14,000	3.0
	Purified carbonic anhydrase	398	908	2.5

added hemin on the translation of endogenous mRNA and of exogenous globin mRNA in the Krebs II ascites tumor-cell extract.

In the intact reticulocyte, in the presence of added hemin, there is enhancement of the synthesis of carbonic anhydrase which is similar to that observed in the synthesis of globin (Table I). The low levels of radioactivity observed in the carbonic anhydrase fractions are consistent with the addition of relatively large amounts of nonisotopic carbonic anhydrase carrier. The identity and purity of the carbonic anhydrase were established by chromatographic and electrophoretic procedures. These findings support the conclusion that the synthesis of a nonheme protein is enhanced by the addition of hemin to the intact reticulocyte.

The studies with intact Krebs II ascites tumor cells indicate that the effect of hemin is not restricted to erythroid cells. Figure 6 shows

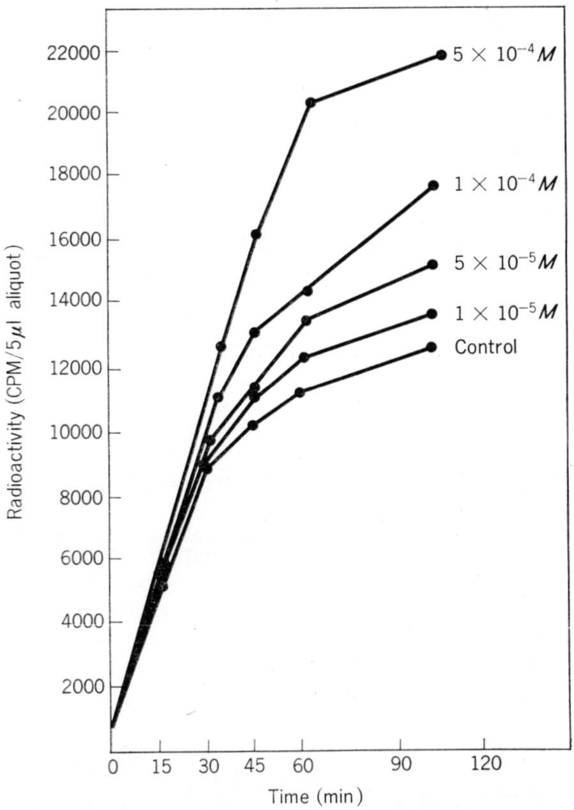

Fig. 6. Effect of various concentrations of hemin on protein synthesis in intact ascites tumor cells.

that protein synthesis in these cells is a function of the concentration of hemin. At the concentrations of hemin added, the initial rate of synthesis does not change. After several minutes, however, the effect of various concentrations of added hemin is reflected in various degrees of maintenance of protein synthesis. Figure 7 illustrates similar findings in an extract of ascites tumor cells. These findings are similar to those observed in the intact reticulocyte and reticulocyte lysate.

The translation of exogenous rabbit globin mRNA in extracts of ascites tumor cells is also enhanced by the addition of hemin (TableII).

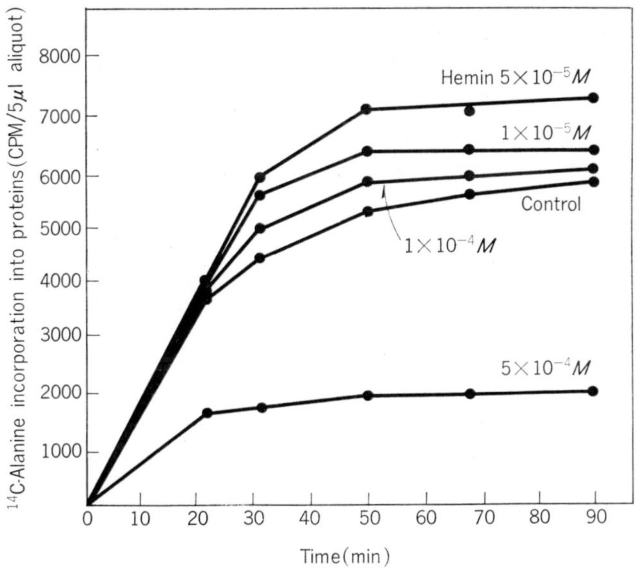

Fig. 7. Effect of various concentrations of hemin on the translation of rabbit reticulocyte mRNA in ascites tumor cell extracts.

TABLE II. Effect of hemin on the translation of 0.5 μgm of rabbit reticulocyte 10 S mRNA in Krebs II ascites cell extract. The final volume is 12 μl and contains: KCl, 100 mmole; $MgCl_2$, 2.7 mmole. The incorporation of ^{14}C-alanine (150 mC/mmole) in proteins is expressed in CPM/10 μl.

Hemin final concentration	Rabbit reticulocyte 10 S mRNA
0	2,900
6×10^{-6} mole	2,900
1.25×10^{-5} mole	3,600
2.5×10^{-5} mole	4,400
5×10^{-5} mole	4,600

When hemin is added at a concentration of 5×10^{-5} *M*, a 60% increase in the translation of the exogenous mRNA occurs; at lower concentrations of added hemin, smaller increments in protein synthesis are observed. Similar findings have been observed on addition of hemin to ascites tumor cell extracts to which mouse globin mRNA or encephalomyocarditis virus mRNA has been added.[38)]

The role of hemin in the synthesis of proteins is not restricted to globin or to erythroid cells. The evidence from our studies, and from studies carried out independently by Hunt[35)] and by Lodish[39)] in reticulocytes, indicates an effect of hemin on protein synthesis more generally. In light of the evidence presented earlier in this paper, it seems likely that hemin can affect the initiation of protein synthesis in erythroid and at least certain nonerythroid cells. This more general effect of hemin has significant implications for an understanding of the hematologic and systemic consequences of iron deficiency and disorders of heme synthesis.

REFERENCES

1 Kruh, J. and Borsook, H., Hemoglobin synthesis in rabbit reticulocytes *in vitro*. *J. Biol. Chem.*, **220**, 905 (1956).

2 Nizet, A., Recherches sur les relations entre les biosyntheses de l'heme et de la globine. *Bull. Soc. Chim. Biol.*, **39**, 265 (1967).

3 Kassenaar, A., Morell, H. and London, I. M., The incorporation of glycine into globin and the synthesis of heme *in vitro* in duck erythrocytes. *J. Biol. Chem.*, **229**, 423 (1957).

4 Morell, H., Savoie, J-C. and London, I. M., The biosynthesis of heme and the incorporation of glycine into globin in rabbit bone marrow *in vitro*. *J. Biol. Chem.*, **233**, 923 (1958).

5 Dresel, E. I. B. and Falk, J. E., Haem and porphyrin formation in intact chicken erythrocytes. *Biochem. J.*, **63**, 72 (1956).

6 Brown, E. G., Evidence for the involvement of ferrous iron in the biosynthesis of δ-aminolevulinic acid by chicken-erythrocyte preparations. *Nature*, **182**, 313 (1958).

7 Karibian, D. and London, I. M., Control of heme synthesis by feedback inhibition. *Biochem. Biophys. Res. Comm.*, **18**, 243 (1965).

8 Bruns, G. P. and London, I. M., The effect of hemin on the synthesis of globin. *Biochem. Biophys. Res. Comm.*, **18**, 236 (1965).

9 Kaplan, B., Synthesis of heme, in Hematology, ed. by Williams, W. J., Beutler, E., Erslev, A. J. and Rundles, R. W. (McGraw-Hill, N. Y., 1972), p. 113.

10 Grayzel, A. I., Horchner, P. and London, I. M., The stimulation of

globin synthesis by heme. *Proc. Nat. Acad. Sci. U.S.*, **55**, 650 (1966).

11 Waxman, H. S. and Rabinovitz, M., Control of reticulocyte polyribosome content and hemoglobin synthesis by heme. *Biochim. Biophys. Acta*, **129**, 369 (1966).

12 Tavill, A. S., Grayzel, A. I., London, I. M., Williams, M. K. and Vanderhoff, G. A., The role of heme in the synthesis and assembly of hemoglobin. *J. Biol. Chem.*, **243**, 4987 (1968).

13 Tavill, A. S., Vanderhoff, G. A. and London, I. M., A comparison of the role of heme in rabbit bone marrow and reticulocytes. *J. Biol. Chem.*, **247**, 326 (1972).

14a London, I. M., Tavill, A. S., Vanderhoff, G. A., Hunt, T. and Grayzel, A. I., Erythroid-cell differentiation and the synthesis and assembly of hemoglobin. *Devel. Biol. Suppl.*, **1**, 227 (1967).

14b London, I. M., The biosynthesis of hemoglobin and its control in relation to some hypochromic anemias in man. *Series Hematologica*, **2**, 1 (1965).

15 Zucker, W. V. and Schulman, H. M., Stimulation of globin-chain initiation by hemin in the reticulocyte cell-free system. *Proc. Nat. Acad. Sci. U.S.*, **59**, 582 (1968).

16 Hunt, T., Vanderhoff, G. A. and London, I. M., Control of globin synthesis: the role of heme. *J. Mol. Biol.*, **66**, 471 (1972).

17 Adamson, S. D., Herbert, E. and Godchaux, W., Factors affecting the rate of protein synthesis in lysate systems from reticulocytes. *Arch. Biochem. Biophys.*, **125**, 671 (1968).

18 Adamson, S. D., Herbert, E. and Kemp, S. F., Effects of hemin and other porphyrins on protein synthesis in a reticulocyte lysate cell-free system. *J. Mol Biol.*, **42**, 247 (1969).

19 Howard, G. A., Adamson, S. D. and Herbert, E., Studies on cessation of protein synthesis in a reticulocyte lysate cell-free system. *Biochim. Biophys. Acta*, **213**, 237 (1970).

20 Mizrahi, I. J., On the relationship between a post-microsomal fraction and polynucleotide-directed amino acid incorporation by rat-liver ribosomes. *Biochim. Biophys. Acta*, **108**, 419 (1965).

21 Beard, N. S. and Armentrout, S. A., Protein synthesis by reticulocyte ribosomes, III. Description of a ribonucleoprotein fraction which stimulates messenger RNA-ribosomal interaction. *Proc. Nat. Acad. Sci. U.S.*, **58**, 750 (1967).

22 Fuhr, J. E., London, I. M. and Grayzel, A. I., A factor promoting the initiation of globin synthesis in a rabbit-reticulocyte cell-free system. *Proc. Nat. Acad. Sci. U.S.*, **63**, 129 (1969).

23 Miller, R. L. and Schweet, R., Isolation of a protein fraction from reticulocyte ribosomes required for *de novo* synthesis of hemoglobin. *Arch. Biochem. Biophys.*, **125**, 632 (1968).

24 Cohen, B. B., A factor converting monoribosomes into polyribosomes during protein synthesis *in vitro*. *Biochem. J.*, **110**, 231 (1968).

25 Shafritz, D. A. and Anderson, W. F., Isolation and partial characterization of reticulocyte factors M_1 and M_2. *J. Biol. Chem.*, **245**, 5553 (1970).

26 Prichard, P. M., Picciano, D. J., Laycock, D. G. and Anderson, W. F., Translation of exogenous messenger RNA for hemoglobin on reticulocyte and liver ribosomes. *Proc. Nat. Acad. Sci. U. S.*, **68**, 2752 (1971).

27 Maxwell, C. R. and Rabinovitz, M., Evidence for an inhibitor in the control of globin synthesis by hemin in a reticulocyte lysate. *Biochem. Biophys. Res. Comm.*, **35**, 79 (1969).

28 Rabinovitz, M., Freedman, M. L., Fisher, J. M. and Maxwell, C. R., Translational control in hemoglobin synthesis. *Cold Spring Harbor Symp. Quant. Biol.*, **34**, 567 (1969).

29 Gross, M. and Rabinovitz, M., Control of globin synthesis in cell-free preparations of reticulocytes by formation of a translational repressor that is inactivated by hemin. *Proc. Nat. Acad. Sci. U.S.*, **69**, 1565 (1972).

30 Adamson, S. D., Yau, P. M-P., Herbert, E. and Zucker, W. V., Involvement of hemin, a stimulating fraction from ribosomes and a protein synthesis inhibitor in the regulation of hemoglobin synthesis. *J. Mol. Biol.*, **63**, 247 (1972).

31 Legon, S., Jackson, R. J. and Hunt, T., How haemin controls protein synthesis in reticulocyte lysates. (submitted for publication).

32 Kaempfer, R. and Kaufman, J., Translational control of hemoglobin synthesis by an initiation factor required for recycling of ribosomes and for their binding to messenger RNA. *Proc. Nat. Acad. Sci. U.S.*, **69**, 3317 (1972).

33 Heywood, S., Specificity of mRNA binding factor in eukaryotes. *Proc. Nat. Acad. Sci. U.S.*, **67**, 1782 (1970).

34 Darnbrough, C., Hunt, T. and Jackson, R. J., A complex between met-$tRNA_F$ and native 40 S subunits in reticulocyte lysates and its disappearance during incubation with double-stranded RNA. *Biochem. Biophys. Res. Comm.*, **48**, 1556 (1972).

35 Hunt, T., (personal communication).

36 Kosower, N. S., Vanderhoff, G. A. and Kosower, E. M., Glutathione VIII. The effects of glutathione disulfide on initiation of protein synthesis. *Biochim. Biophys. Acta.*, **272**, 623 (1972).

37 Beuzard, Y., Rodvien, R. and London, I. M., The effect of hemin on the synthesis of hemoglobin and other proteins in mammalian cells. *Blood*, **40**, 961 (1972).

38 Matthews, M. B., Further studies on the translation of globin mRNA and encephalomyocarditis virus RNA in a cell-free system from Krebs II ascites cells. *Biochim. Biophys. Acta*, **272**, 108 (1972).

39 Lodish, H., (personal communication).

Erythroid-Cell Differentiation by Erythropoietin *in vitro*

F. TAKAKU and Y. MIURA

Professor of Medicine, Head of Hematology Division, Jichi Medical School, Minamikochi-machi, Tochigi-ken, Japan

An *in vitro* method for the study of erythroid cell differentiation, in which spleen of the polycythemic mouse was cultured with erythropoietin, was developed in our laboratory. Using this method, the following characteristics of the erythropoietin-responsive stem cells were demonstrated; sensitivity to irradiation and to actinomycin D, response to initial exposure to erythropoietin, DNA synthesis, appearance in the hematopoietic organ after bone-marrow cell transplantation into an irradiated animal, and regional distribution in the spleen. The presence of erythropoietin in the tissue or cystic fluid of the tumors associated with erythrocytosis was also demonstrated by using this *in vitro* method. Bone marrow cells from patients with various hematological disorders were incubated with erythropoietin. In aplastic anemia and polycythemia vera, different response to erythropoietin were observed in each case. In 2 cases of lymphoblastic leukemia and 1 case of pure red cell aplasia, the bone marrow cells apparently responded *in vitro* to erythropoietin, while no erythroblasts were detected in bone marrow smears. From these observations, it is speculated that some disturbances in hematopoietic-inductive microenvironments, which can be eliminated by transferring the bone marrow cells to the *in vitro* system, may be present in these disorders.

INTRODUCTION

The presence of a factor which is involved in maintaining a stable red-cell concentration by regulating the rate of erythropoiesis, has been well-documented. The speculation that erythropoietin operates only in case of emergency and plays no regulatory role in normal states has prevailed for some time. However, verification of the presence of erythropoietin in normal plasma[1–5] and urine,[6–9] depression of normal erythropoiesis by an administration of antierythropoietin,[10] and other findings have finally invalidated this view of the physiological role of erythropoietin. In these days, no one doubts the importance of this humoral substance in regulating erythropoiesis in normal, as well as in pathological states.

Moreover, series of experiments to elucidate the mechanism of erythroid-cell differentiation by erythropoietin have attracted the attention of many investigators to the problem of hematopoietic stem cells and their differentiation. The results of many studies have indicated that erythropoietin works on erythroid-committed stem cells to differentiate them into erythroblasts.[11–16]

The problem of the differentiation of the hematopoietic stem cell has been discussed for decades. However, many studies have been performed by conventional morphological techniques, the results of which are often too subjective, differing according to individual investigators.[17–21] Thus, erythropoietin provided a first objective and a quantitative method to investigate this classic and still very important subject in hematology.

It is beyond the scope of this short article to cover all the problems related to erythropoietin. Therefore, in this paper, the authors intend to discuss only the subject of the differentiation of erythroid stem cells by erythropoietin *in vitro*, and to introduce the studies which have been performed in our laboratory during the past 8 years.

When we started our work, a number of papers had been published on the *in vitro* effect of erythropoietin on hematopoietic tissue.[22–30] However, most of the studies had been performed using bone marrow cells which contained differentiated erythroblasts as well as undifferentiated stem cells.

At that time, the absence of erythroblasts in the spleen of the polycythemic mouse and the subsequent appearance of these cells after an injection of erythropoietin had been well-documented.[14,31,32] Moreover, the effect of erythropoietin on the differentiated erythroblasts, *i.e.*, to increase heme synthesis or accelerate their maturation, had already been pointed out by several workers.[33–37] Therefore, for observation of the *in vitro* differentiation of erythroblasts by erythropoietin, we planned to use the spleen of the polycythemic mouse as the hematopoietic organ to be cultured under the influence of erythropoietin.

Human bone-marrow cells also have been used for culture under the influence of erythropoietin. Since we have been working in the hematology laboratory in the department of medicine, opportunities to obtain bone-marrow cells from patients with various hematological disorders are abundant.

Therefore, the results of our study will be divided into 2 parts according to the cells cultured.

EFFECT OF ERYTHROPOIETIN ON THE SPLEEN OF THE POLYCYTHEMIC MOUSE *IN VITRO*

In 1964, Miura succeeded in demonstrating the appearance of erythroblasts in the spleen of the polycythemic mouse on addition of erythropoietin *in vitro*.[38] For this demonstration, the spleen had to be incubated for 24 to 48 hr with erythropoietin. As had been already published, the method consisted of taking small fragments from the spleen and attaching them to the wall of the incubation tube with serum containing extract of chick embryo. The incubation mixture consisted of tissue-culture medium NCTC 109 (Difco), calf serum, and erythropoietin which was prepared from the urine of patients with aplastic anemia by acetone precipitation. The appearance of erythroblasts was detected only after 24 hr incubation with erythropoietin, while no erythroblasts were observed in spleen cultured in the absence of erythropoietin. The appearance of erythroblasts due to erythropoietin was also demonstrated by measuring the incorporation of radioactive iron into heme. Apparent heme synthesis was demonstrated in

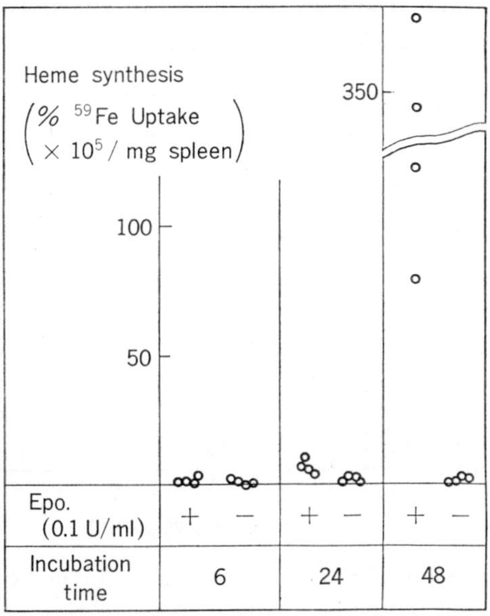

Fig. 1. Effect of erythropoietin on heme synthesis in the spleen of polycythemic mouse *in vitro*.

Spleen fragments were cultured at 37°C for 6–48 hr. ^{59}Fe was added 6 hr before the termination of incubation. Heme was extracted for the radioactivity count.

the spleen of the polycythemic mouse after 48 hr incubation with erythropoietin, while no heme synthesis was observed in the absence of erythropoietin, as shown in Fig. 1. The dose-response relationship between the amounts of erythropoietin added and the resulting heme synthesis was observed. Although this appearance of heme synthesis by erythropoietin is not quantitatively accurate as compared to the erythropoietin-induced increase in heme synthesis observed in a suspension culture of hematopoietic cells, our *in vitro* system was considered to be unique in assaying erythropoietin activity *in vitro* with a system which is very close to the *in vivo* assay system in which the polycythemic mouse is conventionally used as the assay animal.

By using this system, Miura *et al.* measured the *in vivo* and *in vitro* radiosensitivity of erythroid-committed stem cells, obtaining D_{37} values of approximately 70 r and 120 r respectively.[39] Marked sensitivity of the erythropoietin effect to actinomycin D, which had been demonstrated by *in vivo* or *in vitro* assay systems[40–44] was also shown in our *in vitro* system. 0.01 μg/ml of actinomycin D completely blocked erythropoietin-induced heme synthesis in the spleen of the polycythemic mouse.[45] When spleen fragments of the polycythemic mouse were exposed to erythropoietin for 6 hr, transferred to an incubation

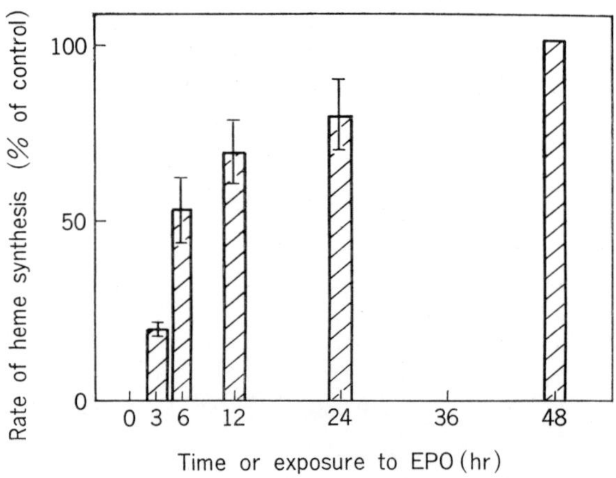

Fig. 2. Effect of limited exposure to erythropoietin on heme synthesis in polycythemic mouse spleen *in vitro*.

Spleen fragments of polycythemic mouse were incubated with erythropoietin for the indicated number of hours, and were then cultured in a medium without erythropoietin until 48 hr later. The rate of heme synthesis in fragments incubated with erythropoietin for 48 hr was regarded as 100%. ^{59}Fe was added on hour 18 of incubation.

medium containing no erythropoietin, and then further incubated for 42 hr, the rate of heme synthesis in the fragments partially exposed to erythropoietin was about 50% of that in the control fragments, which were incubated for 48 hr in constant contact with erythropoietin[45] (Fig. 2). This result is considered to indicate that the necessary events for the differentiation of erythroid stem cells are completed within a short period of time.

Mizoguchi *et al.*[46] cultured the spleen of polycythemic mouse which was lethally irradiated and transfused with isologous bone-marrow cells. When the spleen was removed from the irradiated and bone marrow-transplanted mice after the treatments, erythroid-committed stem cells which were responsive to erythropoietin were first detected on the second day after bone-marrow transplantation, as shown in Fig. 3. Since colony-forming cells (Till and McCulloch[47]) are con-

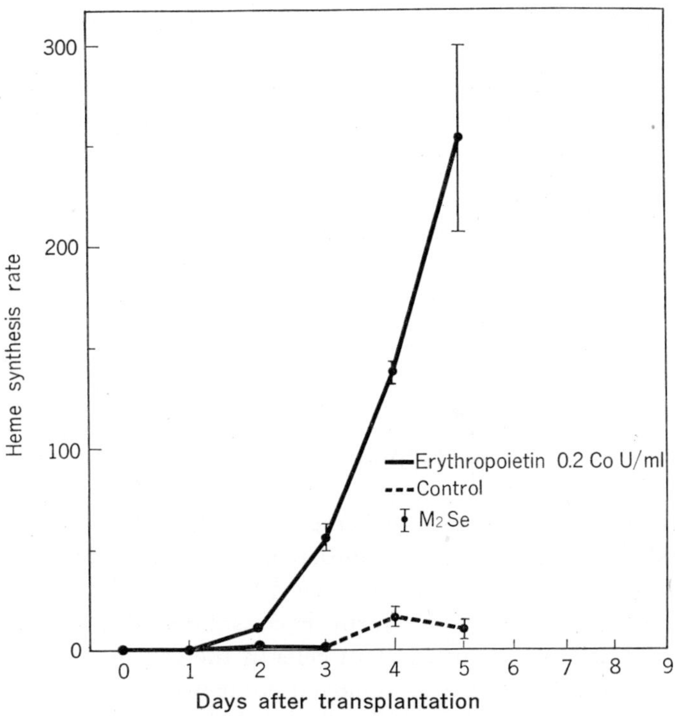

Fig. 3. *In vitro* response of transplanted bone-marrow cells to erythropoietin in the spleen of irradiated polycythemic mice.

Spleen fragments were cultured for 48 hr with erythropoietin. ^{59}Fe was added 6 hr before termination of the culture.

sidered to be present in the spleen of the irradiated mouse soon after the bone-marrow transplantation, the later appearance of measurable amounts of erythropoietin-responsive stem cells is considered to indicate that about 48 hr are necessary for the transplanted colony-forming cells to yield measurable numbers of erythropoietin-responsive stem cells.

Recently, Suzuki *et al.*[48] in our laboratory incubated the capsule of the spleen of polycythemic mouse. The spleen cells were squeezed out from the tissue against a stainless steel mesh. The remaining capsule was washed well with saline, and cut out for incubation by the method which was used for the incubation of spleen fragments. When heme synthesis was compared among the fragments removed from the outer and inner parts, as well as from the capsule of the spleen of polycythemic mouse after 48 hr incubation with erythropoietin, the fragments made from the capsular part of the spleen gave the highest rate of heme synthesis in response to erythropoietin, as shown in Table I.

TABLE I. The rate of heme synthesis in various parts of the spleen of polycythemic or anemic mouse. Capsule, outer and inner layers of the spleen were cultured for 48 hr. Spleen of polycythemic mouse was incubated with 0.2U/ml of erythropoietin. ^{59}Fe was added 6 hr before termination of the culture.

	Erythropoietin	"Capsule"	Outer layer	Inner layer
Polycythemic mouse spleen (48 hr)	+	210±13.0	97±12.9	41± 8.1
	−	0± 0	1± 0.9	0± 0
Anemic mouse spleen (24 hr)	+	167±23.9	408±30.8	272±24.5
				(mean±s.e.)

Rate of heme synthesis=C.P.M./10 γ DNA

In this experiment, the rate of heme synthesis in the fragments was compared among the groups by measuring the radioactivity of radioactive iron incorporated into heme per 10 μg of DNA extracted from the incubated fragments. This result is considered to indicate the presence of erythroid-committed stem cells in the capsular region of the spleen. When the spleen was removed from bled anemic mouse and fragments were prepared from the capsular, outer, and inner portions of the spleen to incubate for 24 hr with radioactive iron, the rate of heme synthesis per DNA was highest in the fragments obtained from the outer part of the spleen (Table I). In this case also, erythropoietin was added to the incubation medium. The rate of heme synthesis in spleen fragments from bled mice measured by short incubation in the presence of erythropoietin is considered to represent mainly the response of erythroblasts present in the fragments. Thus, the erythroblasts are present in the highest concentrations in the outer portion of the spleen, while the erythroid-committed stem cells are located in the capsular region. Figure 4 shows a schematic representation of the move-

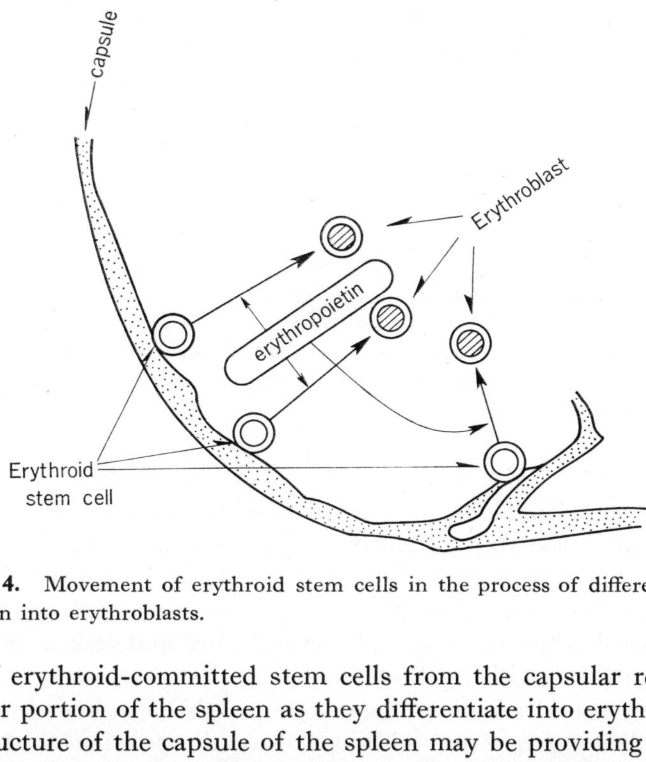

Fig. 4. Movement of erythroid stem cells in the process of differentiation into erythroblasts.

ment of erythroid-committed stem cells from the capsular region to the outer portion of the spleen as they differentiate into erythroblasts. The structure of the capsule of the spleen may be providing suitable hematopoietic-inductive microenvironments (Trentin)[49,50] for the proliferation and differentiation of the erythroid-committed stem cells.

Proliferation of erythroid-committed stem cells in the spleen of the polycythemic mouse had been demonstrated by Miura *et al.*[51] using our *in vitro* system. The incubated spleen fragments were pulsed with ^{3}H-thymidine for 2 hr at times of −2, 0, 6, 22, and 46 hr after the addition of 0.4U/ml of erythropoietin. They were the nchased in a medium containing excess cold thymidine until 48th hr of culture. After incubation, stamps were prepared from the fragments on a glass slide, and the labeling index of the small erythroblasts was counted on the autoradiographed stamp preparation. By this method, we could determine the percentages of differentiated as well as undifferentiated erythroid cells synthesizing DNA during the pulse with ^{3}H-thymidine.

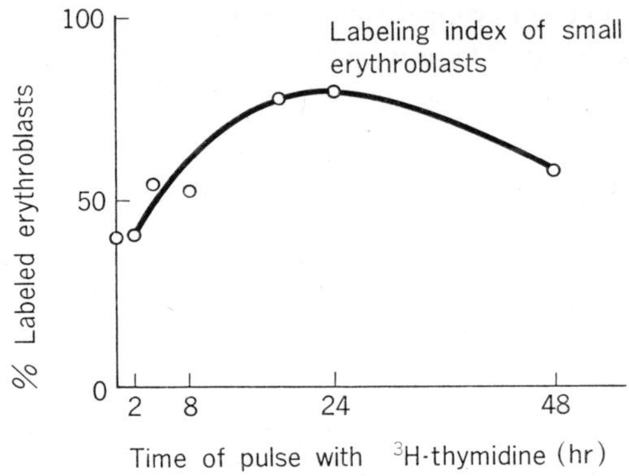

Fig. 5. Labeling index of small erythroblasts in the spleen of polycythemic mouse cultured for 48 hr with erythropoietin.
Spleen fragments were pulsed with ^{3}H-thymidine for 2 hr prior to the indicated time of incubation and then chased in a medium containing excess thymidine.

As shown in Fig. 5, about 40% of the small erythroblasts were labeled when the fragments were exposed to ^{3}H-thymidine for 2 hr before and at the start of culture with erythropoietin. The labeling index increased in proportion to the increase of the contact time with erythropoietin. More than three-fourths of the small erythroblasts were labeled when labeling and chasing were undertaken after 18 to 24 hr incubation with erythropoietin.

An increased mitotic index or rate of DNA synthesis in erythroblasts following *in vitro* addition of erythropoietin has been reported.[52–54] However, autoradiographic studies *in vivo* failed to show any direct increase in the percentages of ^{3}H-thymidine-labeled erythroblasts by erythropoietin.[55–57] When the incorporation of labeled precursors into DNA was measured, the times necessary for the detection of an increased rate of DNA synthesis after addition of erythropoietin markedly differed from 1 to 45 hr according to various investigators.[15,29,58–60] They used different *in vivo* or *in vitro* methods and obtained various results. In spite of these facts, it is generally considered that the increase in DNA synthesis or mitotic index is not an essential initial event taking place after administration of erythropoietin. The increased DNA synthesis is considered to occur mainly as a result of the proliferation of erythroblasts subsequent to differentiation from erythroid stem cells by erythropoietin.

Reports by Hodgson and Eskuche[61] in which they observed a block of the effect of erythropoietin when colchicine or radiation was given before administration of erythropoietin, or the results of thymidine suicide experiments by Lajtha,[62] indicated that the erythropoietin-responsive stem cells are cyclic. Our present experiments, therefore, were also considered to indicate that erythropoietin-responsive stem cells incorporate ^{3}H-thymidine into DNA. Considering the fact that the present experiments were performed using the spleen of polycythemic mouse in which no actual differentiation of erythroblasts from erythropoietin-responsive stem cells is taking place, we may suspect that these stem cells are synthesizing DNA when they are not differentiating. If the erythropoietin-responsive stem cells continue to synthesize DNA while they are not differentiating and undifferentiated stem cells do not die *in situ*, the pool of these stem cells must have been increasing during polycythemia, and the degree of response to erythropoietin could be increased in proportion to the prolongation of the time of polycythemia. It should be noted that DNA synthesis in erythroid stem cells started to increase soon after the addition of erythropoietin *in vitro*, as shown in Fig. 5. From this result it is suggested that the erythroid stem cells try to maintain their pool size by multiplication in the process of differentiation into erythroblasts.

Our method of culturing the spleen of polycythemic mouse was applied for the study of the mechanism of production of erythropoietin in the cells of tumors accompanying erythrocytosis. In this study, Miura *et al.*[63] obtained tumor tissue of cerebellar hemangio-

TABLE II. The rate of heme synthesis* in the mouse spleen cultured with or without tumor fragments.

Spleen of normal mouse was cultured for 48 hr in direct contact with tumor fragments. ^{59}Fe was added 6 hr before termination of the culture.

Tumor+	426±35
Tumor−	196±38

Normal mice were used.

Figures are the mean and one standard error of 3 experiments.

* $\frac{\text{cpm in the heme layer/cpm in 1 ml medium}}{\text{mg spleen}} \times 10^{9}$

blastoma under fresh and sterile conditions from the operating room. The tumor was cut into small fragments and incubated in contact with the spleen of normal mouse. Polycythemic mouse was not available at the time when the surgeons informed us of the operation on the patient. As shown in Table II, in spleen incubated in direct contact with tumor fragments, an apparent increase in the rate of heme synthesis was observed as compared to the control spleen fragments cultured alone. In the cystic fluid of the patient, obtained at the same time during the operation, the presence of erythropoietin was demonstrated *in vitro*. When the spleen of polycythemic mouse was cultured in medium containing the cystic fluid, the appearance of heme synthesis was evident. Moreover, as shown in the Table III, this increase in the rate of heme synthesis was reversed to the control level by adding an antierythropoietin. There is no doubt that the presence of the

TABLE III. Effect of cystic fluid on the rate of heme synthesis* in the spleen of polycythemic mouse *in vitro*.

Spleen fragments of polycythemic mouse were cultured for 48 hr. ^{59}Fe was added before termination of the culture.

Cystic fluid ml/2ml medium	No. of experiments	Heme synthesis rate* Cystic fluid (+) (M±Se)	Cystic fluid (−) (M±Se)
0.2	4	90.5±8.5	14.8±3.4
0.1	1	38.0	0

$$* \ \frac{\text{cpm in the heme layer/cpm in 1 ml medium}}{\text{mg spleen}} \times 10^9$$

tumor cells is closely related to the erythropoietin activity in the cystic fluid. Whether the tumor cells are producing erythropoietin, or whether they produce an enzyme similar to the renal erythropoietic factor (REF)[64,65] which reacts with substrate in the serum to make erythropoietin, is conjectural. It is also possible that the tumor is producing a substrate for this enzyme. However, it seems less likely that, in the patient with cerebellar hemangioblastoma, the REF-like enzyme or substrate produced in the tumor cell react with the substrate or the enzyme in the plasma in the blood vessel to make erythropoietin, and then the erythropoietin formed is concentrated in the cystic fluid. We are inclined, therefore, to consider that erythropoietin itself is produced in the hemangioblastoma cells and excreted into the cyst.

The appearance of heme synthesis in the spleen of polycythemic mouse was also observed by Miura[66] on incubating the spleen in direct contact with hepatoma tissue which was obtained surgically. This patient had erythrocytosis and increased erythropoietin level in his plasma. Contact of the spleen fragments with non-hepatoma tissue from the same patient did not induce any heme synthesis. The presence of erythropoietin in the incubation medium of the hepatoma tissue was demonstrated by the conventional *in vivo* assay using polycythemic mouse. When the spleen of polycythemic mouse was attached to the wall of the incubation tube away from the hepatoma tissue and incubated, apparent heme synthesis was observed. These two tissues could come into contact only through the incubation medium. This fact also shows the presence of erythropoietin in the incubation medium. In culture medium incubated without hepatoma tissue, no erythropoietin activity was detectable.

Incubation of kidney-tissue fragments under the same conditions as for the culture of tumor tissue, failed to demonstrate erythropoietin in the tissue-culture medium.[67] It is considered, therefore, that in the cells of tumors accompanying erythrocytosis, erythropoietin or related substance(s) is produced by a different mechanism from the REF-substrate interaction demonstrated by Gordon and his co-workers.[68]

EFFECT OF ERYTHROPOIETIN ON HUMAN BONE-MARROW CELLS *IN VITRO*

The effect of erythropoietin on human bone-marrow cells has been reported by several investigators.[23,25] However, a clear quantitative effect of erythropoietin on human erythroid cells in the bone marrow was first demonstrated by Krantz.[69] Dose-responsive increase in the rate of synthesis on adding erythropoietin was clearly demonstrated.

After trying several other methods, we finally adopted the same method as that described by Krantz, in which the effect of erythropoietin was measured by the increase in the rate of heme synthesis. This method apparently differed from the above *in vitro* method of culturing the spleen of polycythemic mouse in that in human bone-marrow cells, undifferentiated stem cells and differentiated erythroid cells are mixed. The increase in the rate of heme synthesis due to erythropoietin may not correlate with the numbers of erythroid-committed stem cells. It is possible that the increased rate of heme synthesis is a summation of the response of erythroid-committed stem cells and of differentiated erythroblasts to erythropoietin. Although, in the following discussion, we presume that the increase in the rate of heme synthesis due to erythropoietin represents the number of erythroid-committed stem cells contained in the bone-marrow, the cells measurable by this method are considered to be best called erythropoietin-responsive cells.

The first disorder in which we studied bone-marrow cells for their responsiveness to erythropoietin *in vitro* was aplastic anemia. It was demonstrated by Mizoguchi *et al.*[70] that, in some patients with this disorder, no response to erythropoietin was observed. However, in other cases, a response to erythropoietin similar to that in normal bone-marrow cells was noted (Fig. 6). Even in patients with no demonstrable erythropoietin-responsive cells, when they recovered, response to erythropoietin close to normal was observed on incubating their bone-marrow cells.

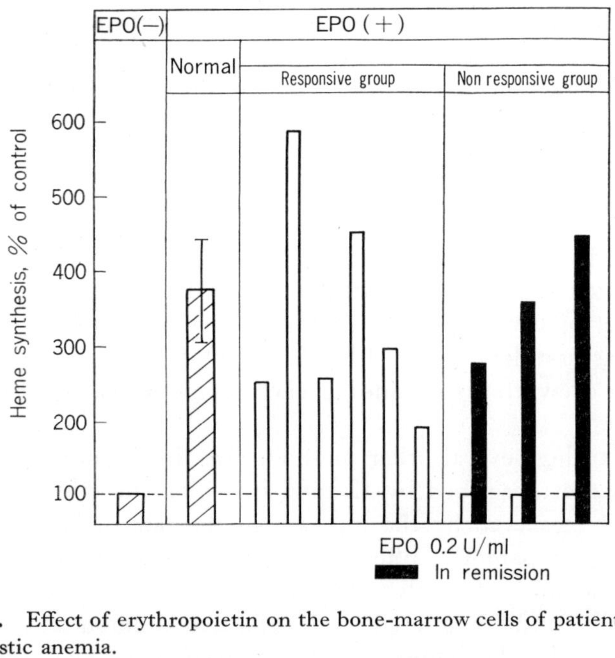

Fig. 6. Effect of erythropoietin on the bone-marrow cells of patients with aplastic anemia.

Bone-marrow cells were incubated with 0.2 U/ml of erythropoietin for 72 hr. ^{59}Fe was added 6 hr before termination of the culture. Solid bars represent the rate of heme synthesis measured in the same patients at the stage of remission.

It has been well-recognized that aplastic anemia is a heterogenous disorder with different etiologies. Our findings of different responses to erythropoietin by case is also suggestive of the heterogeneity of this disorder. Only bone-marrow cells taken from patients with remaining hematopoietic activity, measured by routine hematological methods or by using plasma clearance and red blood-cell utilization of radioactive iron, responded to erythropoietin. However, the difference of hematopoietic activity between the responsive and nonresponsive groups was not marked as compared to the apparent difference in the response to erythropoietin. In consideration of the different responses to erythropoietin observed in patients with aplastic anemia, we have to consider not only the numbers of erythropoietin-responsive cells remaining, but also the microenvironments around these cells. As shown later in this paper, erythropoietin-responsive cells which are suppressed from differentiating *in vivo* can be freed from the suppression when they are transferred to the *in vitro* culture system. Therefore, in patients with aplastic anemia whose bone-marrow cells could respond to erythropoietin *in vitro*, the hematopoietic-inductive microenvironments in the bone marrow might be inhibitory to the differentiation of erythropoietin-responsive cells, while in patients whose bone-marrow cells did not respond to erythropoietin *in vitro*, the numbers of erythropoietin-

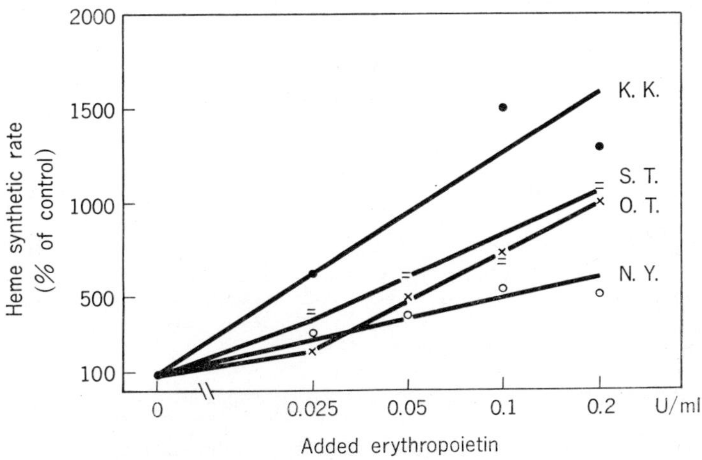

Fig. 7. Effect of erythropoietin on the bone-marrow cells of patients with uremic anemia.

Bone-marrow cells of patients with uremic anemia were incubated for 72 hr with various amounts of erythropoietin. ^{59}Fe was added 6 hr before termination of the culture.

responsive cells were really decreased, or the disorder of the hemato-poietic-inductive microenvironments in the bone marrow of these patients was not eliminated by transferring to the *in vitro* system.

The response of the bone-marrow cells to erythropoietin *in vitro* was also studied in patients with uremic anemia. In all patients, anemia was severe with increased serum urea nitrogen level. In all cases we have studied so far, an apparent increase in heme synthesis in response to added erythropoietin was demonstrated (Fig. 7). The degree of response to erythropoietin was not different from that observed in normal bone-marrow cells. This result shows that although hemato-poiesis is reduced in uremic anemia patients, erythropoietin-responsive cells are present and can respond to erythropoietin as in normal bone-marrow cells. It may be speculated, therefore, that when erythro-

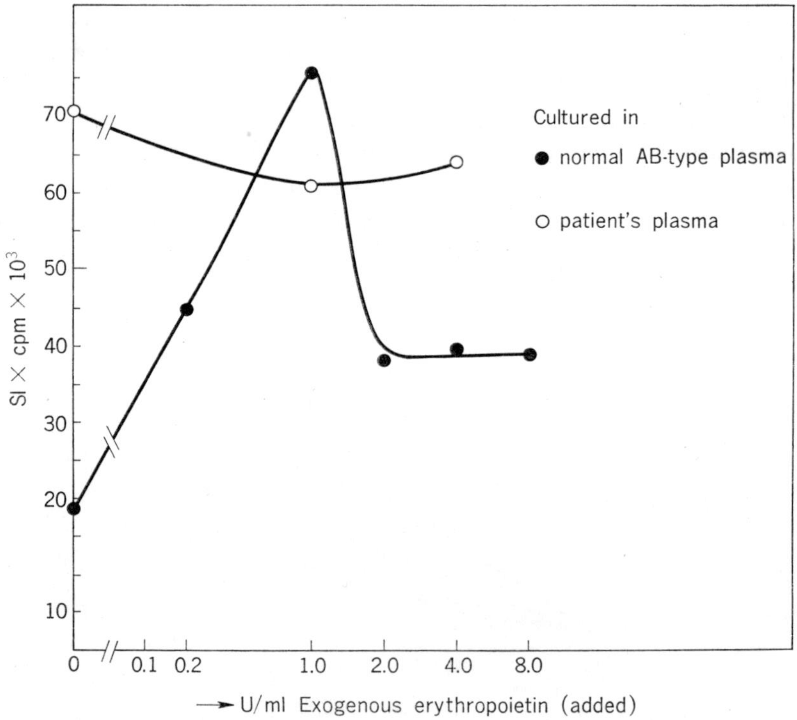

Fig. 8. Effect of exogenous erythropoietin on the rate of heme synthesis in the bone-marrow cells of a patient with pure red-cell aplasia cultured in the patient's or normal plasma.

Bone-marrow cells were cultured for 72 hr with erythropoietin. ^{59}Fe was added 6 hr before termination of the culture.

poietin has become available for clinical use, uremic anemia will be one of the first disorders to be treated.

The presence of an antibody to immature red cells especially directed to the nucleus in the serum of patients with pure red-cell aplasia had been reported by Krantz.[71] When Miura *et al.* incubated for 72 hr the bone-marrow cells of a patient with pure red-cell aplasia in medium containing her own plasma, marked heme synthesis was observed in the absence of exogenous erythropoietin. When her bone-marrow cells were cultured for 72 hr in normal plasma, very slight heme synthesis was detected. However, addition of large amounts of erythropoietin resulted in an increase in the rate of heme synthesis as shown in Fig. 8.[72] It is noteworthy that in a smear of the bone-marrow cells of this patient, the number of erythroblasts was quite few and yet marked heme synthesis was observed on incubation *in vitro* for 72 hr in her own plasma, which contained approximately 5 units/ml of erythropoietin. In this patient, some defects in the differentiation process of erythropoietin-responsive cells to erythroblasts were considered to be present *in vivo*. This defect could have been eliminated when the bone-marrow cells were transferred to the *in vitro* system. Addition of the plasma of the patient to a bone-marrow cell suspension obtained from a normal person with the same ABO typing resulted in an apparent increase in heme synthesis, probably because of the presence of large amounts of erythropoietin in the patient's plasma. Further increase in the amount of the patient's plasma added, however, caused a decrease of heme synthesis in normal bone-marrow cells. The mechanism which makes the patient's bone-marrow cells unable to respond to erythropoietin *in vivo* is unknown.

Similar *in vitro* response to erythropoietin was observed in bone-marrow cells from 2 patients with acute lymphoblastic leukemia by Chiyoda *et al.*[73] in our group. In these patients too, almost no erythroblasts were detected on a smear preparation of bone-marrow cells. However, when bone-marrow cells of these patients were incubated in the presence of erythropoietin, a marked, dose-responsive increase in the rate of heme synthesis was observed, as shown in Fig. 9. In these cases too, erythropoietin-responsive cells which could not be differentiated in the bone marrow *in vivo* were releaed from some inhibition, and became responsive to erythropoietin *in vitro*. These observations on the recovery of responsiveness of erythropoietin-responsive cells to erythropoietin on transferring the bone-marrow cells from the tissue and suspending them in the tissue-culture medium can be

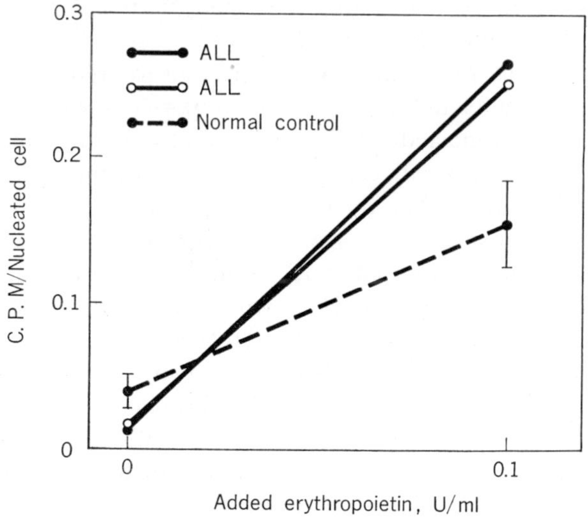

Fig. 9. Effect of erythropoietin on the bone-marrow cells of 2 patients with acute lymphoblastic leukemia.

Bone-marrow cells were cultured for 72 hr with erythropoietin. ^{59}Fe was added 6 hr before termination of the culture.

explained by supposing the presence of some disorder in the hematopoietic-inductive microenvironments in the bone marrow of these patients.

Krantz reported a poor response to erythropoietin *in vitro* in the bone-marrow cells of patients with polycythemia vera.[74] Similar results have also been reported recently by Zucker *et al.*[75] However, when we studied the *in vitro* response to erythropoietin in 4 patients with this disorder, bone-marrow cells from 3 patients responded normally, and only in 1 case was the response poor as compared to normal. From clinical observations on changes of hematopoiesis after bleeding and iron treatment in patients with polycythemia vera, DeGowin and Gurney postulated the presence of 2 kinds of erythroid-committed stem cells, 1 of which is responsive to erythropoietin and the other not.[76] Similar suggestions were also put forward by other people.[77,78] It is possible, therefore, that the present discrepancy in the *in vitro* response to erythropoietin of bone-marrow cells of polycythemia vera is due to the existence of 2 kinds of erythropoietin-responsive cells. If normal stem cells, which are responsive to erythropoietin, predominate in the bone-marrow cell suspension, the effect of adding erythropoietin will appear as an increased rate of heme synthesis. On the other hand, if abnormal stem cells with autonomous differentiation are predominant, no response to erythropoietin will be observed. It is conjectured that in patients with polycythemia vera, because of reduced or absent production of erythropoietin, only pathologic stem cells are differentiated.

Regarding the effect of erythropoietin on the synthesis of different kinds of hemoglobins, Necheles[79)] found that erythropoietin exerts a stimulating effect on hemoglobin A, while the synthesis of hemoglobin F was not affected. Gabuzda *et al.*[80)] observed, by long-term incubation of human bone-marrow cells, a persistence of hemoglobin A synthesis in the presence of erythropoietin, and of hemoglobin F in the absence of erythropoietin. Several investigators, however, found that red-cell transfusion resulted in suppression of the synthesis of hemoglobin F, and that the recurrence of anemia in the same patients induced increased formation of hemoglobin F, indicating that the synthesis of hemoglobin F *in vivo* is under the control of erythropoietin.

Mizoguchi[81)] in our group, incubating human bone-marrow cells in the presence of urinary erythropoietin, found increased incorporation of ^{14}C-isoleucine into hemoglobin. Therefore, the erythropoietin-responsive cells are considered to be differentiated, with a resulting increase of hemoglobin A as well as hemoglobin F.

DISCUSSION

In the initial part of this paper, the results of our *in vitro* studies obtained by incubating the spleen of polycythemic mouse were introduced. As discussed already, this method of culture is unique in that we can observe the differentiation of erythroblasts from erythropoietin-responsive stem cells, morphologically as well as by measuring the rate of heme synthesis. The highest rate of heme synthesis in the capsule of the spleen after incubating with erythropoietin, presented in this report, gives us an important clue to investigate the problem of hematopoietic-inductive microenvironments using an *in vitro* system.

Incubation of the hematopoietic organ in direct contact with tumor tissue from patients with tumors accompanying erythrocytosis provided interesting results concerning the mechanism of erythropoietin production in the tumor tissue. Whether the enzyme-substrate interaction, which has been reported to be necessary for the normal production of erythropoietin, is also operative in the tumor tissue is unknown. However, it is our postulate that the tumor tissue produces erythropoietin itself.

In the latter part of this paper, our work on the *in vitro* response to erythropoietin in human bone-marrow cells from various hematological disorders is presented. The response to erythropoietin has been suggested to represent the number of erythroid stem cells present in the bone marrow of the patients. However, the results of our studies on bone-marrow cells from patients with pure red-cell aplasia or acute lymphoblastic leukemia lead us to a seriously doubt on the possibility that the *in vitro* response to erythropoietin represents the *in vivo* state in the bone marrow of the patient. By removing the bone-marrow cells and suspending them in tissue-culture medium, we are releasing the hepatopoietic cells from the hematopoietic-inductive microenvironments which play an important role in the regulation of differentiation of stem cells.

The problem of stem cells has been attracting the attention of many hematologists, and the pathophysiology of many hematological disorders have been explained based on changes in the nature or the numbers of stem cells. However, changes in the hematopoietic-inductive microenvironments around stem cells in the bone marrow could be as important as changes in the stem cells themselves. Several of our studies related to the problems of hematopoietic-inductive microenvironments, as presented in this article, seem to indicate the importance of the microenvironments in normal as well as in various hematological states. However, for the study of hematopoietic-inductive microenvironments in human bone marrow, organ culture of the bone marrow will be more suitable than suspension culture. The development of new techniques to culture bone-marrow tissue may provide a potent tool for the further progress of studies of this problem.

REFERENCES

1 Reichlin, M. and Harrington, W. J., Studies on erythropoietin. I. Demonstration of erythropoietin in normal plasma. *Blood*, **16**, 1298 (1960).

2 Kuratowska, Z., Kowalski, E., Lipinski, B. and Michalak, E., Human blood as a source for preparation of erythropoietin. *in* Erythropoiesis, ed. by Jacobson, L. O. and Doyle, M. (Grune and Stratton, New York, 1962), p. 58.

3 Gordon, A. S., Weintraub, A. H. and Camiscoli, J. F., Plasma and urinary levels of erythropoietin in Cooley's anemia. *Ann. N.Y. Acad.*

Sci., **119**, 561 (1964).

4 Mirand, E. A., Weintraub, A. H., Gordon, A. S., Prentice, T. C. and Grace, J. T., Jr., Erythropoietic activity of untreated and deproteinized normal human plasma. *Proc. Soc. Exptl. Med.*, **118**, 823 (1965).

5 Goldwasser, E., Biochemical control of erythroid cell development. *in* Current Topics in Developmental Biology. ed. by Monroy, A. and Moscona, A. A. (Academic Press, 1966), p. 173.

6 Finne, P. H., Erythropoietin in concentrates of urine from healthy persons. *Brit. Med. J.*, **1**, 697 (1965).

7 Van Dyke, D. C., Nohr, M. L. and Lawrence, J. H., Erythropoietin in the urine of normal and erythropoietically abnormal human beings. *Blood*, **28**, 535 (1966).

8 Adamson, J. W., Alexanian, R., Martinez, C. and Finch, C. A., Erythropoietin excretion in normal man. *Blood*, **28**, 354 (1966).

9 Alexamian, R., Urinary excretion of erythropoietin in normal men and women. *Blood*, **28**, 344 (1966).

10 Schooley, J. C. and Garcia, J. F., Some properties of serum obtained from rabbits immunized with human urinary erythropoietin. *Blood*, **25**, 204 (1965).

11 Althoff, H. and Werner, H., Zum Angriffspunkt der Erythropoietine am Erythron. *Folia Haematol.* (Frankfurt), **3**, 102 (1958).

12 Alpen, E. L. and Cranmore, D., Observations on the regulation of erythropoiesis and on cellular dynamics by ^{59}Fe autoradiography. *in* Kinetics of Cellular Proliferation. ed. by Stohlman, F., Jr. (Grune & Stratton, New York, 1959), p. 290.

13 Erslev, A. J., The effect of anemic anoxia on the cellular development of nucleated red cells. *Blood*, **14**, 386 (1959).

14 Filmanowicz, E. and Gurney, C. W., Studies on erythropoiesis. XVI. Response to a single dose of erythropoietin in polycythemic mouse. *J. Lab. Clin. Med.*, **57**, 65 (1961).

15 Nakao, K., Takaku, F., Fujioka, S. and Sassa, S., The effect of erythropoietin on hematopoietic organs of the polycythemic mouse. *Blood*, **27**, 537 (1966).

16 Hanna, I. R. A., Response of early erythroid precursors to bleeding. *Nature*, **214**, 355 (1967).

17 Maximow, A. A., Relation of blood cells to connective tissue and endothelium. *Physiol. Rev.*, **4**, 533 (1924).

18 Doan, C. A., Current views on the origin and maturation of the cells of the blood. *J. Lab. Clin. Med.*, **17**, 887 (1932).

19 Sabin, F. R., Miller, F. R., Smithburn, K. C., Thomas, R. M. and Hunmel, L. E., Changes in the bone marrow and blood cells of developing rabbits. *J. Exper. Med.*, **64**, 97 (1936).

20 Downey, H., Handbook of Hematology (New York, Paul B. Hoeber,

Inc., 1938).

21 Bloom, W. and Bartelmez, G. W., Hematopoiesis in young human embryos. *Amer. J. Anat.*, **67**, 21 (1940).

22 Friederici, L., Über den nachweis des erythropoetins in der gewebekultur. *Klin. Wochschr.*, **36**, 132 (1958).

23 Matoth, Y., Biezunski, N. and Szabo, G., Effect of sera from patients with anoxia on the proliferative activity of human erythropoietic tissue *in vitro*. *J. Lab. Clin. Med.*, **51**, 420 (1958).

24 Rosse, W. F. and Gurney, C. W., Studies on erythropoiesis. X. The use of bone-marrow tissue culture in demonstrating erythropoietin. *J. Lab. Clin. Med.*, **53**, 446 (1959).

25 Powsner, E. R. and Berman, L., Erythroblast maturation in bone-marrow culture: Effect of erythropoietin. *Blood*, **18**, 781 (1961).

26 Erslev, A. J., Erythropoietin *in vitro*. *in* Erythropoiesis, ed. by Jacobson, L. O. and Doyle, M. (New York, Grume & Stratton, 1962), p. 275.

27 Krantz, S. B., Gallien-Lartigue, O. and Goldwasser, E., The effect of erythropoietin upon heme synthesis by marrow cells *in vitro*. *J. Biol. Chem.*, **238**, 4085 (1963).

28 Dukes, P. P., Takaku, F. and Goldwasser, E., The effect of erythropoietin upon utilization of glucosamine by marrow cells in culture. *Biochem. Biophys. Res. Comm.*, **13**, 223 (1963).

29 Erslev, A. J., Erythropoietin *in vitro*. II. Effect on " stem cells ". *Blood*, **24**, 331 (1964).

30 Gallien-Lartigue, O. and Goldwasser, E., Hemoglobin synthesis in marrow-cell culture. The effect of rat plasma on rat cells. *Science*, **145**, 277 (1964).

31 Jacobson, L. O., Goldwasser, E., Plzak, L. and Fried, W., Studies on erythropoiesis. IV. Reticulocyte response of hypophysectomized and polycythemic rodents to erythropoietin. *Proc. Soc. Exptl. Biol. Med.*, **94**, 243 (1957).

32 Gurney, C. W., Wackman, N. and Filmanowicz, E., Studies on erythropoiesis. XVII. Some quantitative aspects of the erythropoietic response to erythropoietin. *Blood*, **17**, 531 (1961).

33 Fischer, S., Studies on the mechanism and site of action of erythropoietin. *in* Erythropoiesis. ed. by Jacobson, L. O. and Doyle, M. (New york, Grume & Stratton, 1962), p. 204.

34 Gordon, A. S., Lo Bue, J., Dornfest, B. S. and Cooper, G. W., Reticulocyte and leukocyte release from isolated rat legs and femurs. *in* Erythropoiesis. ed. by Jacobson, L. O. and Doyle, M. (New York, Grune & Stratton, 1962), p. 321.

35 Hodgson, G. and Eskuche, I., Time course of effects of erythropoiesis-stimulating factor(s) (ESF) on ^{59}Fe distribution. *in* Erythropoiesis. ed. by Jacobson, L. O. and Doyle, M. (New York, Grume & Stratton, 1962),

p. 222.

36 Gallagher, N. I., Seifert, G. L., Callinan, J. L., Maes, A. A. and Lange, R. D., Influence of erythropoietin on erythropoiesis in polycythemic rats. *J. Lab. Clin. Med.*, **61**, 258 (1963).

37 Stohlman, F., Jr., Shortened survival of erythrocytes produced by erythropoietin or severe anemia. *Proc. Soc. Exptl. Biol. Med.*, **107**, 884 (1971).

38 Nakao, K., Miura, Y. and Takaku, F., *In vitro* effect of erythropoietin on the spleen of the polycythemic mouse. I. *Blood*, **27**, 646 (1966).

39 Miura, Y., Takaku, F. and Nakao, K., *In vitro* effect of erythropoietin on the spleen of the polycythemic mouse. II. Radiosensitivity of stem cells. *Blood*, **29**, 852 (1967).

40 Gurney, C. W. and Hofstra, D., Assessment of actinomycin and radiation damage of stem cells by the erythropoietin-tolerance test. *Rad. Res.*, **15**, 599 (1963).

41 Gallien-Lartigue, O. and Goldwasser, E., On the mechanism of erythropoietin-induced differentiation. Effect on RNA synthesis. *Biochim. Biophys. Acta*, **103**, 325 (1965).

42 Keighley, G. and Lowy, P.H., Actinomycin and erythropoiesis and production of erythropoietin in mice. *Blood*, **28**, 637 (1966).

43 Reissmann, K. R. and Ito, K., Selective inhibition of erythroid-cell differentiation in the mouse by low doses of actinomycin D. *Ann. N.Y. Acad. Sci.*, **149**, 193 (1968).

44 Hodgson, G. and Eskuche, I., Dose-response relationships for the " early " and " late " response to erythropoietin. *Proc. Soc. Exptl. Biol. Med.*, **170**, 1094 (1968).

45 Miura, Y., Mizoguchi, H., Takaku, F. and Nakao, K., *In vitro* effect of erythropoietin on the spleen of the polycythemic mouse. III. Limited exposure to erythropoietin and actinomycin D. *Blood*, **31**, 433 (1968).

46 Mizoguchi, H., Miura, Y., Takaku, F. and Nakao, K., Effect of erythropoietin on polycythemic mouse spleen *in vitro*. IV. Response of the colony-forming cell to erythropoietin. *Blood*, **32**, 271 (1968).

47 Till, J. E. and McCulloch, E. A., A direct measurement of the radiation sensetivity of normal mouse bone marrow cells. *Rad. Res.*, **14**, 213 (1961).

48 Suzuki, S., Miura, Y., Mizoguchi, H. and Takaku, F., Effect of erythropoietin on the spleen of the polycythemic mouse *in vitro*. V. Localization of erythropoietin-responsive cells in the spleen. to be published in *Exp. Cell Res.* (1973).

49 Curry, J. L. and Trentin, J. J., Hemopoietic spleen colony studies. I. Growth and differentiation. *Develop. Biol.*, **15**, 395 (1967).

50 Trentin, J. J., Influence of hematopoietic organ stroma (Hematopoietic-inductive microenvironment) on stem-cell differentiation. *in* Regulation

of hematopoiesis, Vol. 1. ed. by Gordon, A. S. (Appleton-Century-Crofts, New York, 1970), p. 159.

51 Miura, Y., Takaku, F. and Nakao, K., Effect of erythropoietin on polycythemic mouse spleen. *in* The regulation of erythropoiesis and hemoglobin synthesis. ed. by Travnicek, T. and Neuwirt, J. (Universita Karlova, Praha, 1971), p. 285.

52 Matoth, Y. and Ben-Porath (Arkin), E., Effect of erythropoietin on mitotic rate of erythroblasts in bone marrow cultures. *J. Lab. Clin. Med.*, **54**, 722 (1959).

53 Powsner, E. R. and Berman, L., Effect of erythropoietin on DNA synthesis by erythroblasts *in vitro*. *Blood*, **30**, 189 (1967).

54 Necheles, T. F., Sheehan, R. G. and Meyer, H. J., Studies on the control of hemoglobin synthesis, nucleic acid synthesis and normoblast proliferation in the presence of erythropoietin. *Ann. N. Y. Acad. Sci.*, **149**, 449 (1968).

55 Schooley, J. C. and Garcia, J. F., Immunologic studies on the mechanism of action of erythropoietin. *Proc. Soc. Exptl. Biol. Med.*, **110**, 636 (1962).

56 Nielson, N. O., Feinendegen, L. E., Bond, V. P., Odartchenko, N. and Cottier, H., *In vitro* uptake of tritiated thymidine by erythrocytic precursors following hemorrhage in the dog. *Proc. Soc. Exptl. Biol. Med.*, **116**, 498 (1964).

57 Monette, F. C., LoBue, J., Gordon, A. S. and Chan, P. C., Erythropoiesis in transfusion-induced polycythemic rats studied with ^{3}H-thymidine autoradiography. *Proc. Soc. Exptl. Biol. Med.*, **119**, 445 (1965).

58 Hodgson, G., Synthesis of RNA and DNA at various intervals after erythropoietin injection in transfused mice. *Proc. Soc. Exptl. Biol. Med.*, **124**, 1045 (1967).

59 Dukes, P. P., *In vitro* studies on DNA synthesis of bone-marrow cells stimulated by erythropoietin. *Ann. N. Y. Acad. Sci.*, **149**, 437 (1968).

60 Paul, J. and Hunter, J. A., DNA synthesis is essential for increased hemoglobin synthesis in response to erythropoietin. *Nature*, **219**, 1362 (1968).

61 Hodgson, G. and Eskuche, I., Changes in the erythropoietin-responsive cell after exposure to irradiation. *Ann. N. Y. Acad. Sci.*, **149**, 230 (1968).

62 Lajtha, J. G., Bone-marrow stem-cell kinetics. *Semin. Hematol.*, **4**, 293 (1967).

63 Miura, Y., Suzuki, S., Mizoguchi, H., Takaku, F., Sano, K. and Sato, O., Stimulation of the mouse-spleen erythropoiesis by direct contact with cerebellar hemangioblastoma tissue *in vitro*. in preparation.

64 Contrera, J. F. and Gordon, A. S., Erythropoietin: Production by a par-

ticulate fraction of rat kidney. *Science*, **152**, 653 (1966).
65 Gordon, A. S. and Zanjani, E. D., Some aspects of erythropoietin physiology. *in* Regulation of hematopoiesis, ed. by Gordon, A. S., Vol. 1. (Appleton-Century-Crofts, New York, 1970), p. 413.
66 Miura, Y., personal communication.
67 Suzuki, S., personal communication.
68 Gordon, A. S., Fisher, J. W. (ed.) and Zanjani, E. D., Studies on the renal erythropoietic factor (REF). *in* Kidney hormones, ed. by Fisher, J. W. (Academic Press, London, 1971), p. 295.
69 Krantz, S. B., The effect of erythropoietin on human bone-marrow cells *in vitro*. *Life Sci.*, **4**, 2393 (1965).
70 Mizoguchi, H., Miura, Y., Takaku, F., Sassa, S., Chiba, S. and Nakao, K., The effect of erythropoietin on human bone-marrow cells *in vitro*. I. Studies of nine cases of bone-marrow failure. *Blood*, **37**, 624 (1971).
71 Krantz, S. B. and Kao, V., Studies on cell aplasia. I. Demonstration of a plasma inhibitor to heme synthesis and an antibody to erythroblast nuclei. *Proc. Natl. Acad. Sci.*, **58**, 493 (1967).
72 Miura, Y., Kikuchi, H., Yotsumoto, H., Mizoguchi, H. and Takaku, F., A case of pure red-cell aplasia with bone-marrow cells responsive to erythropoietin *in vitro*. 14th Congress of Japanese Clinical Hematology (Sapporo, 1972).
73 Chiyoda, S., Suzuki, S., Mizoguchi, H., Miura, Y. and Takaku, F., Erythropoietin-responsive cells in acute leukemia. 14th Congress of Japanese Clinical Hematology (Sapporo, 1972).
74 Krantz, S. B., Response of polycythemia vera marrow to erythropoietin *in vitro*. *J. Lab. Clin. Med.*, **71**, 999 (1968).
75 Zucker, S., Howe, D. M. and Weintraub, L. R., Bone-marrow response to erythropoietin in polycythemia vera and chronic granulocytic leukemia. *Blood*, **39**, 341 (1972).
76 DeGowin, R. L. and Gurney, C. W., Hemopoiesis in polycythemia vera after phlebotomy and iron therapy. *Arch. Int. Med.*, **114**, 424 (1964).
77 Stohlman, F., Jr., Pathogenesis of erythrocytosis. *Semin. Hematol.*, **3**, 181 (1966).
78 Adamson, J. W. and Finch, C. A., Erythropoietin and the polycythemia, *Ann. N. Y. Acad. Sci.*, **149**, 560 (1968).
79 Necheles, T. F., Sheehan, R. G. and Meyer, H. J., Effect of erythropoietin and oxygen tension on *in vitro* synthesis of hemoglobin A and F by adult human bone marrow. *Proc. Soc. Exptl. Biol. Med.*, **119**, 1207 (1965).
80 Gabuzda, T. G., Lewis, H. B. and Silver, R. K., Biochemical studies of cultured erythroid cell. *in* The regulation of erythropoiesis and hemo-

globin synthesis. ed. by Travnicek, T. and Neuwirt, J. (Universita Karlova, Praha, 1971), p. 384.

81 Mizoguchi, H., personal communication.

The Formation and Reduction of Methemoglobin in Human Erythrocytes*

E. R. JAFFÉ

Department of Medicine Albert Einstein College of Medicine, New York, U.S.A.

Although the general characteristics of methemoglobin have been known for over a century, the nature of the alterations in the hemoglobin molecule have only recently been identified. Hemoglobin is protected against oxidation to methemoglobin by its inherent structure and by reactions within erythrocytes that can destroy hydrogen peroxide or equivalent free radicals. Oxidation of hemoglobin can occur spontaneously, but is accelerated by certain drugs and chemicals. The change in electron pattern from the low-spin ferric state of oxyhemoglobin to the high-spin ferric state of methemoglobin is reversible in normal human erythrocytes. Reduction of methemoglobin to hemoglobin is dependent upon the structural integrity of the erythrocytes, is associated with the metabolism of carbohydrate substrates, and requires the generation of reduced pyridine nucleotides. The reduction of methemoglobin is carried out primarily by the NADH-methemoglobin reductase, which is subject to genetically determined polymorphism, and which is deficient in the erythrocytes of certain patients with hereditary methemoglobinemia. The NADH-dependent reaction appears to be catalyzed by an enzyme system distinct from NADPH-dehydrogenases. The structural characteristics of the methemoglobin reductases remain to be determined and the sequence of electron transfer from reduced pyridine nucleotides to methemoglobin remains to be defined.

DEFINITION

Methemoglobin (ferrihemoglobin, hem*i*globin, ferriprotoporphyrin IX-globin) is hemoglobin in which the iron of the heme moiety is in the high-spin ferric state. Five unpaired electrons are present in methemoglobin and the ferric heme can no longer bind oxygen reversibly. The sixth coordination position, normally available to oxygen, is occupied by water or anionic ligands such as chloride, azide, or

* The investigations in the author's laboratory are supported by United States Public Health Service grants AM-13698, PO2 AM-13430, and T01 AM-5435.

cyanide. The change in the oxidation state of the heme iron and the formation of complexes with ligands are reflected in alterations in the absorption spectra that are utilized in the determination of the concentrations of hemoglobin and methemoglobin.[1] Methemoglobin probably represents the "mildest" alteration that can occur in hemoglobin, other than the physiological change between oxyhemoglobin and deoxyhemoglobin that takes place repeatedly within the normal human erythrocyte. The heme moiety of methemoglobin is more loosely bound to the globin than is the heme of oxyhemoglobin or ligand-bound methemoglobin.[2] Further modification of the hemoglobin molecule may result from the action of certain denaturing agents that produce hemichromes in which both the fifth and sixth coordination positions are bound to a nitrogenous base.[3] Additional changes occur with greater oxidation of the hemoglobin molecule that lead to denaturation and precipitation. Precipitated hemoglobin may appear in erythrocytes as Heinz bodies[4] that probably represent irreversibly denatured protein aggregates which may have lost their heme moieties.[5] While methemoglobin is readily reversible to hemoglobin under suitable conditions, hemichromes and denatured hemoglobin (choleglobin) are essentially irreversible forms under physiological conditions.

HISTORICAL REVIEW

The general nature of altered hemoglobin pigments, including methemoglobin, and the occurrence of drug-induced cyanosis were well-known and frequently described during the nineteenth century. The first description of a patient with long-standing congenital cyanosis without obvious cardiac or pulmonary disease probably was the report of François[6] in 1845. In 1891, Dittrich[7] established that the methemoglobinemia which developed in dogs after the administration of "Blutgifte," such as nitroglycerine and acetanilide, disappeared without a change in the number of circulating erythrocytes. He emphasized that the methemoglobinemia with cyanosis which developed in patients given certain medicines tended to disappear and he suggested that methemoglobin was reduced to hemoglobin within the erythrocytes. Stokvis[8] and Talma[9] in 1902 described patients with "autotoxic enterogenous cyanosis" which was attributed to the formation of intracellular methemoglobin by toxic substances absorbed from an inflamed or ulcerated gastrointestinal tract. In 1905, van den Bergh[10] differentiated methemoglobin from sulfhemoglobin in the erythrocytes of patients with "enterogenous cyanosis." Slosse and Wybauw[11] in 1912 and Litarczek and associates[12] in 1930 described patients with spectroscopically identified methemoglobinemia of several years duration without gastrointestinal tract disease or known ingestion of methemoglobin-producing agents. In 1928, Conant and Scott[13] demonstrated the difference in the valence of the heme iron that characterizes methemoglobin. Thus, it was established that methemoglobinemia could result from exposure to certain drugs and chemicals, could be associated with gastrointestinal or other disorders and could occur without apparent cause.

During the first third of the twentieth century, toxic methemoglobinemia became a significant clinical problem. The advent of sulfonamides and other drugs as chemotherapeutic agents, the production of aniline dyes and their derivatives, and the use of nitrates, nitrites, and chlorates provided numerous instances of drug-induced, toxic methemoglobinemia. Changing social and medical practices have reduced the incidence of this disorder, but it might reappear with the development of new medicines or manufacturing processes. The subject of toxic methemoglobinemia has been reviewed in great detail[14,15] and will not be considered further in the present discussion.

Hitzenberger[16] in 1932 probably was the first to describe a familial incidence of idiopathic cyanosis. He suggested the possibility of congenital, familial methemoglobinemia. At the same time, Dieckmann[17] described a woman with congenital cyanosis that increased in intensity during a pregnancy. He postulated that the constant methemoglobinemia probably was due to the continued presence or production of a substance capable of oxidizing hemoglobin. In 1938, Bensley and associates[18] documented familial, idiopathic methemoglobinemia in 2 French-Canadian siblings. One year later, Lian *et al.*[19] described French siblings whose methemoglobinemia they attributed to an abnormal resistance of the methemoglobin to reduction, although it responded to the administration of ascorbic acid. Between 1943 and 1945, Gibson,[20] Barcroft and his associates[21] and Sievers and Ryon[22] proposed that the erythrocytes of patients with familial, idiopathic methemoglobinemia were deficient in their capacity to reduce the methemoglobin which was formed normally in the cells. Sievers and Ryon[22] demonstrated that an abnormality in the plasma was not responsible. The classic investigations of Gibson[23] in 1948 provided substantial evidence that there was a deficiency in coenzyme factor I (diaphorase, a methemoglobin reductase) in the erythrocytes of patients with this disorder. An unusually high incidence of hereditary methemoglobinemia among Alaskan Eskimos and Indians was noted by Scott and Hoskins.[24] In 1959, Scott and Griffith[25] reported the absence in erythrocytes of these patients of an enzyme which catalyzed the reduction of methemoglobin by NADH. These observations have now been confirmed by many investigators.[26,27] More recently, the NADH-dependent methemoglobin reductase has been demonstrated by various electrophoretic techniques[28,29] and a number of electrophoretic variants have been described.[27] Thus, the concept that an abnormality in the metabolic capacity of human erythrocytes could cause methemoglobinemia was well established.

The family histories of subjects with hereditary methemoglobinemia usually were compatible with the thesis that the abnormality was transmitted as an autosomal, recessive characteristic.[21] In 1948, however, Hörlein and Weber[30] described a German family in which hereditary methemoglobinemia appeared to be transmitted as a dominant characteristic through 4 generations. They demonstrated an abnormality in the globin of their patients' hemoglobin, but were unable to detect a defect in the capacity of the erythrocytes to reduce methemoglobin. This disorder, the first hemoglobinopathy described, was designated as hemoglobin M by Singer.[31] Several distinct types of hemoglobin M and the associated amino acid substitutions have been reported.[32] The difference between this type of methemoglobinemia and that associated with a failure in the reducing systems of the erythrocytes was demonstrated clearly in the studies of Rossi-Fanelli and his associates[33] in 1957.

These investigations provided a basis for differentiating hereditary, often congenital, methemoglobinemia into 2 major categories. In one, methemoglobinemia of 10 to 50% was due to a significant decrease in the capacity of the erythrocytes to reduce methemoglobin to hemoglobin and was often associated with a deficiency in the activity of an NADH-methemoglobin reductase system. In the other, methemoglobinemia was due to an alteration in the structure of 2 of the 4 polypeptide chains of the hemoglobin. This change enhanced the tendency of the hemoglobin to be oxidized and decreased the susceptibility of the abnormal methemoglobin to reduction by the normal mechanisms present in the erythrocytes.[32]

OXIDATION OF HEMOGLOBIN TO METHEMOGLOBIN

One percent or less of the total hemoglobin in normal human erythrocytes is in the form of methemoglobin.[14] This relatively constant concentration may be considered to result from an equilibrium between the rate at which hemoglobin is oxidized and the rate at which methemoglobin is reduced.[32] Scott[34] has reviewed these assumptions and has noted that the reducing capacity of the erythrocyte may be about 250 times greater than its oxidizing capacity. An increase in the concentration of methemoglobin can result from exposure to noxious agents which increase greatly the rate of oxidation and which may overwhelm intraerythrocytic protective mechanisms. Alternatively, methemoglobinemia can occur as a consequence of abnormalities in the mechanisms available to the cell to reduce methemoglobin to hemoglobin or in the structure of the hemoglobin molecule (hemoglobin M's).

The presence of a small, but constant, amount of methemoglobin in normal human blood is compatible with the concept that oxidation of hemoglobin takes place *in vivo*. Further support for this thesis is derived from the observations that methemoglobin reappears at a linear rate of 0.5 to 3% of the total hemoglobin per day in the erythrocytes of patients whose cells are deficient in the NADH-dependent methemoglobin reductase system, after all of the methemoglobin has been converted to hemoglobin by appropriate therapy.[35–37] The rate of oxidation of hemoglobin to methemoglobin *in vitro* is slow. Intact human erythrocytes, incubated at 37°C in the absence of added substrate, will contain about 70% methemoglobin after 7 days, while a solution of crystalline human hemoglobin is essentially completely oxidized in the same period of time.[38] In hemolysates, oxidation proceeds to completion in about 5 days.[35]

The iron of the heme moiety of hemoglobin was for long considered to be in the ferrous state to permit the reversible binding and transportation of oxygen.[39] Weiss[40] challenged this concept for oxyhemoglobin and suggested that the heme iron of oxyhemoglobin was in the ferric low-spin state. Peisach *et al.*[41] and Wittenberg *et al.*[42] provided evidence in support of this hypothesis. They proposed that oxygen was bound as the superoxide anion to the sixth coordination position. Deoxyhemoglobin would then be the only known high-spin form of ferrous hemoglobin. Upon oxygenation, 1 unpaired electron would be given up (partial transfer) to oxygen to form a superoxide anion and low-spin ferric iron. The bound superoxide would not be reactive, probably because the oxygen-binding site resides in a very hydrophobic region of the globin polypeptide chain[43,44] where the superoxide would have the stability that characterizes this anion in nonaqueous media. The diamagnetism characteristic of oxygenated hemoglobin, despite the presence of ferric iron, could be explained by spin coupling between the unpaired electrons resident on the heme iron atom and the superoxide ligand. If the hydrophobic region about the heme moiety has been disturbed, the iron may be readily oxidized to the high-spin ferric state that characterizes methemoglobin.

Despite extensive investigations and many postulates, the mechanism by which hemoglobin is oxidized to methemoglobin is still not completely understood.[15,45] Changes in the superoxide anion, perhaps simple dissociation, might lead to methemoglobin formation. Spontaneous autoxidation of hemoglobin occurs slowly, the rate depending upon the relative concentrations of deoxyhemoglobin and oxyhemoglobin.[46] The rate of autoxidation is maximal at a fairly low oxygen pressure, close to that at which hemoglobin is half-saturated.[47] George[48] has postulated a mechanism involving the formation of a radical and the presence of an electron-accepting group in the hemoglobin. If oxyhemoglobin contains a superoxide anion, hydrogen peroxide or OH radicals might be formed. Although contradictory observations have been reported about the effect of the addition of catalase on the rate of autoxidation,[49,50] careful analyses have failed to provide any direct evidence for the production of hydrogen peroxide.[15]

Methemoglobin formation is accelerated by some chemicals, such as ferricyanide, which directly oxidizes the ferrous heme of deoxyhemoglobin, and by many drugs and chemicals or their metabolites that can undergo coupled oxidation and reduction in the presence of oxyhemoglobin.[15,45] In these latter reactions, generation of hydrogen peroxide (peroxyhemoglobin or equivalent free radicals) is thought to cause the formation of methemoglobin.[51,52] Some of these agents also can induce alterations which lead to hemolysis *in vivo*, especially in individuals whose erythrocytes are deficient in glucose-6-P dehydrogenase (G-6-PD) activity.[53] Nitrite, commonly used to prepare methemoglobin-containing erythrocytes *in vitro* and often responsible for toxic methemoglobinemia in infants and children, may form complexes with hemoglobin that dissociate to yield methemoglobin.[15,54] Generation of hydrogen peroxide during the reaction of nitrite with oxyhemoglobin in lysates, however, has also been reported.[55]

The role of methemoglobin in the irreversible denaturation of hemoglobin has been the subject of considerable discussion.[56] Because the heme moiety of methemoglobin is loosely bound[2] and because globin devoid of heme is more susceptible to denaturation,[57] methemoglobin formation has been considered to predispose to the oxidative denaturation of hemoglobin.[58] Some of the hereditary unstable hemoglobins appear to have an increased tendency to form methemoglobin.[44] Methemoglobin formation, therefore, has been postulated to be a necessary intermediate in the sequence of oxidative degradation of hemoglobin.[5,58] There is evidence, however, that irreversible denaturation of hemoglobin can occur without an intermediate methemoglobin state.[59,60] Nitrite-induced methemoglobinemia in rats does not enhance the hemolytic properties of phenylhydrazine and may even protect against this type of oxidative hemolysis.[59] Methemoglobin, as an isolated alteration in the erythrocytes of patients with hereditary methemoglobinemia, does not appear to shorten significantly the life span of these erythrocytes.[61,62] Thus, there may be several pathways for the oxidative denaturation of hemoglobin, only one of which requires the formation of methemoglobin.

PROTECTION AGAINST OXIDATION OF HEMOGLOBIN

The inherent structure of hemoglobin, with the heme moiety in an intensely hydrophobic pocket, tends to shield the iron against oxidation. The erythrocyte membrane may also serve as a permeability barrier to exogenous hydrogen peroxide.[63] If hydrogen peroxide generation within the erythrocyte is involved in the formation of methemoglobin, reduced glutathione (GSH) peroxidase activity can serve to protect the hemoglobin by destroying hydrogen peroxide when it is generated at a low, steady rate.[64] Slightly elevated levels of methemoglobin have been reported in the erythrocytes of some patients with hereditary nonspherocytic hemolytic anemia associated with a partial deficiency in GSH peroxidase activity.[65] Catalase also can destroy hydrogen peroxide and is capable of destroying almost all that enters from the exterior.[63] Catalase, however, appears to be physiologically important only when hydrogen peroxide concentrations are very high or are maintained in the absence of the metabolic activity required for the regeneration of GSH.[66] The concentration of methemoglobin in the blood of patients with acatalasemia is normal.[67] One Japanese patient, however, has been noted to have a slight increase in methemoglobin when fatigued or suffering from a cold, even without administration of methemoglobin-forming medicines.[67]

Direct protective effects of such reducing agents as GSH, NADPH ergothioneine, and cysteine have been postulated, but not proved.[68]

These protective mechanisms depend upon the ability of the compounds or enzymes to serve as reducing systems capable of destroying hydrogen peroxide or the equivalent free radicals. In addition, there is an electron hiatus between molecular oxygen and intracellular electron donors, such as heme, in mature mammalian erythrocytes because these cells lack cytochrome oxidase and an intact cytochrome system.[69] These observations explain the stability of normal human hemoglobin as long as the erythrocyte is intact and the increased tendency for methemoglobin formation upon hemolysis of the cell or purification of the hemoglobin.

REDUCTION OF METHEMOGLOBIN TO HEMOGLOBIN

Extensive studies utilizing erythrocytes from patients with hereditary methemoglobinemia and normal human erythrocytes containing nitrite-induced methemoglobin have provided considerable information about the mechanisms involved in the reduction of methemoglobin. The initial studies on the reduction of methemoglobin *in vitro* were performed with erythrocytes obtained from animals[70] and demonstrated considerable quantitative species variation. The basic pathways, however, appeared to be the same. Smith and Beutler[71] examined the rate of methemoglobin formation upon the addition of nitrite to hemoglobin solutions and the reduction of methemoglobin by intact erythrocytes obtained from man, sheep, horse, cattle, and pigs. In general, a rapid methemoglobin formation rate was offset by a rapid methemoglobin reduction rate. Normal reduction of methemoglobin depended upon the structural integrity of the erythrocytes,[72] was associated with the metabolism of carbohydrate substrates,[70] and required the generation of reduced pyridine nucleotides.[73]

The pathways by which methemoglobin is reduced by human erythrocytes and the manner in which these processes are related to metabolic activity are summarized in Fig. 1. The reduction of methemoglobin upon incubation of erythrocytes with glucose or lactate is accompanied by the formation of an amount of pyruvate approximately equivalent to the amount of methemoglobin reduced.[23] With glucose as substrate, approximately 1 μmole of heme is reduced per hr per ml cells.[74,75] Addition of iodoacetate, which probably inactivates GAPD,

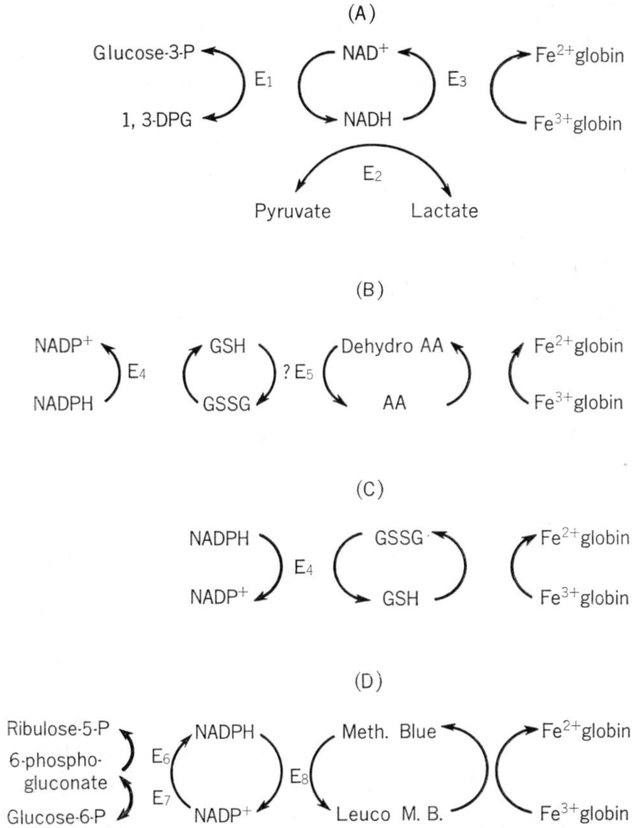

Fig. 1. Metabolic pathways in human erythrocytes related to the reduction of methemoglobin (Fe^{3+} globin) to hemoglobin (Fe^{2+} globin). *Substrates:* GAP=glyceraldehyde-3-phosphate; 1,3-DPG=1,3-diphosphoglycerate; GSH=reduced glutathione; GSSG=oxidized glutathione; DehydroAA =dehydroascorbic acid; AA=ascorbic acid; Meth. Blue=methylene blue; Leuco. M. B.=leucomethylene blue; *Enzymes:* E_1=glyceraldehyde-3-P dehydrogenase; E_2=lactate dehydrogenase; E_3=NADH-methemoglobin reductase; E_4=oxidized glutathione reductase; E_5= dehydroascorbic acid reductase; E_6=6-phosphogluconate dehydrogenase; E_7=glucose-6-P dehydrogenase; E_8=NADPH-dehydrogenase (methemoglobin reductase). Reproduced from 27 with permission from the publisher, Grune and Stratton.

inhibits the reduction of methemoglobin with glucose as substrate, but not with lactate.[23)] Addition of fluoride, which strongly inhibits the activity of enolase, does not inhibit reduction with either substrate. High concentrations of pyruvate inhibit reduction when lactate is the substrate, but do not affect reduction with glucose. The reaction catalyzed by GAPD (Fig. 1, A), and requiring triose phosphate derived from glucose, therefore, appears to be of major importance for the reduction of methemoglobin in human erythrocytes.[76] Under certain conditions, the level of 2,3-DPG increases during the reduction of methemoglobin and it has been suggested that the diversion of glucose into 2,3-DPG serves to conserve NADH for the reduction of methemoglobin.[77] Lactate, when present in great excess, can serve to provide NADH through the activity of lactate dehydrogenase. Incubation of nitrite-treated, normal human erythrocytes with fructose, galactose, fumarate, formaldehyde, purine nucleosides, ribose, deoxyribose, sorbitol, and xylitol will also result in the reduction of methemoglobin.[68,78–80] Metabolism of these substrates results in the generation of NADH. For example, utilization of the ribose moiety of inosine bypasses the initial reactions of the Embden-Meyerhof pathway of glycolysis and does not require ATP for phosphorylation, but permits the generation of NADH through the activity of GAPD. During the reduction of methemoglobin with inosine, pyruvate does not accumulate,[76] probably because the accumulation of ATP or the depletion of ADP promotes the diversion of 1,3-DPG to 2,3-DPG. The coupling of methemoglobin reduction to the oxidation of xylitol to xylulose has indicated the existence of xylitol dehydrogenase activity in human erythrocytes.[80] Recently, it has been suggested but not proved that the formation of NADH through the polyol pathway may provide the reduced pyridine nucleotide required for physiologic methemoglobin reduction.[81] When these various compounds have been employed in studies of the reduction of methemoglobin *in vitro* by erythrocytes from patients with hereditary methemoglobinemia, they have not been able to support significant reduction.

Ascorbic acid will promote the reduction of methemoglobin in the erythrocytes of patients with hereditary methemoglobinemia *in vivo* and *in vitro*, and in normal erythrocytes and their hemolysates *in vitro*.[68] The pathway postulated to explain this reaction (Fig. 1, B) involves the direct reduction of methemoglobin by ascorbic acid with the formation of hemoglobin and dehydroascorbic acid. The dehydroascorbic acid is then reduced to ascorbic acid through a GSH-dependent dehydroascorbic acid reductase.[82–84] The rate at which ascorbic acid reduces methemoglobin is so slow that it is unlikely that it plays a major physiologic role, but Scott[34] has calculated that it could account for 16% of the reducing capacity of normal human erythrocytes.

Significant methemoglobinemia has not been described in scurvy, but it is of interest that low serum ascorbic acid levels have been reported in some patients with hereditary methemoglobinemia.[32]

GSH reduces methemoglobin to hemoglobin *in vitro* slowly.[68] Direct nonenzymatic reduction of methemoglobin by GSH has been invoked to explain whatever reduction of methemoglobin results from the activity of the hexose monophosphate shunt pathway[85] (Fig. 1, C). The GSSG formed during this reaction is reduced to GSH by GSSG-reductase activity. GSH does not appear to be required for the reduction of methemoglobin in nitrite-treated erythrocytes incubated with inosine even when the GSH is bound with N-ethyl maleimide.[86] The inhibition of reduction by N-ethyl maleimide when glucose is the substrate can be explained by the impairment of glycolysis with decreased generation of NADH. Scott[34] has calculated that the GSH normally present in erythrocytes can account for about 12% of the reducing capacity. A few patients with hereditary methemoglobinemia have been noted to have a low concentration of GSH in their erythrocytes.[32] Patients with hereditary nonspherocytic hemolytic anemia and extremely low concentrations of GSH in their erythrocytes, secondary to a deficiency in GSH synthetase activity, however, do not have significant methemoglobinemia.[87,88]

Methylene blue greatly accelerates the reduction of methemoglobin *in vitro* and *in vivo* in both normal erythrocytes and cells from patients with hereditary methemoglobinemia. These observations have been invoked to postulate the existence of a NADPH-dependent methemoglobin reductase system.[68] This system is linked to the NADPH-generating steps of the hexose monophosphate shunt pathway and appears to involve a NADPH-dehydrogenase that can reduce methylene blue to leucomethylene blue (Fig. 1, D). Although Scott[34] has attributed as much as 5% of the normal reducing capacity of human erythrocytes to NADPH-dehydrogenase activity, it seems unlikely that this system plays a significant role in the absence of an artificial electron carrier. Hexose monophosphate shunt pathway activity is not increased in the erythrocytes of patients with hereditary methemoglobinemia, despite the presence of significant amounts of methemoglobin.[26] The failure of methylene blue to accelerate the reduction of methemoglobin in erythrocytes deficient in G-6-PD activity as much as it does in normal erythrocytes is consistent with the dependence of this system on the generation of NADPH.[89,90]

Thus, there are at least 4 pathways by which methemoglobin can be reduced to hemoglobin in normal human erythrocytes: a NADH-dependent methemoglobin reductase (NADH-methemoglobin reductase), direct nonenzymatic reduction by ascorbic acid and GSH, and an NADPH-methemoglobin reductase (NADPH-dehydrogenase). The major pathway, however, appears to involve the NADH-methemoglobin reductase.

The rate of reduction of methemoglobin may not be determined solely by the level of activity of NADH-methemoglobin reductase.[91] The increased glycolytic rate that results from the addition of Pi to a glucose-containing medium is associated with a slight increase in the rate of reduction.[26] The rate of reduction by normal erythrocytes is also accelerated by the addition of fluoride which may increase the diversion of glycolytic intermediates into 2,3-DPG and conserve NADH by decreasing the need for the reduction of pyruvate to lactate.[26] A more striking increase in rate can be induced by enhancing the intracellular concentration of NAD^+ and, presumably, of NADH by preincubating erythrocytes with nicotinic acid, glucose, glutamine, and Pi.[86] The very low rate of reduction of methemoglobin manifested by erythrocytes severely deficient in NADH-methemoglobin reductase activity is not influenced significantly by the presence of increased concentrations of NAD^+. Erythrocytes from heterozygous subjects with intermediate levels of NADH-methemoglobin reductase activity demonstrate increased rates of reduction when the NAD^+ content is elevated, but the rates never attain those observed with erythrocytes from normal individuals. The rate of reduction may, therefore, be somewhat dependent upon the availability of NADH. The ability of erythrocytes deficient in the activity of G-6-PD, GSSG reductase, pyruvate kinase, phosphoglycerate kinase, or triosephosphate isomerase to reduce nitrite-induced methemoglobin *in vitro*, however, is normal or elevated in relation to the degree of reticulocytosis[90,92–95] (unpublished observations). The level of metabolic activity required to reduce methemoglobin, therefore, does not appear to be curtailed by these enzymatic deficiencies. Recently, it has also been suggested that the rate may be influenced by the availability of cytochrome b_5.[96,97]

In the normal individual, modest changes in the rate of oxidation of hemoglobin or in the level of activity of the NADH-methemoglobin reductase system will have minimal effects on the concentration of methemoglobin in the cells. Significant methemoglobinemia (greater than about 5 to 10%) will then occur only in the presence of a severe deficiency in the NADH-methemoglobin reductase system or in the face of massive intoxication that overwhelms the protective and reductive capacities of the erythrocytes. A deficiency in the content of NAD^+ and in the capacity to generate NADH from NAD^+ might also lead to methemoglobinemia, but such disorders have not yet been documented. A hemoglobin with an abnormal structure (hemoglobin M, an unstable hemoglobin) may be an unsuitable substrate for the reductase system.

THE METHEMOGLOBIN REDUCTASES OF HUMAN ERYTHROCYTES

A universally accepted concept of the enzyme or enzymes involved in the reduction of methemoglobin cannot be presented. The discrepant observations which have been reported probably reflect differences in the methods employed for the isolation of the enzymes, the terminal electron acceptors used to measure the enzymatic activities, and the assay conditions. In addition, the various terminologies that have been used have contributed to the confusion. The NADH-dependent system has been called a diaphorase, NADH-dehydrogenase (I and II), coenzyme factor I, ferrihemoglobin reductase, and NADH-methemoglobin reductase. NADH-methemoglobin reductase will be used in this discussion. The NADPH-dependent system has been called Hämiglobinreduktase, coenzyme factor II, NADPH-methemoglobin reductase, and methemoglobin reductase. Because this enzyme system appears to catalyze the reduction of a dye, such as methylene blue, rather than methemoglobin itself, it will here be called NADPH-dehydrogenase.

1) NADH-Methemoglobin Reductases

Scott and his associates[98–100] isolated 2 NADH-methemoglobin reductases from normal human erythrocytes by ammonium sulfate and calcium phosphate gel fractionation. The enzyme (NADH-dehydrogenase I) with sufficient activity to account for about 61% of the capacity of normal erythrocytes to reduce methemoglobin *in vitro* was absent from the erythrocytes of an Eskimo with hereditary methemoglobinemia.[101] Scott[34] calculated that this enzyme could account for over 95% of the capacity of normal human erythrocytes to reduce methemoglobin *in vivo*. The enzyme appeared to contain flavin adenine dinucleotide and was quite specific for NADH, for the activity with NADPH was only about 1.5% of that with NADH. The final electron acceptor could be oxygen, cytochrome c, ferricyanide, methemoglobin, or any one of several dyes. The lowest activity was observed with methemoglobin and the highest with 2,6-dichlorophenolindophenol (DCIP). Because the rate with the dye was so much greater than that with methemoglobin, the reduction of the dye has been utilized to measure the activity of this system in hemolysates of nitrite-treated erythrocytes.[98,102] Although a 50,000-fold purification of the enzyme was achieved, its molecular weight was not defined and heme was a variable, but persistent, impurity. The reaction catalyzed by this enzyme was considered to involve the formation of binary complexes of substrate and enzyme with reduction of flavin by NADH and then reduction of the final acceptor, dye or methemoglobin. The residual ability of the erythrocytes of a patient with hereditary methemoglobinemia to reduce methemoglobin *in vitro* was attributed to the activity of NADH-dehydrogenase II which differed from I in chromatographic behavior and kinetic properties, and lacked flavin. NADH-dehydrogenase II could not be prepared free of activity with NADPH.

Hegesh and his associates[103–105] employed DEAE-cellulose adsorption, elution, and fractionation with CM-cellulose columns to prepare a ferrocyanide-dependent methemoglobin reductase that was absolutely specific for NADH when assayed with methemoglobin or cytochrome c as the acceptor. This enzyme was free of NADPH-dehydrogenase activity, although it had some activity with NADPH when other acceptors, such as DCIP, methylene blue, or ferricyanide, were used. A 300- to 1,500-fold purification was achieved, but there was persistent and variable contamination with methemoglobin and the flavin content was extremely low or questionable. The purest enzyme preparation had a homogeneous, symmetrical peak on ultracentrifugation with a sedimentation constant of $S_{20}W$, 9.2×10^{-13}. A molecular weight of about 300,000 was postulated from the position of elution from a Sephadex column.[105] While the enzyme did not reduce pure methemoglobin, activation by ferrocyanide was thought to involve a slight modification of the structure of the methemoglobin which permitted the enzyme to approach the site of reduction more readily.[103] Ferrocyanide was not thought to be acting as an artificial electron carrier. The K_m for the methemoglobin-ferrocyanide complex was about 8 μM. Because the purified enzyme catalyzed the reduction of cytochrome c directly, it was defined as a cytochrome c reductase. These observations were utilized to devise a more rapid and somewhat less cumbersome assay for NADH-methemoglobin reductase activity in hemolysates of human erythrocytes than the procedure employing DCIP.[106] The correlation between the 2 methods has been excellent.[106–108]

A particulate form of NADH-cytochrome c reductase (NADH-dehydrogenase) has been demonstrated in the stroma of human erythrocytes.[109] The enzyme, anchored in the structural phospholipoprotein complex of the membrane, was thought not to represent residual catalytic activity of the soluble NADH-methemoglobin reductase of whole hemolysates. Neither the particulate nor the solubilized form appeared to reduce methemoglobin at more than a barely detectable rate.[97]

Hultquist and Passon[97] have reported the isolation and purification of a cytochrome b_5 and a cytochrome b_5 reductase from the soluble fraction of hemolysates of mature human erythrocytes. The reductase appeared to be identical to the NADH-methemoglobin reductase (NADH-dehydrogenase I) described by Scott *et al.*,[100] and its properties differed from those of the particulate NADH-cytochrome c reductase. The reaction catalyzed by the enzyme was completely dependent upon the presence of the reductase and NADH, for there was no measurable rate when NADPH replaced NADH. The quantity of cytochrome b_5 appeared to decrease with the maturation of reticulocytes and upon storage of whole blood under blood-bank conditions. Hultquist and Passon proposed that cytochrome b_5 might serve as the natural cofactor to transfer electrons from the NADH-methemoglobin reductase to methemoglobin and that this latter reaction might be the rate-limiting step in the reduction of methemoglobin in the intact erythrocyte.

Recently, Sugita *et al.*[110] achieved a 44,000-fold purification of NADH-methemoglobin reductase from human erythrocytes with ammonium sulfate fractionation, calcium phosphate gel chromatography, Sephadex G-100 gel filtration, and isoelectric focusing. This preparation considered to be identical to the NADH-dehydrogenase I of Scott *et al.*,[100] had a molecular weight of about 28,000, but did not contain flavin nucleotides or heme. Addition of ferrocyanide to the enzyme preparation greatly accelerated the reduction of methemoglobin, but ferrocyanide did not serve as an electron carrier. The rate of reduction of methemoglobin in the presence of cytochrome b_5 was approximately equal to the rate of reduction of cytochrome b_5 alone. The authors suggested that cytochrome b_5 was reduced enzymatically with NADH and that methemoglobin was reduced nonenzymatically by reduced cytochrome b_5. The enzyme, therefore, was defined as a reduced cytochrome b_5 dehydrogenase.

Since the levels of cytochrome b_5 and cytochrome b_5 reductase in human erythrocytes have not been investigated extensively, their exact function in the reduction of methemoglobin must await further study at the cellular level. Assuming that as much as 3% of the circulating hemoglobin is oxidized to methemoglobin each day[32)] and that the reducing capacity of normal erythrocytes is about 250 times greater than their oxidizing capability,[34)] one would expect to find about 227 μmoles of cytochrome b_5 per liter of whole blood in order to maintain a low, steady-state level of methemoglobin. This concentration of cytochrome b_5 is considerably greater than the concentration of NAD^+ in human erythrocytes. Further studies, especially with erythrocytes from patients with hereditary methemoglobinemia and normal levels of NADH-methemoglobin reductase activity, will be required to establish the physiological role of cytochrome b_5.

2) *NADPH-Dehydrogenases*

NADPH-dehydrogenases have been isolated and partially purified from mammalian erythrocytes by several investigators. Considerable variation in the properties and activities of these enzymes was noted, but all required an artificial electron carrier, such as methylene blue, to promote the rapid reduction of methemoglobin to hemoglobin. Kiese *et al.*[111)] isolated an enzyme (Hämiglobinreduktase) that appeared to contain flavin adenine dinucleotide as the prosthetic group. Huennekens *et al.*[112)] obtained 180-fold purification of a NADPH-dehydrogenase by treatment of hemolysates with ethanol-chloroform, acid precipitation, and fractionation with ammonium sulfate. This enzyme, with a minimum molecular weight of 185,000, required methylene blue, contained a large amount of bound heme, but no flavin, and was almost completely dependent upon added NADPH, having with NADH only about 20% of the activity with NADPH. Shrago and Falcone[113)] found that the heme-containing component was not required for activity, and that some activity was demonstrable without added methylene blue. Kajita, Kerwar, and Huennekens[114)] recently purified 3 pyridine nucleotide-dependent methemoglobin reductases from human erythrocytes that were devoid of flavin, but contained variable amounts of heme. They employed batchwise treatment of hemolysate with DEAE-cellulose to remove hemoglobin, fractionation with ammonium sulfate and acetone, and chromatography on DEAE-cellulose. Each of the enzymes, purified about 1,800-fold, exhibited both NADH- and NADPH-methemoglobin reductase activities with a constant ratio of about 4: 1, but methylene blue was always required. The K_m values for NADPH, however, were much lower than for NADH. The authors concluded that NADH- and NADPH-methemoglobin reductase activities were carried out by separate electron transport systems on the same enzyme protein. Since NADH could be generated at a rate 9 to 14 times greater than NADPH under the usual conditions that obtain in erythrocytes, they believed that the reduction of methemoglobin might be largely NADH-dependent when glycolysis was dominant in the cell and NADPH-dependent when glucose was metabolized via the hexose monophosphate shunt pathway. Most recently, Niethammer and Huennekens[115)] have again modified the procedure for the isolation of methemoglobin-reducing systems. They utilized CM-Sephadex to remove residual hemoglobin and to separate the enzyme into 2 principal forms I and II, which corresponded to the first 2 forms previously obtained by chromatography with DEAE-cellulose. The molecular weight of these proteins was about 21,000 and they reduced methemoglobin in the presence of NADH or NADPH and methylene blue with a ratio of 3: 1. Only traces of heme were present and it was evident that no heme protein was required for either catalytic activity or structural integrity. Form II contained 1 mole of noncovalently bound $NADP^+$ per mole of protein and incubation of form I with $NADP^+$, but not NAD^+, at neutral pH resulted in the formation of form II.[116)] The authors suggested that the 2 principal forms of the enzyme differed because of the presence or absence of an equimolar amount of $NADP^+$ and that this difference might explain the polymorphism demonstrated in methemoglobin reductases. This enzyme(s) was not the same as the enzyme isolated by Hegesh and Avron[104)] which was strictly NADH-specific and had a slightly different mobility on polyacrylamide gel.[117)] Forms I and II, redesignated B-I and B-II, were normal in the erythrocytes of a patient with severe methemoglobinemia, while the NADH-dependent enzyme was almost totally deficient.

Scott *et al.*[100)] isolated and chracterized 2 NADPH-dehydrogenases, designated A and B. They contained heme, but not flavin, were weak methemoglobin reductases even in the absence of methylene blue, could account for about 5% of the normal ability of human erythrocytes to reduce methemoglobin, and were present in the erythrocytes of patients with hereditary methemoglobinemia. Losses of natural cofactors, alterations in activities due to differences in isolation procedures, nonoptimal assay conditions, and the use of different dyes as electron acceptors were advanced as explanations for these discrepant observations.[34,92] Shimizu and Matsuura[118] isolated from the erythrocytes of the blue-white dolphin a homogeneous enzyme protein that reduced methemoglobin, metmyoglobin and cytochrome c with NADPH or NADH in the presence of methylene blue. The enzyme was reported to contain neither heme nor flavin, had a molecular weight of 23,000 to 28,000, and was more specific for NADPH than for NADH. In the presence of methylene blue, the NADH-methemoglobin reductase isolated by Hegesh *et al.*[105] reduced methemoglobin at a more rapid rate with NADPH than with NADH. They, therefore, again suggested that one enzyme might be responsible for both NADPH-dehydrogenase and NADH-methemoglobin reductase activities.

The studies of Beutler and Baluda[119] and of Sass and his associates[120] demonstrated that when NADPH-dehydrogenase activity was involved in the reduction of methemoglobin, the enzyme served to reduce methylene blue to the leuco form which, in turn, reduced methemoglobin directly and non-enzymatically. A deficiency in the activity of NADPH-dehydrogenase was not associated with methemoglobinemia, impaired ability of erythrocytes to reduce methemoglobin *in vitro*, or decreased stimulation of hexose monophosphate shunt pathway activity by such agents as primaquine, acetylphenylhydrazine, ascorbic acid, and DCIP.[121,122]

The observations summarized here are most consistent with the thesis that a NADH-methemoglobin reductase system is the major pathway for the reduction of methemoglobin in human erythrocytes. NADH-methemoglobin reductase activity appears to be catalyzed by a distinct enzyme that is subject to considerable electrophoretic and functional heterogeneity upon a genetic basis.[27] The NADPH-dehydrogenase system may be a reserve pathway for the reduction of methemoglobin that becomes active only when an artificial electron carrier, such as methylene blue, is added. NADPH-dehydrogenase activity appears to be carried out by an enzyme protein different from that responsible for NADH-methemoglobin reductase activity.

ELECTROPHORETIC VARIANTS OF NADH-METHEMOGLOBIN REDUCTASE

Several groups of investigators have described electrophoretic variants of the NADH-methemoglobin reductase system.[105,108,123–129] Multiple structural aberrations of this enzyme in human erythrocytes probably exist, some with differences in charge and some with alterations in functional or stability characteristics. Hereditary methemoglobinemia, therefore, may be due to decreased synthesis or increased instability of a normal NADH-methemoglobin reductase enzyme protein, or to the synthesis of an abnormal enzyme protein with altered catalytic activity or stability. Schwartz and his associates[130)] examined the NADH-methemoglobin reductase isolated from the erythrocytes of patients with herditary methemoglobinemia who were members of 3 apparently unrelated Puerto Rican kindreds. The electrophoretic mobility of these enzymes was essentially the same as that described previously as characteristic of the Puerto Rican variant.[108)] Decreased affinity for NADH, increased affinity for the dye, DCIP, retarded utilization of deamino-NADH, and moderately reduced thermal stability were noted. The activity of NADH-methemoglobin reductase did not decline greatly with ageing of normal human erythrocytes *in vivo*, losing only about 17% of its activity.[130)] The abnormal enzyme, on the other hand, appeared to lose activity at a 20-fold greater rate. These authors, therefore, suggested that the deficient activity of NADH-methemoglobin reductase resulted from accelerated inactivation of the variant enzyme during the life span of the erythrocyte. A similar age-dependent decline in activity has also been observed in the erythrocytes of a patient with the Boston Fast variants.[131)]

In most electrophoretic studies with starch gel, a single band with NADH-methemoglobin reductase activity has been observed with normal hemolysates.[108,123,126–129)] Not infrequently, and especially after concentration, partial purification, or prolonged storage of hemolysates *in vitro*, an inconstant, minor, more anodic band has been noted.[108,126,128,129)] This minor band may represent a degradation product or subunits of the major component with NADH-methemoglobin reductase activity. It has been suggested that this minor sub-band may arise from hydrolysis of amide groups on the protein during purification or storage.[116)] The electrophoretic mobility of this minor band in normal hemolysates differs from that observed with 6 different electrophoretic variants.[108)] The minor band, therefore, probably does not correspond to the NADH-dehydrogenase II of Scott. Similar results have been obtained with agarose electrophoresis.[126)]

A comparison of the electrophoretic migration of bands with NADH-methemoglobin reductase activity after electrophoresis on starch gel at alkaline pH described in 2 recent publications.[108,127)] has permitted the tentative designation of at least 8 different variants.

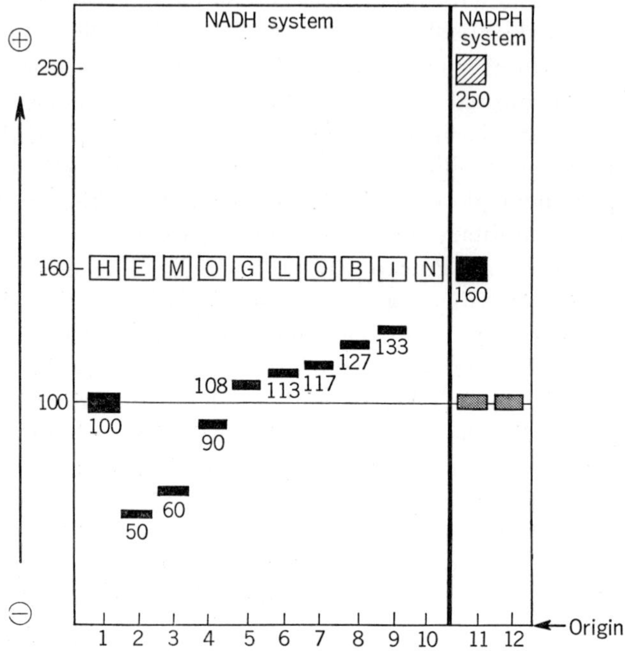

Fig. 2. Schematic representation of electrophoretic mobilities of human erythrocyte NADH-methemoglobin reductase and NADPH-dehydrogenase (methemoglobin reductase) on starch gel at pH 8.6–9.3. The migration of hemoglobin A is indicated, and relative mobilities of variants of NADH-methemoglobin reductase are represented in relation to the mobility of the common type or Dia 1 of Hopkinson *et al.*[127)] (channel 1) taken as 100; channel 2=Dia 3 of Hopkinson *et al.*; channel 3=Dia 4 of Hopkinson *et al.*; channel 4=Boston Slow; channel 5=Duarte; channel 6=Princeton; channel 7=Puerto Rico or Dia 6 or Dia 5 of Hopkinson *et al.*; channel 8=Boston Fast or Dia 2 of Hopkinson *et al.*; channel 9=California; channel 10=no demonstrable NADH-methemoglobin reductase band. Staining for NADPH-dehydrogenase activity is represented in the right-hand portion of the figure. Channel 11=partially purified (hemoglobin-free) enzyme extract of normal erythrocytes with 2 NADPH-dehydrogenase bands, 1 with the mobility of hemoglobin A and a more diffuse band with more rapid migration. Some staining of NADH-methemoglobin reductase occurs with NADPH. Channel 12=partially purified enzyme extract of erythrocytes from patient with NADPH-dehydrogenase deficiency. Note absence of both bands normally staining with NADPH and cross-reactivity of normal NADH-methemoglobin reductase with NADPH. Reproduced from 27 with permission from the publisher, Grune and Stratton.

These possible variants are shown schematically in Fig. 2 in which the relative migration of the abnormal bands is related to that of the normal or common band. Hopkinson *et al.*[127] discovered 1 common and 5 rare electrophoretic variants in a survey of 2,783 individuals, and an incidence of abnormal bands of about 1 per 100 in a European, Indian, Negro, Greek Cypriot, and unspecified population group. All of their variants were found as a second band with NADH-methemoglobin reductase activity, along with a band with normal mobility, in hemolysates of erythrocytes from apparently asymptomatic individuals. In their Dia 6–1 variant, the faster band stained with appreciably weaker intensity and it was of interest that this abnormal band appeared to have the same relative mobility as the Puerto Rico variant which was associated with decreased activity.[108] Dia 2, the most common variant, appeared to have the same mobility as the Boston Fast variant. Recently, Feig *et al.*[131] have noted that the hemolysate originally thought to have a single NADH-methemoglobin reductase band with the mobility of Boston Fast may have 2 separate bands with similar, but not identical, mobilities. Brewer *et al.*,[124] Detter *et al.*,[128] West and Prankerd,[125] and Hsieh and Jaffé[108] have also reported abnormal or double-band patterns in hemolysates of erythrocytes obtained from asymptomatic individuals. The activity of these NADH-methemoglobin reductases was only slightly decreased, if at all. Thus, there may be many variants of NADH-methemoglobin reductase that are not expressed as significant deficiencies in activity and, therefore, are not clinically apparent. Patients with transient and atypical methemoglobinemia may have had variants with only minimal decreases in activity. Precise correlations between levels of NADH-methemoglobin reductase activity, electrophoretic mobility, and clinical severity have not been established. In most cases with significant methemoglobinemia and an electrophoretically abnormal enzyme, however, the activity of NADH-methemoglobin reductase has been 25% of normal or less. An exception to this was noted with the Boston Slow variant where methemoglobinemia was associated with 40% of normal activity.[108]

Two other variants of NADH-methemoglobin reductase with altered electrophoretic mobilities have been reported. Because they have not been examined under comparable experimental conditions, their relationships to those described above have not been established. West *et al.*[28] described 2 bands in normal hemolysates and a single less intense band with intermediate mobility in the partially purified extract of the hemolysate of the erythrocytes of a patient with hereditary methemoglobinemia and NADH-methemoglobin reductase deficiency. The erythrocytes of the patient's mother had 2 normal bands and a faint band with the same abnormal mobility. Brewer *et al.*[124] noted a band with abnormal migration in the hemolysate of a Negro male's erythrocytes, but further studies were not possible.

Polyacrylamide gel electrophoresis at pH 9.0 was used by Hegesh *et al.*[132] to demonstrate 4 (occasionally 5) bands with NADH-methemoglobin reductase activity in hemolysates of normal erythrocytes. Two of these bands, NADH-3 and NADH-4, were absent from the hemolysate of the erythrocytes of the Puerto Rican patient with NADH-methemoglobin reductase deficiency and hereditary methemoglobinemia.[79,133] After starch gel electrophoresis, this patient's NADH-methemoglobin reductase migrated as a single, consistent abnormal band.[108]

Different patterns of migration were observed after isoelectric focusing of hemolysates of human erythrocytes and staining for NADH-methemoglobin reductase and NADH-dehydrogenase activity.[134] The NADH-specific enzyme (D_{II}) appeared to stain with decreased intensity and to have an abnormal component upon examination of a hemolysate from a subject heterozygous for hereditary methemoglobinemia. Further studies, comparing the patterns obtained with the different electrophoretic techniques, will be required to permit definition of the precise characteristics of the various enzymes that have been identified.

When NADH in the staining mixture was replaced by an equimolar amount of NADPH, 2 bands were observed after electrophoresis on starch gel (Fig. 2). One ill-defined band migrated to a position more anodal than hemoglobin. The second, sharper, band migrated with hemoglobin A and, therefore, was obscured on electrophoresis of whole hemolysates. These bands were normal in all hemolysates with electrophoretically abnormal NADH-methemoglobin reductases. Although NADH-methemoglobin reductase showed some cross-reactivity with NADPH after electrophoresis of partially purified enzyme extracts, NADPH-dehydrogenase (methemoglobin reductase) did not show appreciable staining with NADH. Both bands with NADPH-dehydrogenase activity were absent after electrophoresis of hemolysate and partially purified enzyme extract of the erythrocytes of the patient reported by Sass *et al.*[121] to be deficient in NADPH-dehydrogenase activity.[108] This patient did not have methemoglobinemia, the ability of his erythrocytes to reduce methemoglobin *in vitro* in the absence of added methylene blue was normal, and the activity and electrophoretic mobility of NADH-methemoglobin reductase were normal. The electrophoretic patterns attributed to NADPH-dehydrogenase activity will have to be reevaluated in the light of the recent finding of alterations in mobility after incubation with $NADP^+$.[116]

These observations have provided additional evidence for the thesis that NADH-methemoglobin reductase is an enzyme system distinct from the NADPH-dehydrogenases and is the major system for the reduction of methemoglobin to hemoglobin in normal human erythrocytes. Further studies will be required to define accurately the nature of the NADH-methemoglobin reductase and the sequence of the reactions involved in the transfer of electrons from reduced pyridine nucleotides to the ferric heme moiety of methemoglobin.

REFERENCES

1 Evelyn, K. A. and Malloy, H. T., Microdetermination of oxyhemoglobin, methemoglobin, and sulfhemoglobin in a single sample of blood. *J. Biol. Chem.*, **126**, 655 (1938).

2 Bunn, H. F. and Jandl, J. H., Exchange of heme among hemoglobin molecules. *Proc. Nat. Acad. Sci. U. S.*, **56**, 974 (1966).

3 Keilin, J., Nature of the haem-binding groups in native and denatured haemoglobin and myoglobin. *Nature* (London), **187**, 365 (1960).

4 Dacie, J. V., Grimes, A. J., Meisler, A., Steingold, L., Hemsted, E. H., Beaven, G. H. and White, J. C., Hereditary Heinz-body anaemia. *Br. J. Haematol.*, **10**, 388 (1964).

5 Jacob, H. S., Mechanisms of Heinz-body formation and attachment to red cell membrane. *Semin. Hematol.*, **7**, 341 (1970).

6 François, D., Cas de cyanose congéniale sans cause apparente. *Bull. Acad. Roy. Med. Belg.*, **4**, 698 (1845).

7 Dittrich, P., Ueber methämoglobinbildende Gifte. *Naunyn Schmiedeberg's Arch. Exper. Path. Pharmakol.*, **29**, 247 (1891).

8 Stokvis, B. J., Zur Casuistik der autotoxischen enterogenen Cyanosen. (Methaemoglobinaemia (?) et enteritis parasitaria). *Internat. Beitr. Inn. Med.*, **1**, 597 (1902).

9 Talma, S., Intraglobulaire methaemoglobinaemie bij den mensch. *Nederl. Tijdschr. Geneesk.*, **2**, 721 (1902).

10 van den Bergh, A. A. H., Enterogene Cyanose. *Deutsches Arch. Klin. Med.*, **83**, 86 (1905).

11 Slosse, A. and Wybauw, R., Un cas de méthémoglobinémie idiopathique. *Ann. Soci. Roy. Sci. Méd. Natur. Brux.*, **70**, 206 (1912).

12 Litarczek, G., Aubert, H., Cosmulesco, I., Comanesco, V. and Litarczek, S., Sur un cas de cyanose auto-toxique par méthémoglobinémie

intra-globulaire. *Le Sang*, **4**, 188 (1930).
13 Conant, J. B. and Scott, N. D., A spectrophotometric study of certain equilibria involving the oxidation of hemoglobin to methemoglobin. *J. Biol. Chem.*, **76**, 207 (1928).
14 Bodansky, O., Methemoglobinemia and methemoglobin-producing compounds. *Pharmacol. Rev.*, **3**, 144 (1951).
15 Kiese, M., The biochemical production of ferrihemoglobin-forming derivatives from aromatic amines, and mechanisms of ferrihemoglobin formation. *Pharmacol. Rev.*, **18**, 1091 (1966).
16 Hitzenberger, K., Autotoxische Zyanose. (Intraglobuläre Methämoglobinämie.) *Wien. Arch. Inn. Med.*, **23**, 85 (1932).
17 Dieckmann, W. J., Methemoglobinemia. *Arch. Intern. Med.*, **50**, 574 (1932).
18 Bensley, E. H., Rhea, L. J. and Mills, E. S., Familial idiopathic methaemoglobinaemia. *Quar. J. Med.* (New Series), **7**, 325 (1938).
19 Lian, C., Frumusan, P. and Sassier, D., Méthémoglobinémie congénitale et familiale. Action favorable de l'acide ascorbique. *Bull. Mém. Soc. Méd. Hosp. Paris*, **55**, 1194 (1939).
20 Gibson, Q. H., The reduction of methaemoglobin by ascorbic acid. *Biochem. J.*, **37**, 615 (1943).
21 Barcroft, H., Gibson, Q. H., Harrison, D. C. and McMurray, J., Familial idiopathic methaemoglobinaemia and its treatment with ascorbic acid. *Clin. Sci.*, **5**, 145 (1945).
22 Sievers, R. F. and Ryon, J. B., Congenital idiopathic methemoglobinemia. Favorable response to ascorbic acid therapy. *Arch. Inter. Med.*, **75**, 299 (1945).
23 Gibson, Q. H., The reduction of methaemoglobin in red blood cells and studies on the cause of idiopathic methaemoglobinaemia. *Biochem. J.*, **42**, 13 (1948).
24 Scott, E. M. and Hoskins, D. D., Hereditary methemoglobinemia in Alaskan Eskimos and Indians. *Blood*, **13**, 795 (1958).
25 Scott, E. M. and Griffith, I. V., The enzymic defect of hereditary methemoglobinemia: diaphorase. *Biochim. Biophys. Acta*, **34**, 584 (1959).
26 Keitt, A. S., Hereditary methemoglobinemia with deficiency of NADH-methemoglobin reductase. *in*: The Metabolic Basis of Inherited Disease, Third Edition. ed. by, Stanbury, J. B., Wyngaarden, J. B. and Fredrickson, D. S. (McGraw-Hill Book Company, New York, 1972), pp. 1389–1397.
27 Jaffé, E. R. and Hsieh, H.-S., DPNH-methemoglobin reductase deficiency and hereditary methemoglobinemia. *Semin. Hematol.*, **8**, 417 (1971).
28 West, C. A., Gomperts, B. D., Huehns, E. R., Kessel, I. and Ashby, J. R., Demonstration of an enzyme variant in a case of congenital

methaemoglobinaemia. *Br. Med. J.*, **4**, 212 (1967).

29 Kaplan, J.-C., Studies on NADH and NADPH diaphorases in blood cells from normal subjects and in congenital methaemoglobinaemia. *in*: Red Cell Structure and Metabolism. ed. by Ramot, B. (Academic Press, New York, 1971), pp. 125–134.

30 Hörlein, H. and Weber, G., Über chronische familiäre Methämoglobinämie und eine neue Modifikation des Methämoglobins. *Deutsche Med. Wochenschr.*, **73**, 476 (1948).

31 Singer, K., Hereditary hemolytic disorders associated with abnormal hemoglobins. *Amer. J. Med.*, **18**, 633 (1955).

32 Jaffé, E. R. and Heller, P., Methemoglobinemia in man. *Prog. Hematol.*, **4**, 48 (1964).

33 Rossi-Fanelli, A., Antonini, E. and Mondovì, B., Ferrihemoglobin reduction in normal and methemoglobinemic subjects. *Clin. Chim. Acta*, **2**, 476 (1957).

34 Scott, E. M., Congenital methemoglobinemia due to DPNH-diaphorase deficiency. *in*: Hereditary Disorders of Erythrocyte Metabolism. ed. by Beutler, E. (Grune and Stratton, New York and London, 1968), pp. 102–108.

35 Eder, H. A., Finch, C. and McKee, R. W., Congenital methemoglobinemia. A clinical and biochemical study of a case. *J. Clin. Invest.*, **28**, 265 (1949).

36 Waisman, H. A., Bain, J. A., Richmond, J. B. and Munsey, F. A., Laboratory and clinical studies in congenital methemoglobinemia. *Pediatrics*, **10**, 293 (1952).

37 Jaffé, E. R. and Neumann, G., A comparison of the effect of menadione, methylene blue and ascorbic acid on the reduction of methaemoglobin *in vivo*. *Nature* (London), **202**, 607 (1964).

38 Jandl, J. H., Engle, L. K. and Allen, D. W., Oxidative hemolysis and precipitation of hemoglobin. I. Heinz-body anemias as an acceleration of red-cell aging. *J. Clin. Invest.*, **39**, 1818 (1960).

39 Roughton, F. J. W. and Kendrew, J. C., Haemoglobin (Butterworths Scientific Publications, London, 1949), p. 57.

40 Weiss, J. J., Nature of the iron-oxygen bond in oxyhaemoglobin. *Nature* (London), **202**, 83 (1964).

41 Peisach, J., Blumberg, W. E., Wittenberg, B. A. and Wittenberg, J. B., The electronic structure of protoheme proteins. III. Configuration of the heme and its ligands. *J. Biol. Chem.*, **243**, 1871 (1968).

42 Wittenberg, J. B., Wittenberg, B. A., Peisach, J. and Blumberg, W. E., On the state of the iron and the nature of the ligand in oxyhemoglobin. *Proc. Nat. Acad. Sci. U.S.*, **67**, 1846 (1970).

43 Perutz, M. F. and Lehmann, H., Molecular pathology of human haemoglobin. *Nature* (London), **219**, 902 (1968).

44 Carrell, R. W. and Lehmann, H., The unstable haemoglobin haemolytic anaemias. *Semin. Hematol.*, **6**, 116 (1969).
45 Lemberg, R. and Legge, J. W., Hematin Compounds and Bile Pigments (Interscience Publishers, New York, 1949).
46 Brooks, J., The oxidation of haemoglobin to methaemoglobin by oxygen. *J. Physiol.* (London), **107**, 332 (1948).
47 Brooks, J., The oxidation of haemoglobin to methaemoglobin by oxygen. II. The relation between the rate of oxidation and the partial pressure of oxygen. *Proc. Roy. Soc. London, Ser.* B, **118**, 560 (1935).
48 George, P., The specific reactions of iron in some hemoproteins. *Adv. Catal.*, **4**, 367 (1952).
49 Kikuchi, G., Shukuya, R., Suzuki, M. and Nakamura. C., On the mechanism of the activation of molecular oxygen by hemoglobin. *J. Biochem.*, **42**, 267 (1955).
50 Keilin, D., Reactions of haemoproteins with hydrogen peroxide and the supposed formation of hydrogen peroxide during the autoxidation of haemoglobin. *Nature* (London), **191**, 769 (1961).
51 Cohen, G. and Hochstein, P., Generation of hydrogen peroxide in erythrocytes by hemolytic agents. *Biochemistry* (Washington), **3**, 895 (1964).
52 Kosower, N. S., Vanderhoff, G. A., Kosower, E. M. and Huang, P.-K. C., Decreased glutathione content of human erythrocytes produced by methyl phenylazoformate. *Biochem. Biophys. Res. Comm.*, **20**, 469 (1965).
53 Beutler, E., Drug-induced hemolytic anemia. *Pharmacol. Rev.*, **21**, 73 (1969).
54 Van Assendelft, O. W. and Zijlstra, W. G., The formation of haemiglobin using nitrites. *Clin. Chim. Acta*, **11**, 571 (1965).
55 Cohen, G., Martinez, M. and Hochstein, P., Generation of hydrogen peroxide during the reaction of nitrite with oxyhemoglobin. *Biochemistry* (Washington), **3**, 901 (1964).
56 Beutler, E., Abnormalities of the hexose monophosphate shunt. *Semin. Hematol.*, **8**, 311 (1971).
57 Rossi-Fanelli, A., Antonini, E. and Caputo, A., Studies on the structure of human hemoglobin. I. Physicochemical properties of human globin. *Biochim. Biophys. Acta*, **30**, 608 (1958).
58 Allen, D. W. and Jandl, J. H., Oxidative hemolysis and precipitation of hemoglobin. II. Role of thiols in oxidant drug action. *J. Clin. Invest.*, **40**, 454 (1961).
59 Beutler, E. and Baluda, M. C., The role of methemoglobin in oxidative degradation of hemoglobin. *Acta Haematol.*, **27**, 321 (1962).
60 Rentsch, G., Genesis of Heinz bodies and methemoglobin formation. *Biochem. Pharmacol.*, **17**, 423 (1968).

61 Hurley, T. H., Weisman, R., Jr. and Pasquariello, A. E., The determination of the survival of transfused red cells by a method of differential hemolysis. *J. Clin. Invest.*, **33**, 835 (1954).

62 Harris, J. W. and Kellermeyer, R. W., The Red Cell. Production, Metabolism, Destruction: Normal and Abnormal. Revised edition (Harvard University Press, Cambridge, Mass., 1970), p. 495.

63 Nicholls, P., Activity of catalase in the red cell. *Biochim. Biophys, Acta*, **99**, 286 (1965).

64 Mills, G. C., Hemoglobin catabolism. I. Glutathione peroxidase, an erythrocyte enzyme which protects hemoglobin from oxidative breakdown. *J. Biol. Chem.*, **229**, 189 (1957).

65 Boivin, P., Galand, C., Hakim, J. and Blery, M., Déficit en glutathionperoxydase érythrocytaire et anémie hémolytique médicamenteuse. Une nouvelle observation. *La Presse Medicale*, **78**, 171 (1970).

66 Aebi, H., Bossi, E., Cantz, M., Matsubara, S. and Suter, H., Acatalas(em)ia in Switzerland. *in*: Hereditary Disorders of Erythrocyte Metabolism. ed. by Beutler, E. (Grune and Stratton, New York, 1968), pp. 41–61.

67 Takahara, S., Acatalasemia and hypocatalasemia in the Orient. *Semin. Hematol.*, **8**, 397 (1971).

68 Jaffé, E. R., Metabolic processes involved in the formation and reduction of methemoglobin in human erythrocytes. *in*: The Red Blood Cell. A Comprehensive Treatise. ed. by Bishop, C. and Surgenor, D. M. (Academic Press, New York, 1964), pp. 397–422.

69 Rubinstein, D., Ottolenghi, P. and Denstedt, O. F., The metabolism of the erythrocyte. XIII. Enzyme activity in the reticulocyte. *Canad. J. Biochem. Physiol.*, **34**, 222 (1956).

70 Kiese, M., Die Reduktion des Hämiglobins. *Biochem. Z.*, **316**, 264 (1944).

71 Smith, J. E. and Beutler, E., Methemoglobin formation and reduction in man and various animal species. *Amer. J. Physiol.*, **210**, 347 (1966).

72 Warburg, O., Kubowitz, F. and Christian, W., Über die katalytische Wirkung von Methylenblau in lebenden Zellen. *Biochem. Z.*, **227**, 245 (1930).

73 Gutmann, H. R., Jandorf, B. J. and Bodansky, O., The rôle of pyridine nucleotides in the reduction of methemoglobin. *J. Biol. Chem.*, **169**, 145 (1947).

74 Gibson, Q. H., The reduction of methaemoglobin in red blood cells and studies on the cause of idiopathic methaemoglobinaemia. *Biochem. J.*, **42**, 13 (1948).

75 Keitt, A. S., Smith, T. W. and Jandl, J. H., Red-cell " pseudomosaicism " in congenital methemoglobinemia. *New Eng. J. Med.*, **275**, 398 (1966).

76 Jaffé, E. R., Hereditary methemoglobinemias associated with abnormali-

ties in the metabolism of erythrocytes. *Amer. J. Med.*, **41**, 786 (1966).

77 Schröter, W. and Winter, P., Zur Bedeutung des 2,3-Diphosphoglycerat-Zyklus in Erythrozyten: Beziehungen zwischen Methämoglobin-und 2,6-Dichlorophenolindophenol-Reduktion, Glykolyse, und 2,3-Diphosphoglyceratbildung. *Blut*, **14**, 1 (1966).

78 Matthies, H., Die wirkung von aldehyden auf die methämoglobinrückbildung in erythrocyten. *Biochem. Z.*, **329**, 341 (1957).

79 Jaffé, E. R., The reduction of methemoglobin in human erythrocytes incubated with purine nucleosides. *J. Clin. Invest.*, **38**, 1555 (1959).

80 Asakura, T., Adachi, K., Minakami, S. and Yoshikawa, H., Nonglycolytic sugar metabolism in human erythrocytes. I. Xylitol metabolism. *J. Biochem.*, **62**, 184 (1967).

81 Travis, S. F., Oski, F. A., Morrison, A. D., Clements, R. S., Jr. and Winegrad, A. I., Polyol pathway and methemoglobin reduction in human RBCs. *Blood*, **38**, 831 (1971).

82 Christine, L., Thomson, G., Iggo, B., Brownis, A. C. and Stewart, C. P., The reduction of dehydroascorbic acid by human erythrocytes. *Clin. Chim. Acta*, **1**, 557 (1956).

83 Teruuchi, J. and Mochizuki, H., Metabolism of dehydroascorbic acid in human subjects. *J. Vitaminol.* (Kyoto), **6**, 163 (1960).

84 Hughes, R. E. and Maton, S. C., The passage of vitamin C across the erythrocyte membrane. *Br. J. Hematol.*, **14**, 247 (1968).

85 Strömme, J. H. and Eldjarn, L., The role of the pentose phosphate pathway in the reduction of methaemoglobin in human erythrocytes. *Biochem. J.*, **84**, 406 (1962).

86 Jaffé, E. R. and Neuman G., Hereditary methemoglobinemia, toxic methemoglobinemia and the reduction of methemoglobin. *Ann. N. Y. Acad. Sci.*, **151**, 795 (1968).

87 Prins, H. K., Loos, J. A. and Zürcher, C., Glutathione deficiency. *in*: Hereditary disorders of erythrocyte metabolism. ed. by Beutler, E. (Grune and Stratton, New York, 1968), pp. 165–174.

88 Mohler, D. N., Majerus, P. W., Minnich, V., Hess, C. E. and Garrick, M. D., Glutathione synthetase deficiency as a cause of hereditary hemolytic disease. *New Eng. J. Med.*, **283**, 1253 (1970).

89 Dawson, J. P., Thayer, W. W. and Desforges, J. F., Acute hemolytic anemia in the newborn infant due to naphthalene poisoning: Report of two cases, with investigations into the mechanism of the disease. *Blood*, **13**, 1113 (1958).

90 Jaffé, E. R., The reduction of methemoglobin in erythrocytes of a patient with congenital methemoglobinemia, subjects with erythrocyte glucose-6-phosphate dehydrogenase deficiency, and normal individuals. *Blood*, **21**, 561 (1963).

91 Kanazawa, Y., Hattori, M., Kosaka, K. and Nakao, K., The relation-

ship of NADH-dependent diaphorase activity and methemoglobin reduction in human erythrocytes. *Clin. Chim. Acta*, **19**, 524 (1968).

92 Jaffé, E. R. and Neumann, G., The methemoglobin reductase systems of human erythrocytes. *in*: Metabolism and membrane permeability of erythrocytes and thrombocytes. ed. by Deutsch, E., Gerlach, E. and Moser, K. (Georg Thieme, Stuttgart, 1968), pp. 83–90.

93 Jaffé, E. R., Rieber, E. E., Anderson, H. M., Kosower, N. S. and Penny, J. L., Glutathione reductase activity and hemolysis in hemoglobin C disease. *J. Clin. Invest.*, **47**, 51a (1968).

94 Valentine, W. N., Hsieh, H.-S., Paglia, D. E., Anderson, H. M., Baughan, M. A., Jaffé, E. R. and Garson, O. M., Hereditary hemolytic anemia: Association with phosphoglycerate kinase deficiency in erythrocytes and leukocytes. *Trans. Assoc. Amer. Physicians*, **81**, 49 (1968).

95 Jaffé, E. R., Paglia, D. E., Harris, S. R., Valentine, W. N., Klein, R. L. and Rapin, I., Triosephosphate isomerase deficiency and hemolytic anemia in an adult. Abstracts, XIII International Congress of Hematology, Munich, Germany (1970), p. 122.

96 Petragnani, N., Nogueira, O. C. and Raw, I., Methaemoglobin reduction through cytochrome b_5. *Nature* (London), **184**, 1651 (1959).

97 Hultquist, D. E. and Passon, P. G., Catalysis of methaemoglobin reduction by erythrocyte cytochrome b_5 and cytochrome b_5 reductase. *Nature New Biology*, **229**, 252 (1971).

98 Scott, E. M. and Griffith, I. V., The enzymic defect in hereditary methemoglobinemia: diaphorase. *Biochim. Biophys. Acta*, **34**, 584 (1959).

99 Scott, E. M. and McGraw, J. C., Purification and properties of diphosphopyridine nucleotide diaphorase of human erythrocytes. *J. Biol. Chem.*, **237**, 249 (1962).

100 Scott, E. M., Duncan, I. W. and Ekstrand, V., The reduced pyridine nucleotide dehydrogenases of human erythrocytes. *J. Biol. Chem.*, **240**, 481 (1965).

101 Scott, E. M., Purification of diphosphopyridine nucleotide diaphorase from methemoglobinemic erythrocytes. *Biochem. Biophys. Res. Comm.*, **9**, 59 (1962).

102 Jaffé, E. R., DPNH-methemoglobin reductase (diaphorase). *in*: Biochemical methods in red-cell genetics. ed. by Yunis, J. J. (Academic Press, New York, 1969), pp. 231–253.

103 Hegesh, E. and Avron, M., The enzymatic reduction of ferrihemoglobin. I. The reduction of ferrihemoglobin in red blood cells and hemolysates. *Biochim. Biophys. Acta*, **146**, 91 (1967).

104 Hegesh, E. and Avron, M., The enzymatic reduction of ferrihemoglobin. II. Purification of a ferrihemoglobin reductase from human erythrocytes. *Biochim. Biophys. Acta*, **146**, 397 (1967).

105 Hegesh, E., Calmanovici, N., Lupo, M. and Bochkowsky, R., Dia-

phorases of human erythrocytes. *in*: Red cell structure and metabolism. ed. by Ramot, B. (Academic Press, New York, 1971), pp. 113–124.

106 Hegesh, E., Calmanovici, N. and Avron, M., New method for determining ferrihemoglobin reductase (NADH-methemoglobin reductase) in erythrocytes. *J. Lab. Clin. Med.*, **72**, 339 (1968).

107 Scott, E. M., A comparison of two methods of determining DPNH-methemoglobin reductase. *Clin. Chim. Acta*, **23**, 495 (1969).

108 Hsieh, H.-S. and Jaffé, E. R., Electrophoretic and functional variants of NADH-methemoglobin reductase in hereditary methemoglobinemia. *J. Clin. Invest.*, **50**, 196 (1971).

109 Zamudio, I., Cellino, M. and Canessa-Fischer, M., The relation between membrane structure and NADH: (acceptor) oxidoreductase of erythrocyte ghosts. *Arch. Biochem. Biophys.*, **129**, 336 (1969).

110 Sugita, Y., Nomura, S. and Yoneyama, Y., Purification of reduced pyridine nucleotide dehydrogenase from human erythrocytes and methemoglobin reduction by the enzyme. *J. Biol. Chem.*, **246**, 6072 (1971).

111 Kiese, M., Schneider, C. and Waller, H.-D., Hämiglobinreduktase. *Naunyn-Schmiedeberg's Arch. Exper. Path. Pharmakol.*, **231**, 158 (1957).

112 Huennekens, F. M., Caffrey, R. W., Basford, R. E. and Gabrio, B. W., Erythrocyte metabolism. IV. Isolation and properties of methemoglobin reductase. *J. Biol. Chem.*, **227**, 261 (1957).

113 Shrago, E. and Falcone, A. B., Human-erythrocyte reduced triphosphopyridine nucleotide oxidase. *Biochim. Biophys. Acta*, **67**, 147 (1963).

114 Kajita, A., Kerwar, G. K. and Huennekens, F. M., Multiple forms of methemoglobin reductase. *Arch. Biochem. Biophys.*, **130**, 662 (1969).

115 Niethammer, D. and Huennekens, F. M., Electrophoretic separation and characterization of the multiple forms of methemoglobin reductase. *Arch. Biochem. Biophys.*, **146**, 564 (1971).

116 Niethammer, D. and Huennekens, F. M., Bound TPN as the determinant of polymorphism in methemoglobin reductase. *Biochem. Biophys. Res. Comm.*, **45**, 345 (1971).

117 Niethammer, D. and Huennekens, F. M., DPNH- and TPNH-dependent methemoglobin reducing systems from human erythrocytes. *Blood*, **38**, 831 (1971).

118 Shimizu, C. and Matsuura, F., Purification and some properties of "methemoglobin reductase." *Agric. Biol. Chem.*, **32**, 587 (1968).

119 Beutler, E. and Baluda, M. C., Methemoglobin reduction. Studies of the interaction between cell populations and of the role of methylene blue. *Blood*, **22**, 323 (1963).

120 Sass, M. D., Caruso, C. J. and Axelrod, D. R., Mechanism of the

TPNH-linked reduction of methemoglobin by methylene blue. *Clin. Chim. Acta*, **24**, 77 (1969).

121 Sass, M. D., Caruso, C. J. and Farhangi, M., TPNH-methemoglobin reductase deficiency: A new red-cell enzyme defect. *J. Lab. Clin. Med.*, **70**, 760 (1967).

122 Sass, M. D., Observations on the role of TPNH dehydrogenase in human red cells. *Clin. Chim. Acta*, **21**, 101 (1968).

123 Kaplan, J.-C. and Beutler, E., Electrophoresis of red-cell NADH- and NADPH-diaphorases in normal subjects and patients with congenital methemoglobinemia. *Biochem. Biophys. Res. Comm.*, **29**, 605 (1967).

124 Brewer, G. J., Eaton, J. W., Knutsen, C. S. and Beck, G. C., A starch gel electrophoretic method for the study of diaphorase isozymes and preliminary results with sheep and human erythrocytes. *Biochem. Biophys. Res. Comm.*, **29**, 198 (1967).

125 West, C. A. and Prankerd, T. A. J., The production of methaemoglobinaemia. *in*: Metabolism and membrane permeability of erythrocytes and thrombocytes. ed. by Deutsch, E., Gerlach, E. and Moser, K. (Georg Thieme, Stuttgart, 1968), pp. 147–149.

126 Bloom, G. E. and Zarkowsky, H. S., Heterogeneity of the enzymatic defect in congenital methemoglobinemia. *New Eng. J. Med.*, **281**, 919 (1969).

127 Hopkinson, D. A., Corney, G., Cook, P. J. L., Robson, E. B. and Harris, H., Genetically determined electrophoretic variants of human red-cell NADH diaphorase. *Ann. Hum. Genet.* (London), **34**, 1 (1970).

128 Detter, J. C., Anderson, J. E. and Giblett, E. R., NADH diaphorase: an inherited variant associated with normal methemoglobin reduction. *Amer. J. Hum. Genet.*, **22**, 100 (1970).

129 Schwartz, J. M., Ross, J. M., Paress, P. S., Fagelman, K. and Fogel, L., Electrophoretic and kinetic characterization of a NADH-diaphorase variant in a methemoglobinemic subject. *in*: Red Cell Structure and Metabolism. ed. by Ramot, B. (Academic Press, New York, 1971), pp. 135–146.

130 Schwartz, J. M., Paress, P. S., Ross, J. M., DiPillo, F. and Rizek, R., Unstable variant of NADH-methemoglobin reductase in Puerto Ricans with hereditary methemoglobinemia. *J. Clin. Invest.*, **51**, 1594 (1972).

131 Feig, S. A., Nathan, D. G., Gerald, P. S. and Zarhowrki, H. S., Congenital methemoglobinemia: The result of Age-dependent Decay of methemoglobin reductase. *Blood*, **39**, 407 (1972).

132 Hegesh, E., Calmanovici, N., Lupo, M. and Bochkowsky, R., The diaphorase bands of human erythrocytes. *J. Lab. Clin. Med.*, **77**, 859 (1971).

133 Jaffé, E. R., Neumann, G., Rothberg, H., Wilson, F. T., Webster,

R. M. and Wolff, J. A., Hereditary methemoglobinemia with and without mental retardation. A study of three families. *Amer. J. Med.*, **41**, 42 (1966).

134 Sonnet, J., De Noyette, J. P. and Steichen-Defalque, M., Focalisation isoélectrique de la NADH: methémoglobine réductase et des NAD(P)H: diaphorases de l'érythrocyte humain. *Clin. Chim. Acta*, **32**, 5 (1971).

Metabolic Disorders in Red Blood Cells

H. D. WALLER and H. C. BENÖHR

Department of Internal Medicine, University of Tübingen, Germany

One must mainly distinguish in the red blood cells, enzyme defects in glycolysis and the pentose phosphate cycle. So far autosomal-recessive inherited enzyme defects are known for 9 of the main and side-chain enzymes of glycolysis. These defects lead generally to spontaneous nonspherocytic hemolytic anemia. The cause of hemolysis is probably an ATP deficiency. Enzyme defects in the pentose phosphate cycle cause GSH deficiency and instability. Hemolysis rarely occurs spontaneously, however, but often after exposure to drugs. The same is true for defects in GSH synthesis and in GSSG reduction.

Gibson,[1] in 1948, succeeded for the first time in demonstrating a relationship between an enzymatic defect and a hematologic disorder with the detection of a methemoglobin reductase deficiency. Since then numerous congenital metabolic disorders in erythrocytes have been discovered which indirectly or directly shorten the life span of blood cells. The detection of enzymatic abnormalities led not only to interesting considerations concerning the pathogenesis of hemolytic anemias, but also contributed significantly to the understanding of normal erythrocyte metabolism and its regulation. Above all, we must distinguish between 2 groups of metabolic disorders: those concerned with a defect in ATP-generating glycolysis and in the cleavage of ATP, and those concerned with disturbances in glutathione synthesis and reduction.

The mature human erythrocyte contains neither nucleus, mitochondria, nor ribosomes. The generation of ATP is exclusively dependent on the glycolytic degradation of glucose. The continuous supply of an adequate ATP concentration is necessary for the maintenance of cation equilibrium, as well as for the integrity of the membrane structure. ATP is necessary for the synthesis of glutathione from amino acids, for the generation of pyridine nucleotides from adenine,[2] and for the exchange of cholesterol and phosphatides between the erythrocyte membrane and blood plasma. NADH formed from glycolysis is necessary for the reduction of pyruvate to lactate, in addition to methemoglobin reduction, which is catalyzed by methemoglobin reductase. The major organic phosphate of the erythrocyte, made available by the Rapoport-Luebering cycle, is 2,3-DPG, a compound of great importance for the regulation of glycolysis. In addition, by binding to deoxyhemoglobin, 2,3-DPG affects the affinity of hemoglobin for oxygen.[3,4] Metabolic disorders in glycolysis may lead to a shortened erythrocyte life span mainly by a decrease in the ATP concentration.

Approximately 10% of the glucose is oxidatively metabolized by the pentose phosphate cycle. NADPH formed thereby, is then made available for glutathione reductase-catalyzed glutathione reduction. Methemoglobin reduction, catalyzed by a NADPH-dependent methemoglobin reductase, is of only minor importance. A deficiency of reduced glutathione, as a consequence of a defect in the enzymatic chain for reduction or synthesis of glutathione, can lead to hemolysis when the cell is subjected to the effects of certain drugs, legumes, or radiation. Spontaneous nonspherocytic anemias are observed only rarely in disturbances of glutathione reduction.

DEFECTS IN GLYCOLYSIS IN RED BLOOD CELLS

Absence or decrease in activity, especially of the main glycolytic enzymes, leads for the most part to a decrease in the glycolytic rate and, therefore, also in ATP formation. The consequence is a shortened life span of the erythrocytes. Generally there is a clinical picture of nonspherocytic hemolytic anemia. After a short lifetime the erythrocytes assume a spherical shape and are probably sequestered prematurely in the reticuloendothelial system.

Presently, genetic defects are known in 9 of the total of 13 main and side-chain enzymes of glycolysis (Fig. 1). Biochemical diagnosis is based on the detection of the decrease in actual enzyme activity as measured spectrophotometrically. Homozygous carriers of the defect have residual activities of less than 1 and up to 20%, heterozygotes between 40 and 60%. The transmittance is mostly autosomal recessive. Extensive metabolic studies of the various carriers of enzyme defects have shown, however, that by no means must each enzyme deficiency in the glycolytic chain result in a parallel decrease in the rate of glycolysis and ATP formation. The metabolites produced before the disturbed enzyme reaction are generally increased, while those behind the enzyme block are decreased. The absence of a definite correlation between the

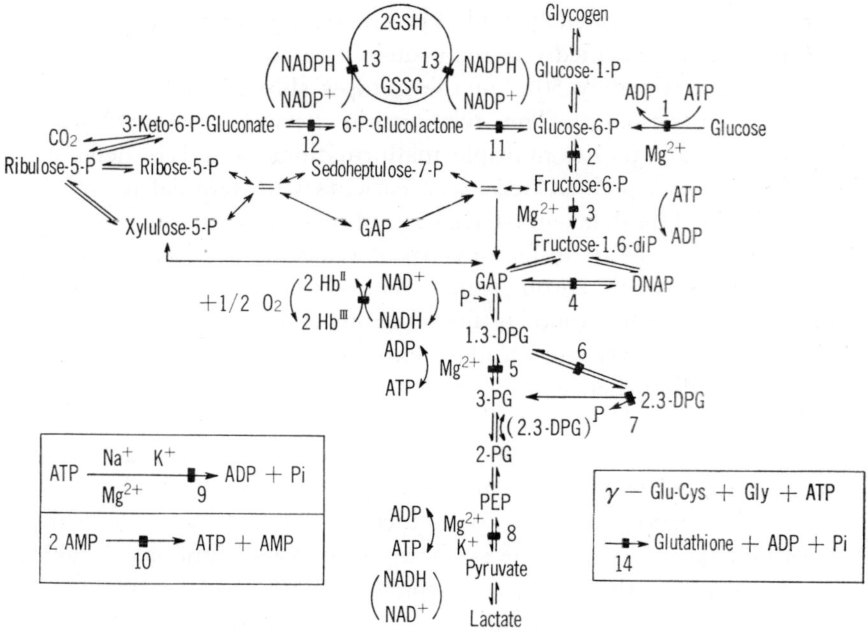

Fig. 1. Pathways by which glucose is metabolized in human erythrocytes. The bars indicate enzymatic deficiencies whose association with hereditary hemolytic anemia is well-established. 1) HK deficiency. 2) PHI deficiency. 3) PFK deficiency. 4) TIM deficiency. 5) PGK deficiency. 6) DPGM deficiency. 7) 2,3-DPGase deficiency. 8) PK deficiency. 9) ATPase deficiency. 10) AK deficiency. 11) GPD deficiency. 12) 6-Phosphogluconate dehydrogenase deficiency. 13) GSSG reductase deficiency. 14) GSH synthetase deficiency.

decrease in enzyme activities and the severity of the clinical picture is remarkable. So far, the precise relationship between an enzymatic block, a metabolic disturbance, and the premature sequestration of erythrocytes has yet to be definitely explained in many enzymopathies.

1) *Hexokinase Deficiency*

HK deficiency was first described in 1965 by Löhr *et al.*[5] in 3 patients from 2 nonrelated families with familial panmyelopathy (Type Fanconi) and multiple malformations. The enzymatic defect was detected in erythrocytes, leukocytes, and thrombocytes. The HK activity was between 24 and 60%, the lactate formation of erythrocytes between 25 and 60%, and the ATP content between 30 and 70% of normal values. The Michaelis constant for glucose of the HK in the erythrocytes was elevated 10-fold. The kinetic measurements, however, need analyses on purified enzyme protein as a control. In lymphocyte cultures, approximately 50% of the mitoses showed numerous chromosomal aberrations.[6] The relationship between panmyelopathy, chromosomal anomalies, multiple malformations, and HK deficiency is so far still unexplained because 2 patients with familial panmyelopathy without HK deficiency have been observed by the same research team. Perhaps there are different types of Fanconi anemias. As a causal relationship between chromosomal anomalies and enzymatic defect one can suggest that there is first a point mutation leading to HK deficiency which may then lead to chromosomal aberrations because of metabolic disturbances.

Valentine *et al.*[7] reported an 11-year-old girl with a severe non-spherocytic hemolytic anemia (Type Dacie I) and HK deficiency. Splenectomy led to minor, temporary improvement of the hemolytic anemia. The enzyme activity was reduced to 30% of its normal value. The ATP concentration in the erythrocytes was also diminished, taking into consideration the young cell population with 15.6% reticulocytes. Glucose utilization was diminished to 30–50%, whereas the glutathione content and stability were normal. The flux through the pentose phosphate cycle was unexpectedly increased. Kinetic and electrophoretic properties of HK were not changed. In a clinically healthy brother with normal red-cell life span, the HK activity was decreased to 50% of the normal value.

Keitt[8] found a 50% decrease in HK activity in the erythrocytes of 2 female patients with macrocytic hemolytic anemia. In the leukocytes the enzyme activity was normal. In the erythrocytes the concentrations of glucose-6-P were decreased to 40%, of ATP to 80%, and of 2,3-DPG to 55 and 80%, respectively. However, the GSH content was normal. The electrophoretic properties (Agarose pH 7.0 with glucose, 2-mercaptoethanol, and EDTA) of HK were not changed. Keitt[8] concluded from the rapid inactivation of the enzyme when warmed or stored in a glucose-deficient medium, that the enzyme protein was altered.

Necheles *et al.*[9] described an HK deficiency which was detectable only with low glucose concentrations (7–10 m*M*) in the erythrocytes and leukocytes of a 4-year-old child with hemolytic anemia. At the same time the glucose metabolism of the erythrocytes was greatly decreased. With higher substrate concentrations (75–150 m*M* glucose), however, the enzyme activity was almost normal and the glucose consumption and ATP content somewhat increased. After electrophoretic separation of the enzyme protein on starch gel the third fraction enzyme which contains the HK with the highest affinity for glucose, was absent. Because the erythrocytes are exposed to very low glucose concentrations during their stay in the plexus of the red spleen pulp, their increased sequestration could be explained by the absence of this enzyme fraction of HK.

Moser *et al.*[10] reported a 22-year-old woman with hemolytic anemia and HK deficiency, in whom the enzyme activity was decreased to half of the normal value. The Michaelis constants of the enzyme for glucose and ATP were slightly increased. The ATP and GSH content, as well as the glycolytic rate in the erythrocytes, decreased to a small extent only.

To summarize, 9 patients with HK deficiency have been reported to date. Three of them had a familial panmyelopathy (Type Fanconi) and most had a macrocytic hemolytic anemia. One boy was clinically healthy, in spite of a definite HK deficiency. In some patients the rate of glycolysis (glucose consumption, lactate formation) and the ATP content in the cells were decreased, but in others no definite abnormality could be detected. We may be dealing with different types of HK deficiencies. In 7 carriers of the defect the kinetic or electrophoretic properties of the HK were altered, and thus the increased sequestration of erythrocytes in the substrate-deficient plexus of the spleen could be explained. The transmittance of HK deficiency is autosomal recessive.

The enzyme defect was also found once in leukocytes and 3 times in leukocytes and platelets. Necheles *et al.*[9] observed a significant decrease in hemolysis in patients after splenectomy.

2) Hexosephosphate Isomerase (PHI) Deficiency

A PHI deficiency in relation to a nonspherocytic hemolytic anemia was described first in 1968 by Baughan *et al.*[11] In the meantime 8 homozygous carriers of this enzymatic defect have been reported by Paglia *et al.*,[12] Cartier *et al.*[13] and Arnold *et al.*[14]

The enzyme activities in erythrocytes and leukocytes were partially decreased to 5% of the normal values. The electrophoretic behavior of the enzyme protein varied. In 2 patients reported by Baughan *et al.*[11] and Paglia *et al.*,[12] only 1, rather than 3 normal bands, was detectable on starch gel.[15] Of these bands, 1 showed a distinctly faster and 1 a slower electrophoretic mobility. In a third subject, 3 normal bands were visible.

Extensive enzymatic and metabolic investigations were conducted by Arnold *et al.*[14] on 2 carriers of the defect. The deficiency was present in erythrocytes, as well as in leukocytes, thrombocytes, and fibroblasts.[16] Platelet functioning was not disturbed by the enzymatic defect.

The heat stability of PHI concentrated from erythrocytes was markedly decreased. The pH dependence of the enzyme reaction and the Michaelis constant for fructose-6-P were normal. Only 1 enzyme fraction, rather than 3 was detectable by high-voltage electrophoresis on starch gel (pH 8.1).[17] In the majority of defect carriers the rate of glycolysis was slightly increased, while the metabolic distribution pattern was hardly changed. The ATP content was normal to slightly increased. This finding could be explained by an increased flux through the pentose phosphate cycle.

Paglia *et al.*[12] described in 1 of their patients not only an improvement in the hemolytic anemia with a decrease in the number of reticulocytes after splenectomy, but also an increase in the PHI activity in the blood cells. No explanation for this observation exists to date. Arnold *et al.*[14] were able to observe a decrease in hemolysis with daily infusions of phosphate (500 ml of 0.22 *M* sodium phosphate in 3 hr).

Schröter *et al.*[18] published in 1971 the simultaneous appearance of PHI deficiency and GPD deficiency in an 18-year-old patient with chronic hemolytic anemia in whom a severe hemolytic crisis led to renal failure after he took Amidopyrin. Metabolite determinations showed a 3-fold increase in glucose-6-P and a 30% increase in 2,3-DPG. All other metabolite concentrations were decreased. Which of the 2 enzyme defects is of more importance in relation to the chronic hemolytic anemia is uncertain. Both enzymes compete for the same substrate, namely, glucose-6-P. The increase in glucose-6-P concentration can inhibit the HK reaction, so that here also a decrease in the glycolytic rate can occur.

To summarize, different types of PHI deficiencies apparently exist. To date the relationship between the enzyme defect and hemolytic anemia is unknown. The transmittance of the enzyme defect is autosomal recessive.

3) *PFK Deficiency*

Tarui *et al.*[19] in 1969 described in Japan 3 patients with glycogen-storage disease type VII and deficiency of PFK. The patients suffered from severe myopathy. Hematologically they showed no or only minor hemolysis. The enzyme defect was significant in the muscle tissue, whereas the enzyme activity in the erythrocytes was only decreased to half. Immunological studies (neutralisation test with rabbit antiserum on purified human muscle PFK) of the heterogenous enzyme proteins showed that only the muscle-type PFK in blood cells was missing. In another young patient of Waterbury and Frenkel[20] with a compensated hemolytic anemia the enzyme activity was decreased to 40% of the normal value. The Michaelis constants of the enzyme were normal, the pH optimum of the enzyme reaction was altered, and the heat stability was clearly decreased. The transmittance of the enzyme defect has not yet been determined. It is probably linked to the X chromosome.

4) Triosephosphate Isomerase (TIM) Deficiency

TIM deficiency was first described in 1965 by Schneider *et al.*[21] in 3 nonrelated persons with chronic nonspherocytic hemolytic anemia and neuromuscular disturbances. In the meantime more cases have been reported by Angelman *et al.*[22] and Jaffé *et al.*[23] Most of the patients had a hemolytic anemia since birth. The physical development was normal during the first months of life. However, after 5 to 6 months severe progressive neuromuscular disturbances with spasticity, muscle weakness and atrophy, dementia and susceptibility to infections appeared. Of the 10 homozygous carriers of the defect known so far, 9 died within the first 5 years of life. An exception is the female patient described by Jaffé *et al.*[23] on whom a splenectomy was performed at the age of 16 months. This woman is now 21 years old and suffers only from a compensated hemolytic anemia. The neuromuscular disturbances have also not progressed.

Deficiency of TIM was demonstrated in erythrocytes, leukocytes, skeletal muscle, serum and spinal fluid.[21] The lowest enzyme activities were less than 10% of the normal values in the homozygotes, whereas the heterozygotes had about half of the normal enzyme activity and were clinically free of symptoms. In characterizing the enzyme protein, Schneider *et al.*[24] showed that the enzyme migrated in 2 peaks on the column after it was purified on DEAE-Sephadex A-25. The first band was identical to the polymerized enzyme protein with the main activity. This was missing in the carriers of the enzyme defect. The K_m values of both enzyme fractions were the same for healthy persons as for carriers of the defect.

Metabolic studies showed unexpectedly a glucose consumption which was not lowered, but increased 3-fold with an increase in the metabolites fructose-1,6-diP, GAP and, above all, DHAP. This was probably caused by the high number of reticulocytes. Lactate formation was only half of the value which was expected from the glucose consumption. So far it is not known what happens to the glucose not metabolized in glycolysis. The possibility that DHAP is converted into glycerol-1-P is excluded, because the erythrocytes of the defect carriers had no glycerol-1-P dehydrogenase activity. The 2,3-DPG content of the erythrocytes was close to normal, the ATP content was normal in 1 patient and decreased by about 40% in another patient who was examined. The transmittance of the enzyme defect is autosomal recessive.

Based on the results of metabolic determinations it is difficult to understand the pathogenic relationship between the enzyme defect and hemolytic anemia. Jaffé *et al.*[23] discuss the possibility that DHAP has a toxic effect on the cell, thus causing hemolysis.

5) *GAPD Deficiency*

Harkness[25] in 1966 reported the simultaneous occurrence of GAPD deficiency and nonspherocytic anemia. A father and son had a compensated hemolysis. The result of the autohemolysis test correlated with type Dacie I. The enzyme activity in the blood cells was decreased to 30% of the normal value. The relationship between the enzyme defect and hemolytic anemia is not yet certain. To date the findings could not be confirmed by the discovery of more defect carriers.

6) *PGK Deficiency*

Kraus *et al.*[26] in 1968, were the first to report a PGK deficiency, in a 63-year-old woman with a mild nonspherocytic hemolytlic anemia. The Michaelis constants of the enzyme were normal. The concentrations of the glycolytic metabolites were not changed significantly. Further communications concerning this enzyme defect came from Valentine *et al.*,[27] Hjelm *et al.*,[28] Mazza *et al.*[29] and Cartier *et al.*[30] To date 6 homozygous defect carriers are known. Valentine *et al.*[27] reported 2 Chinese children with nonspherocytic hemolytic anemia, oligophrenia, speech defects and a PGK deficiency in erythrocytes and leukocytes. The enzyme activities were decreased to 5% of the normal values. The lactate and pyruvate formation in the erythrocytes was normal, the ATP content was slightly decreased, and the 2,3-DPG content was increased by 100%.

Cartier and his associates[30] described a 4-year-old boy with a nonspherocytic hemolytic anemia. The enzyme activities were decreased to 23% of the normal values in the erythrocytes, to 11.5% in the granulocytes, and to 33% in the lymphocytes. In the erythrocytes hexose monophosphates were increased by 50% and 2,3-DPG by 20%. Monophosphoglycerates were decreased by 50%, whereas the ATP content, glucose consumption and lactate formation were almost normal. Based on those findings the authors postulate an increased activity of the Rapoport-Luebering cycle with an activation of 2,3-DPGase. The enzyme defect was not detectable in the parents and relatives of the child.

Hjelm *et al.*[28] and Mazza *et al.*[29] also observed in their defect carriers an increase in the 2,3-DPG concentration in red blood cells. The number and function of the leukocytes and thrombocytes were normal in the carriers of the enzyme defect. Based on genetic studies Valentine *et al.*[27] presume a mosaicism of PGK in the heterozygous female defect carriers and hemizygotism in the affected males, so that the enzyme defect could be linked to the X chromosome. The precise relationship between the metabolic disturbance and hemolytic anemia is not yet known.

7) *2,3-Diphosphoglycerate Mutase* (*DPGM*) *Deficiency*

The deficiency of DPGM in red blood cells as the cause of hemolysis was first suggested by Prankerd[31] and by Bowdler and Prankerd.[32] The authors incubated erythrocytes of 2 patients with nonspherocytic hemolytic anemia at 37°C without substrate addition. They demonstrated an augmented decrease in the 2,3-DPG concentration. This could not be improved by the addition of glucose or inosine. The indirect demonstration of the enzyme defect in several patients with nonspherocytic hemolytic anemia, mesobilifuscinuria and formation of large Heinz bodies was accomplished by Löhr and Waller.[33] They showed that the 2,3-DPG- dependent PGM reaction in the patients was much slower than in normal subjects, whereas the reaction was normal after the addition of 2,3-DPG. From this they concluded that a deficiency of 2,3-DPG existed as a consequence of DPGM deficiency. The ATP content and glycolytic rate were clearly decreased in the erythrocytes.

The first direct demonstration of the enzyme deficiency was accomplished by Schröter[34] in 1965, in the heterozygous parents of a baby who died at the age of 3 months from a severe nonspherocytic hemolytic anemia. Two other defect carriers, a father and son (Labie *et al.*[35]), showed a decrease in DPGM activity in erythrocytes to half the normal value, a decrease in the 2,3-DPG content of the cells to 30%, and an increase in triosephosphates and monophosphate glycerates.[30] The oxygen affinity of the hemoglobin was clearly increased in the defect carriers because of the 2,3-DPG deficiency. The transmittance of the enzyme defect is probably autosomal recessive.

8) 2,3-DPGase Deficiency

Syllm-Rapoport *et al.*[36] observed in 1965, 2 nonrelated babies with spherocytosis, cerebral dysgenesis, developmental disturbances, hypotonia of the muscles, achromotrichia, hyperlipidemia and 2,3-DPGase deficiency in the erythrocytes. The enzyme activity was strongly decreased and could not be increased by the addition of ADP and NADH. The ATP and ADP concentrations in the cells were increased by approximately 50%, whereas the 2,3-DPG content was unchanged. The relationship between the enzyme defect and the clinical disturbances has not yet been clarified.

9) PK Deficiency

The most common enzyme defect in glycolysis is PK deficiency. Homozygous defect carriers most often suffer from a nonspherocytic hemolytic anemia. The majority of the more than 150 homozygotes was described in America and Europe. The first reports of nonspherocytic hemolytic anemia with PK deficiency appeared in 1961 from Valentine and co-workers[37] and in 1962 from Waller and Löhr.[38] Numerous additional publications concerning PK defect carriers can be found in references.[39–76] Homozygous defect carriers show a decrease in PK activity to 5–20% of the normal values. However, patients with nonspherocytic hemolytic anemia and PK activities of 40% have also been described.[39,43,51] Presumably there had not been a complete separation of the leukocytes before the hemolysis of the erythrocytes. In heterozygotes the enzyme activity is decreased to about 50%. These carriers generally have no hematologic abnormalities.[53] The transmittance of PK deficiency is autosomal recessive.

The biochemical properties of PK in carriers of the enzyme defect were diverse, indicating that different types of PK deficiency exist. Waller and Löhr[38] in 1962, have already described in 3 patients with

PK deficiency a 2- to 4-fold increase in Michaelis constants for PEP and normal saturation for ADP and magnesium. Further instances of increased Michaelis constants for PEP were reported by Sachs *et al.*,[65] Paglia *et al.*,[64] and Ohyama *et al.*[70] Decreased Michaelis constants for PEP were reported by Rose and Warms,[56] Boivin and Galand,[61] Oski and Bowman,[71] Tanaka *et al.*,[72] as well as Brandt and Hanel,[76] Tanaka *et al.*,[39] Busch,[45] Wiesmann *et al.*[52] and Koler *et al.*[77] However, they were not able to demonstrate an abnormality in the kinetic constants. Staal *et al.*[74] observed in 1 patient with PK deficiency the absence of allosteric properties. Ohyama *et al.*[70] noted in 1 case after partial purification of the enzyme, a shift of the pH optimum from 7.5 to 6.5.

On the basis of column chromatographic, immunologic, and electrophoretic procedures Koler *et al.*[78,79] found that the organism possesses probably 3 enzyme proteins with PK activity. PK I is found only in erythrocytes and liver, PK II in the kidney, and PK III in the other organs, leukocytes, and thrombocytes. The enzymes PK I and PK III show different kinetics. The K_m(PEP) for the PK III is $1.0 \times 10^{-4}M$ and the K_m(ADP) is $1.8 \times 10^{-4}M$, whereas a 10-fold higher PEP concentration is required for saturation of PK I. The Michaelis constants vary depending on the concentration of the second substrate. According to Cartier *et al.*,[67] Staal *et al.*[74] and Koler *et al.*,[78] the PK I of erythrocytes is an allosteric enzyme. Its reaction kinetics, when both active sites are unoccupied, follow a sigmoidal curve, which assumes a hyperbolic shape in the presence of fructose 1,6-diP, as well as PEP.[78,79]

Each PK is under different genetic control. This explains why the defect in nonspherocytic hemolytic anemia with PK deficiency is detectable only in the erythrocytes and not in the leukocytes, thrombocytes nor in muscle tissue. Why the PK activity was also found to be normal in the liver[33,41] remains unexplained. However, Bigley and associates[80] described in 1 case with PK deficiency a 50% decrease of PK in liver. Using horizontal starch gel electrophoresis Townes[81] could detect 2 PK's in erythrocytes, which had been separated sufficiently from leukocytes and thrombocytes. These kinases were missing in the homozygous defect carriers. From this he concluded there was a monomeric and a dimeric or polymeric enzyme, which are under the same genetic control. Rüdiger *et al.*[82] also demonstrated with the help of high-voltage electrophoresis, 2 PK's in erythrocytes of which the faster migrating fraction contained 60% of the total activity. In some families with PK deficiency and nonspherocytic hemolytic anemia, the faster PK band was missing, whereas in 1 family the slow enzyme band was missing.[83] Based on those findings one could imagine red-cell PK existing as 2 alleles.

Most of the homozygous patients showed a slight decrease in ATP content in the erythrocytes, whereas the glycolytic rate was normal or even slightly increased. The 2,3-DPG content of erythrocytes is reported to be elevated,[84,85] as are the PEP and 3-PG concentrations in most cases. By the increase in the 3-PG concentration a part of the glycolytic metabolism is diverted into the Rapoport-Luebering cycle, so that less ATP, though more 2,3-DPG, is formed. The decrease in glycolysis could to some extent be explained by the inhibition of the HK or PK reaction by the increase in the 2,3-DPG concentration. In addition, PGK is inhibited by increased 3-PG, resulting in a further decrease in ATP.[86,87] There are, however, probably more, partly unknown factors which lead to the disturbance of erythrocyte metabolism, to the ATP decrease, and to hemolysis. One can assume that under the poor metabolic conditions in the spleen there is a critical ATP decrease in erythrocytes with PK deficiency. This can no longer be compensated for in the cell and leads to irreparable changes.

Also according to Keitt[55] and Mentzer *et al.*,[88] the reticulocytes are prematurely hemolyzed in the reticuloendothelial system. The factors which lead to the sequestration are in part unexplained. It is discussed whether the low oxygen pressure in the spleen leads to a rapid ATP decrease in the reticulocytes which regenerate ATP mainly via the mitochondrial respiratory chain. With PK deficiency, the ATP decrease could not be compensated for by increased glycolytic production in these cells. This assumption has been supported by the fact that in some cases there is an increase in the number of reticulocytes and improvement of the hematologic conditions after splenectomy. To summarize, there are several pathogenic causes for the premature destruction of erythrocytes in the reticuloendothelial system. Other causes, as for example membrane changes, have also been discussed.[55,66,86] However, experimentally they have not yet been proven.

An interesting concept in some cases of PK deficiency has been advanced by Blume *et al.*[73] In electrophoretic studies the authors found 2 PK types in the erythrocytes, 1 of which, after purification, showed the usual biochemical properties of normal Michaelis-Menten kinetics. On the other hand, the second type showed allosteric properties and a very low affinity for fructose-1,6-diP. In this type a daily infusion of

500 ml of 200 mM insine and 1 mM adenine solution led to a distinct increase in the intracellular fructose-1,6-diP concentration and a decrease in hemolysis.[73] In numerous patients with PK deficiency the beneficial therapeutic affect of splenectomy has been described.[32,39,40,43,49] The long residence of the cells in the spleen and the increased metabolic stress indicate premature sequestration of the cells. Therefore, one would think that operations in individual cases would influence the disease. A^{51}Cr study is required, however, in each case before splenectomy. A complete disappearance of hemolysis should not be expected.

DEFECTS IN GLUTATHIONE SYNTHESIZING AND REDUCING REACTIONS

The tripeptide glutathione (γ-L-glutamyl-L-cysteyl-glycine) is essential for the integrity of the red blood cells. It is synthesized in erythrocytes by a series of enzymatic reactions. Glutathione can be considered to exist in the cells 99% in the reduced form.[89] The GSH concentration amounts to 2–3 mmole/liter of packed erythrocytes. GSSG reduction results from a specific GSSG reductase which receives its hydrogen from NADPH formed in the pentose phosphate cycle. The reduction of $NADP^+$ occurs via the enzyme GPD and to a lesser degree via 6-phosphogluconate dehydrogenase. GSH is important for the protection of the SH groups of hemoglobin, enzymes and membrane proteins,[90] and probably also of reduced pyridine nucleotides.[91] For the detoxification of peroxides which appear in cell metabolism, or under the influence of drugs, GSH peroxidase, along with catalase, is significant.[92–94]

A deficiency in GSH can appear if synthesis or reduction is disturbed. Nonspherocytic hemolytic anemia seldom appears spontaneously in defect carriers. Most often one first notices a partial severe hemolysis under the influence of drugs, which is connected with the formation of Heiz bodies. Heinz bodies are oxidative denaturation products of hemoglobin which can be stained with basic dyes. The shortening of the life span of erythrocytes can result from intravascular hemolysis, generally even from sequestration of cells in the RES. A diminution of GSH peroxidase activity has the same consequences in the erythrocytes. The research team of Alving and Beutler[95–101] demonstrated for the first time in primaquine-sensitive Negroes in the USA, a decrease in red-cell GSH and their special lability toward acetylphenylhydrazine.

The GSH stability test developed by Beutler[100] produced a large number of studies of patients with drug-induced hemolysis or favism.[102,103] As a result, a familial deficiency and instability of GSH was demonstrated in both groups of patients.

Heinz-body formation in the test of Beutler *et al.*[97] was also clearly elevated. More precise analysis of the causes of the GSH instability and the GSH decrease in the erythrocytes led to the discovery of GPD deficiency. The deficiency of glutathione reductase, glutathione synthetase, and glutathione peroxidase were described later as causes of similar diseases with hemolytic anemia. The relationship between 6-phosphogluconate dehydrogenase and nonspherocytic hemolytic anemia has not yet been proven.

1) *GPD Deficiency*

GPD deficiency in more than 100 million gene carriers[104] is one of the most frequently encountered enzyme deficiencies. It is common particularly in the Mediterranean countries (Sardinia, Italy, Greece), in the Middle East (Jewish population), in Southeast Asia and China, and among the Negroes in the USA and in some areas in Africa, *e.g.*, West Guinea. Defect carriers can be found in almost all races, however.

The enzyme defect was described first in 1956 in the USA by Carson *et al.*[105] in Negroes with primaquine-induced hemolysis and by Waller *et al.*[106] in 1957 in a Persian with spontaneous nonspherocytic hemolytic anemia. Since then a vast number of publications on GPD deficiency and different variants have appeared which are interesting not only for molecular biology, but also for population genetics.

Based on the electrophoretic studies of Marks and Gross[107] on starch gel, essentially 2 types of GPD deficiency can be distinguished. The faster-migrating type B was seen exclusively in Caucasians and in approximately 70% of the American Negroes.[107,108] The slower-migrating type A was detectable in 30% of the Negroes, A^+ in 20%, A^- in 10%. In the following years, with the help of various electrophoretic methods, more electrophoretic variants could be detected in Caucasians[109,110] and later in Negroes.[111–115] Enzymatic kinetic studies on purified enzyme preparations led to the discovery of a large number of variants having different properties.[110–134] Each variant has its own characteristic Michaelis constants for glucose-6-P and $NADP^+$, pH optimum and heat stability, and utilization of substrate analogues as 2-deoxyglucose-6-P, galactose-6-P and deamino-$NADP^+$ (WHO[135]). The diminution in the enzyme activities in hemizygotes differs substantially in the variants. If subdividing GPD into types A and B is still justified today, many variants of type B in Caucasians have particularly low activities of less than 1%. One observes most often in these a spontaneous nonspherocytic hemolytic anemia.[116,117] Hemizygotes of type A most often show only a reduction of the enzyme activities to 5–15% of the normal values.

Systematic studies by Yoshida[136] of the amino acid composition of the crystallized enzyme protein showed that in comparison to type B^+, asparagine was replaced by aspartic acid in type A^+. In the mutant Hektoen the same author noted an exchange of histidine for tyrosine.[137] Kirkman *et al.*[138] discussed an exchange of cysteine in the variant Tel Hashomer. Mainly variants with a decrease in the activity of GPD to less than 20% have erythrocytes sensitive to primaquine and other compounds, above all, the family of aromatic amines and nitro compounds. In heterozygotes there are no clinically manifested sensitivities toward these compounds. With daily exposure to 30 mg primaquine the hemolytic anemia in hemizygous and homozygous enzyme defect carriers will take the following clinical course[96,139]: within the first day the GSH content in the erythrocytes decreases; then after 2–3 days severe hemolysis will occur with a diminution in hemoglobin and the number of erythrocytes, and an augmentation in indirect bilirubin. In the following days the reticulocytes increase and hemolysis ceases in spite of the continuation of the drug. The hematological status normalizes in the following weeks. After 5–6 weeks a new hemolysis will be produced by primaquine. The explanation for this intermittent course is that only the old erythrocytes in which also the remaining activity has been lost are hemolyzed.[98] The young red cells are initially resistant to the drug, but after ageing for several weeks they lyse and are sequestered.

In the Mediterranean countries, especially Sardinia, and also in China severe hemolysis will occur in GPD defect carriers after consumption of fava beans (vicia faba). The hemolysis is not intermittent, but progressive because young erythrocytes are also affected by the absence of the enzyme. Hemolysis will occur within a few minutes after inhalation of the pollen, whereas it is observed only 1–3 days after ingestion of the boiled beans. The mechanism of these 2 forms of hemolysis is probably different. Fava hemolysis is observed mainly in mutant carriers with enzyme activities less than 1–3%. It is unexplained why in some hemizygotes in families with distinct GPD deficiency no hemolysis is caused by fava beans. Razin *et al.*[140] suggest that a rela-

TABLE I. The most important compounds and vegetables known to have induced hemolysis in GPD deficiency.

Acetanilide	Naphthalene
Acetylphenylyhdrazine	Nitrofurantoin
Acetylsalicylic acid	Para-aminosalicylic acid
Aniline derivatives	Phenacetin
Antipyrine	Primaquine
Atebrine	Pamaquine
Azulfidine	Pentaquine
Chloramphenicol	Pyramidone
Chloroquine	Sulfanilamide
Diasone	Sulfoxone
Dimercaprol	Vitamin K
Methylene blue	Fava beans

tionship exists between hemolysis and the content of pyrimidine derivatives in fava beans. In contrast, Kosower and Kosower[141)] and Beutler[142)] relate the L-DOPA content in the legumes to hemolysis. The mechanism for drug-induced hemolysis in the enzyme defect carriers can be considered as a deficiency and/or an instability of GSH. Through this mechanism the reduced pyridine nucleotides[91)] and the SH groups of the membrane, enzymes, and hemoglobin[90,143,144)] are not sufficiently protected against oxidative processes. Compounds and the metabolites of those compounds which catalyze oxidation can be found in Table I. The result of the increased oxidation of hemoglobin is the Heinz-body formation. By means of the indicated compounds H_2O_2, which could be removed in normal cells by a GSH peroxidase[92–94,145)] accumulates in the cell. This process is disturbed in cells which cannot sufficiently regenerate GSH. To date it is unknown whether H_2O_2 directly (or free radicals) causes deleterious alterations in the erythrocytes.[146–148)]

The brilliant cresyl blue dye test of Motulsky and Campbell-Kraut[149)] and the methemoglobin reduction test of Brewer *et al.*[150)] have proven to be valuable as screening tests especially for population genetic studies. Intracellular GSH reduction is detected best by the azoester test of Kosower *et al.*[151)] The transmittance of GPD deficiency is linked incompletely dominantly to the X chromosome.[102,103,105)] In heterozygous defect carriers a genetic mosaicism exists with 2 erythrocytic populations.[153,154)] The penetrance of the gene is very different, so that heterozygous defect carriers have enzyme activities between 20–80%. The demonstration of the mosaicism was accomplished by various methods, first by Beutler *et al.*[155] with the help of the methylene blue test, and later by Sansone *et al.*[156] by the elegant elution method of Kleihauer and Betke[157] on blood smears.

Motulsky *et al.*[104] in 1969, indicated a special frequency of GPD defect carriers in the regions with malaria tropica. Luzatto *et al.*[158] showed that, above all, heterozygous enzyme defect carriers were less susceptible to malaria. GPD deficiency was also found in leukocytes,[159] thrombocytes,[160] liver,[161] saliva,[162] skin,[163] and in eye lenses[164] of Caucasians. In Negroes the enzyme deficiency is limited to the erythrocytes.[165]

The relationship between GPD deficiency and hemolysis leaves many questions unanswered. Unexplained, for example, is the reason why in defect carriers, for instance, psychological stress, diabetic acidosis, and severe infections can cause hemolysis. The cause of the changes in the erythrocytic membrane in enzyme defect carriers as seen in the electron microscope is also unknown to date.[166]

2) *6-Phosphogluconate Dehydrogenase Deficiency*

Based on electrophoretic studies, a genetic polymorphism was found to exist for the 6-phosphogluconate dehydrogenase in erythrocytes.[167] Communications regarding enzyme defect carriers concern mainly heterozygotes without clinical disturbances. Parr and Fitch[168] reported a homozygous enzyme defect carrier with 3% enzyme activity without signs of hemolysis. Lausecker *et al.*[169] and Scialom *et al.*[170] found in 2 patients with spontaneous hemolytic anemia a decrease in enzyme activity to 30 and 70%, respectively, of the normal values. A relationship between hemolysis and drug exposure did not exist. The relationship between enzyme deficiency and hemolysis has not yet been established.

3) *GSSG Reductase Deficiency*

GSSG reductase deficiency in blood cells was first described by Carson *et al.*[171] in 1961, and Löhr and Waller[172] in 1962. The enzyme deficiency occurs mainly in Central Europe. A remarkable frequency was also observed among the Skolt Laps in Finland.[173,174] Blume *et al.*[175] detected 1.9% heterozygous and 0.009% hemozygous defect carriers among healthy students of the University of Marburg by the application of high-voltage gradient electrophoresis. An overwhelming number of enzyme defect carriers is clinically healthy. With clinical manifestations, nonspherocytic hemolytic anemia, granulocytopenia and pancytopenia, as well as occasional erythroleukemia are observed.[176] In some defect carriers EEG changes, spastic symptoms and oligophrenia were also observed.[177] Combinations with hemoglobinopathies and other enzyme defects were also reported.[178–180] Hemolytic anemia and pancytopenia occur spontaneously and also after exposure to drugs. These are the same drugs which can cause hemolysis in GPD deficiency. The course of the disease, mainly if there is a pancytopenia, is always unfavorable even when all drugs are discontinued. The relationship between the enzyme deficiency and clinical disturbances has yet to be explained.

The decline in GSSG reductase activities is detectable in erythrocytes and to a lesser degree in leukocytes and thrombocytes.[176] The activities can be decreased to 10% of the normal values. Most often they are between 40 and 60%. The enzyme deficiency only rarely leads to a pathological Heinz-body test.[176] The GSSG reduction rate is normal in the azoester test of Kosower *et al.*[181] Therefore, GSSG reductase, in contrast to GPD, does not become the limiting enzyme of GSSG reduction even when there is a strong decrease in its activity. Obviously, a biochemical polymorphism could be considered to account for the GSSG reductase deficiency. In a part of the carriers the Michaelis constant for GSSG was moderately raised and the pH optimum shifted from 6.8 to 6.4. These findings were made in the hemolysate as well as in purified enzyme preparations.[182] Staal *et al.*[183] found, on the other hand, only a decrease in the affinity of the enzyme for flavine adenine dinucleotide (FAD). In a greater number of defect carriers the properties of the enzyme were normal. Blume *et al.*[184] with the help of high-voltage gradient electrophoresis could separate the enzyme protein into 2 fractions, of which the faster-moving enzyme band was missing in the defect carriers.

Recent studies have now shown that evidently, in almost all defect carriers, the decrease in GSSG reductase activity has a relationship to riboflavin deficiency.[185] After daily oral administration of 5–10 mg of riboflavin a normalization of activity in most enzyme defect carriers takes place.[186–188] The increase in enzyme activity occurs 3 days after the initiation of riboflavin administration. The activities drop again approximately 2–3 weeks after the termination of substitution therapy.[186] In no enzyme defect carriers was the clinical picture of the disease improved by riboflavin treatment, whereas the Heinz-body test was normalized.[189] We noticed also in our enzyme defect carriers a normalization of the pH optimum of the enzyme reaction after treatment with riboflavin.[188] The normalization of GSSG reductase activity was also found *in vitro* on the addition of FAD to the test mixture,[189] while the activity in leukocytes and thrombocytest remained uninfluenced.[190]

In Skolt Laps investigated by us the decline in GSSG reductase activity in the erythrocytes can be explained by a deficiency of riboflavin in the diet.[174] This is probably also the cause for the seasonal variation of the enzyme in the same tested subjects. Further reasons for a deficiency in GSSG reductase activity could be malabsorption of riboflavin, disturbed FAD synthesis in the erythrocytes[186,191] and, together with the formation of an altered enzyme protein, a diminished synthesis of the normal enzyme protein. In GSSG reductase defect carriers normal methemoglobin reductase activities are always found and these were not enhanced *in vitro* on the addition of FAD.[189,191] An increase of GSSG reductase activities in red blood cells was observed in hemizygous GPD defect carriers.[192,193] Further augmentation of enzyme activity by oral administration of riboflavin and *in vitro* on the addition of FAD to the test mixture did not occur so that the affinity of GSSG reductase for FAD in GPD deficiency seems not to be increased.

4) GSH Synthetase Deficiency

The first observation of familial GSH deficiency resulting from a GSH synthetase disturbance was made by Oort *et al.*[194] in 1961, who found this in 5 homozygous patients of a Dutch family with mild nonspherocytic hemolytic anemia. Further cases were presented later by Boivin *et al.*,[195] Mohler *et al.*,[196] Löhr *et al.*,[197] Waller and Gerok[198] and Lo *et al.*[199] In erythrocytes incubated with acetylphenylhydrazine, increased Heinz-body formation was observed. In some patients the GSH content was diminished to 0–10% of the normal values. In other patients it ranged between 40–60%. An increase in hemolysis appeared in defect carriers exposed to fava beans and primaquine.[194] Also, after poisoning with knee-pine extracts or irradiation with X-rays or radium severe hemolysis was observed in cases of GSH deficiency. Incorporation studies with labeled glycine and glutamin acid showed[195,200] that the cause of the decrease in GSH is a deficiency of GSH synthetase. The absence of this enzyme disturbs the second step of GSH synthesis from γ-glutamyl-cysteine and glycine. The first reaction in glutathione synthesis of γ-glutamyl-cysteine was, on the other hand, normal. The transmittance of GSH synthetase deficiency is probably autosomal recessive.

5) *GSH Peroxidase Deficiency*

A diminution in GSH peroxidase activity in the erythrocytes of newborn infants was described for the first time by Gross *et al.*[201] in 1967. The authors suggested that 1 of the causes of the increased sensitivity of children to oxidizing agents could be the deficiency of this enzyme's activity. The formation of Heinz bodies in the red blood cells was distinctly enhanced by incubating them with acetylphenylhydrazine, whereas the GSH stability was normal. The slight hemolysis clinically improved in some newborn infants as the GSH peroxidase activity normalized during the first 4–6 months of life. The first case of GSH peroxidase deficiency in the erythrocytes and acute hemolysis after a blood transfusion in an adult was described by Necheles *et al.*[202] in 1968. The homozygous defect carrier had an enzyme activity of 25% of the normal values. During the hemolytic crisis numerous erythrocytes had Heinz bodies. In 3 heterozygous family members the clinical findings were normal, but with exposure to acetosalicylic acid, sulfisoxazole, and nitrofurantoin in therapeutic doses, self-limited hemolytic episodes occured. Necheles *et al.*[202] in 1969, observed another 2-month-old baby with homozygous GSH peroxidase deficiency. The erythrocytes of homozygous defect carriers could not split H_2O_2 *in vitro*. Some cases of GSH peroxidase deficiency were also described by Boivin *et al.*[203] and Gharib *et al.*[204] The transmittance of the enzyme defect is probably autosomal recessive. The demonstration of the enzyme defect is difficult mainly in the heterozygous defect carriers because the assays are not very reliable to date.[145]

OTHER ENZYME DEFECTS IN ERYTHROCYTES

1) *ATPase Deficiency*

Harvald *et al.*[205] in 1965 and Cotte *et al.*[206] in 1968 described 3 Danish and 1 French patient, respectively, with mild hemolytic anemia and ATPase deficiency in the erythrocytes. The biochemical and clinical data are too sparse to discuss this disease extensively. With ATPase deficiency one would expect a spherocytosis with altered osmotic resistence, because the enzyme is important for the electrolyte metabolism in order to maintain the osmotic equilibrium. The quoted reports, however, do not indicate spherocytosis.

2) Adenylate Kinase (AK) Deficiency

Szeinberg *et al.*[207] in 1969, published a report on a 10-month-old Arab boy with nonspherocytic hemolytic anemia who had an AK deficiency in addition to a hemizygous GPD deficiency. The AK in the erythrocytes was decreased to 4–10% of the normal values. The adenine nucleotides ATP and AMP, and especially ADP, were increased. The 4-year-old sister of the patient in whom AK was decreased to 0.5–4%, showed signs of nonspherocytic hemolytic anemia with slightly increased reticulocytes and mild hyperbilirubinemia. The girl had no GPD deficiency. Another case was reported by Boivin *et al.*[208] in 1971. This was a 13-year-old boy who had had a compensated hemolytic anemia since birth. The AK activities were decreased to 1–13% of the normal values. Of the adenine nucleotides only AMP was slightly increased. Family studies showed both parents to be heterozygous.

3) Glyoxalase II Deficiency

Valentine *et al.*[209] in 1970, were the first to observe a glyoxalase II deficiency in the red blood cells of a family with hereditary elliptocytosis. In this family 4 homozygous and 5 heterozygous carriers had the enzyme defect. Glyoxalase II catalyzes the hydrolysis of the thioester S-lactoyl-glutathione to GSH and D-lactate. The enzyme activities of the homozygous defect carriers were decreased to 10% of the normal values. The enzyme defect could be demonstrated in 3 generations. The transmittance is probably autosomal recessive. Leukocytes had normal enzyme activities. A relationship between glyoxalase II deficiency and elliptocytosis is unlikely, especially since the clinical symptomatology was the same in members of this family with elliptocytosis without glyoxalase II deficiency as in the enzyme defect carriers.

4) Catalase Deficiency

Catalase deficiency was first reported in Japan in 1948, by Takahara.[210] He found in patients with progressive alveolar pyorrhea, ulcerative stomatitis, gingivitis and necrotizing tonsillitis, a brown discoloring of the tissues and the absence of the usual foam formation when spotting the ulcers with H_2O_2. On addition of H_2O_2 to the blood, no foam formation occurred. In the blood, distinct formation of methemoglobin took place. The catalase deficiency was demonstrated in the red blood cells, in bone marrow, liver, and nasal and pharyngeal mucosa.[211] Aebi *et al.*[212] showed that in the blood cells of defect carriers the activities of the enzymes GSSG reductase and GSH peroxidase were augmented. If one adds ascorbic acid (5 m*M*) as a hydrogen peroxide donor, the oxidative glucose degradation will be increased significantly via the pentose phosphate cycle. Evidently in the cells the deficiency of catalase is compensated for by augmentation of GSSG reducing reactions.[213]

The transmittance according to Takahara[210] is probably autosomal recessive. A clinical manifestation appears only in about half of the homozygotes. Aebi *et al.*[214] differentiate between 5 types of acatalasia with varied penetrance of activity deficiency, enzyme properties, and expression of the gene.

In recent years enzymatic studies in red blood cells have proved to be valuable also for the understanding of metabolic diseases in which no obvious hematologic disorder is evident. The easily accessible erythrocytes serve as indicator cells. In the erythrocytes both forms of galactosemia can be detected by determining the activities of galactokinase[215] and of galactose-1-P uridyl transferase.[216,217] One also can diagnose the Lesch-Nyhan syndrome[218] by assaying for hypoxanthine-guanine phosphoribosyl transferase. For methemoglobin reductase deficiency see chapter by Jaffé.

The above results indicate that a number of inherited hematologic disorders can today be related to defined enzyme defects. The causal relationship between molecular protein defects and clinical symptoms is often still unexplained. Above all, the chain of events of enzymopathies, metabolic disturbances, membrane changes, and sequestration of the erythrocytes in RES is not completely understood. Nevertheless, enzymatic hematology has brought fruitful idea to pathogenic studies and genetics.

ADDENDUM

Since January 1972 when this paper was presented for publishing numerous articles on metabolic disorders in red blood cells have been published. Several new variants of glucose-6-phosphate dehydrogenase are discovered, more cases with glucose-phosphate isomerase deficiency are described (H. Arnold, K. G. Blume, R. Engelhardt and G. W. Löhr: *Blood*, **41**, 691 (1973)).

Most of all we would like to point out the discovery of enolase deficiency (M. Stefanini: *Amer. J. Clin. Path.*, **58**, 408 (1972)), of γ-glutamyl-cysteine synthetase deficiency (P. N. Konrad, F. H. Richards, W. N. Valentine and D. E. Paglia: *New Engl. J. Med.*, **286**, 557 (1972)), and furthermore the demonstration of γ-glutamyl-cysteine cycle in erythrocytes by A. Meister and coll. (first reported on the symposium on glutathione Tübingen March 1973).

REFERENCES

1 Gibson, Q. H., *Biochem. J.*, **42**, 13 (1948).

2 Yoshikawa, H. and Nakao, M., *Folia Haematol.*, **78**, 248 (1962).

3 Benesch, R. and Benesch, R. E., *Biochem. Biophys. Res. Comm.*, **26**, 162 (1967).

4 Chanutin, A. and Curnish, R., *Arch. Biochem. Biophys.*, **121**, 96 (1967).

5 Löhr, G. W., Waller, H. D., Anschütz, F. and Knopp, A., *Klin. Wochenschr.*, **43**, 870 (1965).

6 Schroeder, T. M., Anschütz, F. and Knopp, A., *Humangenetik*, **1**, 194 (1964).

7 Valentine, W. N., Oski, F. A., Paglia, D. E., Baughan, M. A., Schneider, A. S. and Naiman, J. L., *New Engl. J. Med.*, **276**, 1 (1967).

8 Keitt, A. S., *J. Clin. Invest.*, **48**, 1997 (1969).

9 Necheles, T. F., Rai, U. S. and Cameron, D., *J. Lab. Clin. Med.*, **76**, 593 (1970).

10 Moser, K., Ciresa, M. and Schwarzmeier, J., *Med. Welt*, **21**, 1977 (1970).

11 Baughan, M. A., Valentine, W. N., Paglia, D. E., Ways, P. O., Simon, E. R. and Demarsh, Q. B., *Blood*, **32**, 236 (1968).

12 Paglia, D. E., Holland, P., Baughan, M. A. and Valentine, W. N., *New Engl. J. Med.*, **280**, 66 (1969).

13 Cartier, P., Temkine, H. and Griselli, C., Lecture VII. International Congress of Clinical Chemistry, Geneve (1969).

14 Arnold, H., Blume, K. G., Busch, D., Lenkeit, U., Löhr, G. W. and Lübs, E., *Klin. Wochenschr.*, **48**, 1299 (1970).

15 Detter, J. C., Ways, P. O., Giblett, E. R., Baughan, M. A., Hopkinson, D. A., Povey, S. and Harris, H., *Ann. Hum. Genet.*, **31**, 329 (1968).

16 Krone, W., Schneider, G., Schulz, D., Arnold, H. and Blume, K. G., *Humangenetik*, **10**, 224 (1970).

17 Tariverdian, G., Arnold, H., Blume, K. G., Lenkeit, U. and Löhr, G. W., *Humangenetik*, **10**, 218 (1970).

18 Schröter, W., Brittinger, G., Zimmerschmitt, E., König, E. and Schrader, D., *Br. J. Haematol.*, **20**, 249 (1971).

19 Tarui, S., Kono, N., Nasu, T. and Nishikawa, M., *Biochem. Biophys. Res. Comm.*, **34**, 77 (1969).

20 Waterbury, L. and Frenkel, E. P., *Clin. Res.*, **17**, 347 (1969).

21 Schneider, A. S., Valentine, W. N., Baughan, M. A., Paglia, D. E., Shore, N. A. and Heins, H. L., Jr. *in*: Hereditary disorders of erythro-

cyte metabolism, ed. by Beutler, E. (Grune and Stratton, New York/London, 1968), p. 265.

22 Angelman, H., Brain, M. C. and MacIver, J. E., Proceedings XIII. International Congress of Hematology (Munich, 1970), p. 122.

23 Jaffé, E. R., Paglia, D. E., Harris, S. R., Valentine, W. N., Klein, R. L. and Rapin, I., Proceedings XIII. International Congress of Hematology (Munich, 1970), p. 122.

24 Schneider, A. S., Dunn, I., Ibsen, K. H. and Weinstein, I. M., *in*: Hereditary disorders of erythrocyte metabolism, ed. by Beutler, E. (Grune and Stratton, New York/London, 1968), p. 273.

25 Harkness, D. R., *J. Lab. Clin. Med.*, **68**, 879 (1966).

26 Kraus, A. P., Langston, M. F., Jr. and Lynch, B. L., *Biochem. Biophys. Res. Comm.*, **30**, 173 (1968).

27 Valentine, W. N., Hsieh, H. S., Paglia, D. E., Anderson, H. M., Baughan, M. A., Jaffé, E. R. and Garson, O. M., *New Engl. J. Med.*, **280**, 528 (1969).

28 Hjelm, M. and Wadman, B., Proceedings XIII. International Congress of Hematology (Munich, 1970), p. 121.

29 Mazza, U., Arese, P., Bozia, A., Gallo, E. and Pescarmona, G. P., Proceedings XIII. International Congress of Hematology (Munich, 1970), p. 121.

30 Cartier, P., Habibi, B., Leroux, J. P. and Marchand, J. C., *Nouv. Rev. Fr. Hematol.*, **11**, 565 (1971).

31 Prankerd, T. A. J., *in*: Hämolyse und hämolytische Erkrankungen. VII. Freiburger Symposium (Springer-Verlag, Heidelberg / Berlin, 1961), p. 236.

32 Bowdler, A. J. and Prankerd, T. A. J., *Acta Haematol.*, **31**, 65 (1964).

33 Löhr, G. W. and Waller, H. D., *Folia Haematol. N.F.*, **8**, 377 (1963).

34 Schröter, W., *Klin. Wochenschr.*, **43**, 1147 (1965).

35 Labie, D., Leroux, J. P., Najman, A. and Rexrolle, C., *FEBS Letters*, **9**, 37 (1970).

36 Syllm-Rapoport, I., Jacobasch, G., Roigas, H. and Rapoport, S., *Folia Haematol.*, **83**, 363 (1965).

37 Valentine, W. N., Tanaka, K. R. and Miwa, S., *Trans. Amer. Physicians*, **74**, 100 (1961).

38 Waller, H. D. and Löhr, G. W., Proceedings IX. Congress of the International Society of Hematology (Mexiko City, 1962), p. 257.

39 Tanaka, K. R., Valentine, W. N. and Miwa, S., *Blood*, **19**, 267 (1962).

40 Bowman, H. S. and Procopio, F., *Ann. Intern. Med.*, **58**, 567 (1963).

41 Brunetti, P., Puxeddu, A., Nengi, G. and Migliorini, E., *Acta Haematol.*, **30**, 88 (1963).

42 De Gruchy, G. C., *Aust. Ann. Med.*, **12**, 6 (1963).

43 Grimes, A. J., Meisler, A. and Dacie, J. V., *Br. J. Haematol.*, **10**, 403

(1963).
44 Oski, F. A. and Diamond, L. K., *New Engl. J. Med.*, **269**, 763 (1963).
45 Bestetti, A., Rossi, U., Loos, J.A. and Prins, H. J., *Vox Sanguinis*, **9**, 492 (1964).
46 Busch, D., *Folia Haematol. N.F.*, **9**, 89 (1964).
47 Oski, F. A., Nathan, D. G., Sidel, V. W. and Diamond, L.K., *New Engl. J. Med.*, **270**, 1023 (1964).
48 Busch, D., *Folia Haematol.*, **83**, 395 (1965).
49 Loder, P. B. and De Gruchy, G. C., *Br. J. Haematol.*, **11**, 21 (1965).
50 Loos, J. A., Doctoral thesis (University Amsterdam, 1965).
51 Miwa, S. and Nagata, M., *Acta Haematol. Jap.*, **28**, 1 (1965).
52 Wiesmann, U., Tönz, O., Richterich, E. and Verger, P., *Klin. Wochenschr.*, **43**, 1311 (1965).
53 Busch, D., Habilitationsschrift (Albert-Ludwig-Universität Freiburg, 1966).
54 Collier, H. B., Ashford, D. R. and Bell, R. E., *Canad. Med. Assoc. J.*, **95**, 1188 (1966).
55 Keitt, A. S., *Amer. J. Med.*, **41**, 762 (1966).
56 Rose, I. A. and Warms, J. V. B., *J. Biol. Chem.*, **241**, 4848 (1966).
57 Hanel, H. K., Harvald, B., Mov, G., Christensen, N. and Deckert, T., *Scand. J. Haematol.*, **4**, 53 (1967).
58 Moser, K., Schwarzmeier, J. and Deutsch, E., *Wien. Klin. Wochenschr.*, **79**, 542 (1967).
59 Twomey, J. J., O'Neal, F. B., Altrey, C. P. and Moser, R., *Blood*, **30**, 576 (1967).
60 Baughan, M. A., Paglia, D. E., Schneider, A. S. and Valentine, W. N., *Acta Haematol.*, **39**, 345 (1968).
61 Boivin, P. and Galand, C., *Nouv. Rev. Fr. Hematol.*, **8**, 201 (1968).
62 Bossu, M., Dacha, M. and Fornaini, G., *Acta Haematol.*, **40**, 166 (1968).
63 Nathan, D. G., Oski, F. A., Miller, D. R. and Gardner, F. H., *New Engl. J. Med.*, **278**, 73 (1968).
64 Paglia, D. E., Valentine, W. N., Baughan, M. A., Miller, D. R., Reed, C. F. and McIntryre, O. R., *J. Clin. Invest.*, **47**, 1929 (1968).
65 Sachs, J. R., Wicker, D. J., Gilcher, R. O., Conradt, M. E. and Cohen, R. J., *J. Labor. Clin. Med.*, **72**, 359 (1968).
66 Zuelzer, W. W., Robinson, A. R. and Hsu, T. H. J., *Blood*, **32**, 33 (1968).
67 Cartier, P., Najman, A., Leroux, J. P. and Temkine, H., *Clin. Chim. Acta*, **22**, 165 (1969).
68 Jacobasch, G., Helbig, W., Syllm-Rapoport, I., Pester, H., Heine, K. M., Boese, Ch., Otto, F. M. G. and Blau, H. J., *Deutsch. Gesundheitswes.*, **24**, 1441 (1969).

69 Najean, Y., Dresch, C. and Russel, A., *Nouv. Rev. Fr. Hematol.*, **9**, 850 (1963).
70 Ohyama, H., Kumatori, T., Nishima, T. and Miwa, S., *Acta Haematol. Jap.*, **32**, 330 (1969).
71 Oski, F. A. and Bowman, H., *Br. J. Haematol.*, **17**, 289 (1969).
72 Tanaka, K. R., *Jap. J. Genet.*, **44**, Suppl. 1, 286 (1969).
73 Blume, K. G., Busch, D., Hoffbauer, R. W., Arnold, H. and Löhr, G. W., *Humangenetik*, **9**, 257 (1970).
74 Staal, G. E. J., Koster, J. F. and Milligen-Boersma, L. v., *Biochim. Biophys. Acta*, **220**, 613 (1970).
75 Blume, K. G., Busch, D., Arnold, H. and Löhr, G. W., *Klin. Wochenschr.*, **49**, 228 (1971).
76 Brandt, N. J. and Hanel, H. K., *Scand. J. Haematol.*, **8**, 126 (1971).
77 Koler, R. D., Bigley, R. H., Jones, R. T., Rigas, D. A., Vanbellinghen, P. and Thompson, P., *Cold Spring Harbor Symp. Quant. Biol.*, **29**, 213 (1964).
78 Koler, R. D. and Vanbellinghen, P., *Adv. Enzyme Regul.*, **6**, 127 (1968).
79 Koler, R. D., Bigley, R. H. and Stenzel, P., *in*: Hereditary Disorders of Erythrocyte Metabolism, ed. by Beutler, E. (Grune and Stratton, New York/London, 1968) p. 249.
80 Bigley, R. H. and Koler, R. D., *Ann. Hum. Genet.*, **31**, 383 (1968).
81 Townes, P. L., *in*: Hereditary Disorders of Erythrocyte Metabolism, ed. by Beutler, E. (Grune and Stratton, New York/London, 1968), p. 182.
82 Rüdiger, H. W., Blume, K. G., Löhr, G. W. and Schalhorn, A., *Klin. Wochenschr.*, **46**, 397 (1968).
83 Motulsky, A. G., Gabrio, B. W., Burkhardt, J. and Finch, C. A., *Amer. J. Med.*, **19**, 291 (1955).
84 Robinson, M. A., Loder, P. B. and De Gruchy, G. C., *Br. J. Haematol.*, **7**, 327 (1961).
85 Busch, D., *in*: Handbuch der Inneren Medizin, 5. Auflage, 2. Band, 2. Teil (Springer-Verlag Berlin / Heidelberg / New York, 1970), p. 294.
86 Busch, D. and Boie, K., *Folia Haematol.*, **91**, 77 (1968).
87 Blume, K. G., Hoffbauer, R. W., Busch, D., Arnold, H. and Löhr, G. W., *Biochim. Biophys. Acta*, **227**, 364 (1971).
88 Mentzer, W. C., Jr., Baehner, R. L., Schmidt-Schönbein, H., Robinson, S. H. and Nathan, D. G., *J. Clin. Invest.*, **50**, 688 (1971).
89 Srivastava, S. K. and Beutler, E., *J. Biol. Chem.*, **244**, 9 (1969).
90 Benesch, R. E. and Benesch, R., *Arch. Biochem.*, **48**, 38 (1954).
91 Löhr, G. W. and Waller, H. D., *Deutsch. Med. Wochenschr.*, **86**, 27, 87 (1961).
92 Mills, G. C., *J. Biol. Chem.*, **229**, 189 (1957).
93 Cohen, G. and Hochstein, P., *Biochemistry*, **2**, 1420 (1963).

94 Cohen, G. and Hochstein, P., *Biochemistry*, **3**, 895 (1964).
95 Dern, R. J., Weinstein, I. M., LeRoy, G. V., Talmage, D. W. and Alving, A. S., *J. Lab. Clin. Med.*, **43**, 303 (1954).
96 Dern, R. J., Beutler, E. and Alving, A. S., *J. Lab. Clin. Med.*, **44**, 171 (1954).
97 Beutler, E., Dern, R. J. and Alving, A. S., *J. Lab. Clin. Med.*, **44**, 177 (1954).
98 Beutler, E., Dern, R. J. and Alving, A. S., *J. Lab. Clin. Med.*, **44**, 439 (1954).
99 Beutler, E., Dern, R. J., Flanagan, C. L. and Alving, A. S., *J. Lab. Clin. Med.*, **45**, 286 (1955).
100 Beutler, E., *J. Clin. Invest.*, **35**, 690 (1956).
101 Beutler, E., Robson, M. and Buttenwieser, E., *J. Clin. Invest.*, **36**, 617 (1957).
102 Szeinberg, A., Asher, Y. and Sheba, C., *Blood*, **13**, 348 (1958).
103 Larizza, P., Brunetti, P., Grignani, F. and Ventura, S., *Haematol.*, **43**, 205 (1958).
104 Motulsky, A. G., Kraut, J. M., Thieme, W. T. and Musto, D. F., *Clin. Res.*, **7**, 89 (1959).
105 Carson, P. E., Flanagan, C. L., Ickes, C. E. and Alving, A. S., *Science*, **124**, 484 (1956).
106 Waller, H. D., Löhr, G. W. and Tabatabai, M., *Klin. Wochenschr.*, **35**, 1022 (1957).
107 Marks, P. A., Banks, J. and Gross, R. T., *Nature*, **194**, 454 (1962).
108 Boyer, S. H., Porter, I. H. and Weilbacher, R. G., *Proc. Nat. Acad. Sci. U.S.*, **48**, 1868 (1962).
109 Porter, I. H. and Boyer, S. H., Proceedings IXth Congress of the European Society of Haematology (Lisbon, 1963), p. 689.
110 Kirkman, H. N., Riley, H. D., Jr. and Crowell, B. B., *Proc. Nat. Acad. Sci. U.S.*, **46**, 938 (1960).
111 Porter, I. H., Boyer, S. H., Watson-Williams, E. J., Adam, A., Szeinberg, A. and Siniscalco, M., *Lancet*, **1**, 895 (1964).
112 Long, W. K., Kirkman, H. N. and Stutton, H. E., *J. Lab. Clin. Med.*, **65**, 81 (1965).
113 Carson, P. E. and Frischer, H., *Amer. J. Med.*, **41**, 744 (1966).
114 Pinto, P. V. C., Newton, W. A., Jr. and Richardson, K. E., *J. Clin. Invest.*, **45**, 823 (1966).
115 Hook, E. B., Stamatoyannopoulos, G., Yoshida, A. and Motulsky, A. G., *J. Lab. Clin. Med.*, **72**, 404 (1968).
116 Beutler, E., *Pharmacol. Rev.*, **21**, 73 (1969).
117 Beutler, E., *Humangenetik*, **9**, 250 (1970).
118 Kirkman, H. N. and Eng, L. I. L., *Nature*, **221**, 959 (1969).
119 Busch, D. and Boie, K., *Klin. Wochenschr.*, **48**, 74 (1970).

120 Flatz, G. and Tantachamroon, T., *Humangenetik*, **10**, 335 (1970).
121 McCurdy, P. R., Blackwell, R. Q., Todd, D., Tso, S. C. and Tuchinda, S., *J. Lab. Clin. Med.*, **75**, 788 (1970).
122 Pawlak, A. L., Zagorski, Z., Rosynkowa, D. and Horst, A., *Humangenetik*, **10**, 340 (1970).
123 Reys, L., Manso, C. and Stamatoyannopoulos, G., *Amer. J. Hum. Genet.*, **22**, 203 (1970).
124 Snyder, L. M., Necheles, T. F. and Reddy, W. J., *Amer. J. Med.*, **49**, 125 (1970).
125 Staal, G. E. J., Punt, V., Geerdink, R. A., Boos, C. C. and Bartstra, H., *Scand. J. Haematol.*, **7**, 401 (1970).
126 Stamatoyannopoulos, G., Voigtländer, V. and Akrivakis, A., *Humangenetik*, **9**, 23 (1970).
127 Waitz, R., *Nouv. Rev. Fr. Hematol.*, **10**, 312 (1970).
128 Benöhr, H. Chr., Klumpp, F. and Waller, H. D., *Deutsch. Med. Wochenschr.*, **96**, 1029 (1971).
129 Benöhr, H. Chr., Waller, H. D., Arnold, H., Blume, K. G. and Löhr, G. W., *Klin. Wochenschr.*, **49**, 1058 (1971).
130 Kalm, A., Boivin, P., Hakim, J. and Lagneau, J., *Nouv. Rev. Fr. Hematol.*, **11**, 741 (1971).
131 Kaplan, J. C., Hanzlickova-Leroux, A., Nicolas, A. M., Rosa, R., Weiler, C. and Lepercq, G., *Enzyme*, **12**, 25 (1971).
132 Kwiatkowska, J. and Kacprzak-Bergmann, J., *Acta Haematol.*, **46**, 188 (1971).
133 Ratazzi, M. C., Corash, L. M., van Zanen, G. E., Jaffé, E. R. and Piomelli, S., *Blood*, **38**, 205 (1971).
134 Stamatoyannopoulos, G., Voigtländer, V., Kotsakis, P. and Akrivakis, A., *J. Clin. Invest.*, **50**, 1253 (1971).
135 World Health Organization Technical Report Series, 366 (1967).
136 Yoshida, A., *in*: Hereditary disorders of erythrocyte metabolism, ed. by Beutler, E. (Grune and Stratton, New York/London, 1968), p. 126.
137 Yoshida, A., *J. Mol. Biol.*, **52**, 483 (1970).
138 Kirkman, H. N., Ramot, B. and Lee, J. T., *Biochem. Genet.*, **3**, 137 (1969).
139 Kellermeyer, R. W., Tarlov, A. R., Schrier, S. L., Carson, P. E. and Alving, A. S., *J. Lab. Clin. Med.*, **58**, 225 (1961).
140 Razin, A., Hershko, A., Glaser, G. and Mager, J., *Isr. J. Med, Sci.*, **4**, 852 (1968).
141 Kosower, N. S. and Kosower, E. M., *Nature*, **215**, 285 (1967).
142 Beutler, E., *Blood*, **36**, 523 (1970).
143 Jacob, H. S. and Jandl, J. H., *J. Clin. Invest.*, **41**, 1514 (1962).
144 Jacob, H. S. and Jandl, J. H., *J. Biol. Chem.*, **241**, 4243 (1966).
145 Flohé, L., Habilitationsschrift (University of Tübingen, 1970).

146 Liebowitz, J. and Cohen, G., *Biochem. Pharmacol.*, **17**, 983 (1968).
147 Kosower, N. S., Song, K. R. and Kosower, E. M., *Biochim. Biophys. Acta*, **192**, 23 (1969).
148 Kosower, N. S., Marikowsky, Y., Wertheim, B. and Danon, D., *J. Lab. Clin. Med.*, **78**, 533 (1971).
149 Motulsky, A. G. and Campbell-Kraut, J. M., Proceedings Conference of Genetic Polymorphisms and Geographic Variations in Diseases (Grune and Stratton, New York, 1961), p. 159.
150 Brewer, G. J., Tarlov, A. R. and Alving, A. S., *Bull. World. Health. Organ.*, **22**, 633 (1960).
151 Kosower, N. S., Vanderhoff, G. A. and London, I. M., *Blood*, **29**, 313 (1967).
152 Gross, R. T., Hurwitz, R. E. and Marks, P. A., *J. Clin. Invest.*, **37**, 1176 (1958).
153 Beutler, E., *Amer. J. Med.*, **41**, 724 (1966).
154 Lyon, M. F., *Amer. J. Hum. Genet.*, **14**, 135 (1962).
155 Beutler, E. and Baluda, M. C., *Blood*, **22**, 323 (1963).
156 Sansone, G., Rasore-Quartino, A. and Veneziano, G., *Pathologica*, **55**, 371 (1963).
157 Kleihauer, E. and Betke, K., *Nature*, **199**, 1196 (1963).
158 Luzatto, L., Usanga, E. A. and Reddy, S., *Science*, **164**, 839 (1969).
159 Ramot, B., Fisher, S., Szeinberg, A., Adam, A., Sheba, C. and Gafni, D., *J. Clin. Invest.*, **38**, 2234 (1959).
160 Ramot, B., Szeinberg, A., Adam, A., Sheba, C. and Gafni, D., *J. Clin. Invest.*, **38**, 1659 (1959).
161 Panizon, F., *Lancet*, **2**, 1093 (1960).
162 Ramot, B., Sheba, C., Adam, A. and Ashkenasi, I., *Nature*, **185**, 931 (1960).
163 Gartler, S. M., Gandini, E. and Cepellini, R., *Nature*, **193**, 602 (1962).
164 Zinkham, W. H., *Bull. John Hopkins Hosp.*, **109**, 206 (1961).
165 Marks, P. A., Gross, R. T. and Hurwitz, R. E., *Nature*, **183**, 1266 (1959).
166 Danon, D., Sheba, C. and Ramot, B., *Blood*, **17**, 229 (1961).
167 Brewer, G. J., *in*: Biochemical Methods in Red Cell Genetics. ed. by, Yunis, J. J. (Academic Press New York/London, 1969), p. 139.
168 Parr, C. W. and Fitch, L. I., *Ann. Hum. Genet.*, **30**, 339 (1967).
169 Lausecker, C., Heidt, P., Fischer, D., Hartleyb, H. and Löhr, G. W., *Arch. Fr. Pediatr.*, **22**, 789 (1965).
170 Scialom, C., Najean, Y. and Bernard, J., *Nouv. Rev. Fr. Hematol.*, **6**, 442 (1966).
171 Carson, P. E., Brewer, G. J. and Ickes, C., *J. Lab. Clin. Med.*, **58**, 804 (1961).
172 Löhr, G. W. and Waller, H. D., *Med. Klin.*, **57**, 1521 (1962).

173 Eriksson, W., Fellman, J., Forsius, H., Gustafsson, B., Lindström, C., Kirjarinta, L., Kirjarinta, M., Lehmann, W., Benöhr, H. and Waller, H. D., *Bull. Europ. Soc. Hum. Genet.*, **1**, 73 (1967).
174 Waller, H. D., Benöhr, H. Chr., Eriksson, A. W. and Lehmann, W., *Klin. Wochenschr.*, **50**, 462 (1972).
175 Blume, K. G., Lingen, A. v., Löhr, G. W. and Rüdiger, H. W., *Humangenetik*, **6**, 266 (1968).
176 Waller, H. D., *in*: Hereditary Disorders of Erythrocyte Metabolism, ed. by, Beutler, E. (Grune and Stratton, New York/London, 1968), p. 185.
177 Waller, H. D., Löhr, G. W., Zysno, E., Gerok, W., Voss, D. and Strauß, G., *Klin. Wochenschr.*, **43**, 413 (1965).
178 Waller, H. D., Bremer, J., Schönthal, H. and Dorow, W., *Klin. Wochenschr.*, **45**, 824 (1967).
179 Moser, K., Fischer, M., Krepler, P. and Lechner, K., *Klin. Wochenschr.*, **46**, 995 (1968).
180 Schröter, W., *Schweiz. Med. Wochenschr.*, **100**, 1101 (1970).
181 Waller, H. D., Benöhr, H. Chr., Heuer, P. and Nerke, O., *Klin. Wochenschr.*, **48**, 79 (1970).
182 Waller, H. D., *Klin. Wochenschr.*, **45**, 827 (1967).
183 Staal, G. E. J., Helleman, P. W., De Wael, J. and Veeger, C., *Biochim. Biophys. Acta*, **185**, 63 (1969).
184 Blume, K. G., Rüdiger, H. W. and Löhr, G. W., *Biochim. Biophys. Acta*, **151**, 686 (1968).
185 Helleman, P. W., *in*: I. Symposium über Stoffwechsel und Membranpermeabilität der Erythrozyten und Thrombozyten. Georg-Thieme-Verlag Stuttgart (1969), p. 146.
186 Beutler, E., *J. Clin. Invest.*, **48**, 1957 (1969).
187 Glatzle, D., Weber, F. and Wiss, O., *Experientia*, **24**, 1122 (1968).
188 Benöhr, H. Chr. and Waller, H. D., Proceedings XIII. International Congress of Hematology (Munich, 1970), p. 120.
189 Waller, H. D. and Benöhr, H. Chr., *Klin. Wochenschr.*, in press.
190 Waller, H. D. and Benöhr, H. Chr., *Klin. Wochenschr.*, **51**, 769 (1973).
191 Beutler, E., *Experientia*, **25**, 804 (1969).
192 Schrier, S. L., Kellermeyer, R. W., Carson, P. E., Ickes, C. E. and Alving, A. S., *J. Lab. Clin. Med.*, **52**, 109 (1958).
193 Zurcher, C., Kuijlman, F. F., 't Sass, F., Zurcher, T., Loos, J. A. and Prins, H. K., *Clin. Chim. Acta*, **25**, 139 (1969).
194 Oort, M., Loos, J. A. and Prins, H. K., *Vox Sanguinis*, **6**, 370 (1961).
195 Boivin, P., Galand, C., André, R. and Debray, J., *Nouv. Rev. Fr. Hematol.*, **6**, 859 (1966).
196 Mohler, D. N., Majerus, P. W., Minnich, V., Hess, C. E. and Garrick, M. D., *New Engl. J. Med.*, **283**, 1253 (1970).

197 Löhr, G. W., Baum, P. and Kamm, G., *Med. Klin.*, **58**, 2111 (1963).
198 Waller, H. D. and Gerok, W., *Klin. Wochenschr.*, **42**, 948 (1964).
199 Lo, S. S., Marti, H. R. and Hitzig, W. H., *Acta Haematol.*, **46**, 14 (1971).
200 Prins, H. K., Oort, M., Loos, J. A., Zurcher, C. and Beckers, T., *Blood*, **27**, 145 (1966).
201 Gross, R. T., Bracci, R., Rudolph, N., Schroeder, E. and Kochen, J. A., *Blood*, **29**, 481 (1967).
202 Necheles, T. F., Steinberg, M. H. and Cameron, D., *Br. J. Haematol.*, **19**, 605 (1970).
203 Boivin, P., Galand, C., Hakim, J. and Blery, M., *La Presse Medicale*, **78**, 171 (1970).
204 Gharib, H., Fairbanks, V. F. and Bartholomew, L. G., *Proc. Staffs Meet. Mayo Clin.*, **44**, 96 (1969).
205 Harvald, B., Hanel, K. H., Squires, R. and Trap-Jensen, J., *Lancet*, **2**, 18 (1964).
206 Cotte, J., Kissin, C., Mathieu, M., Poncet, J., Monnet, P., Salle, B. and German, D., *Rev. Fr. dÉtud. Clin. Biol.*, **13**, 284 (1968).
207 Szeinberg, A., Kahana, D., Gavendo, S., Zaidman, J. and Ben-Ezzer, J., *Acta Haematol.*, **42**, 111 (1969).
208 Boivin, P., Galand, C., Hakim, J., Simony, D. and Seligman, M., *La Presse Medicale*, **79**, 215 (1971).
209 Valentine, W. N., Paglia, D. E., Neerhout, R. C. and Konrad, P. N., *Blood*, **36**, 797 (1970).
210 Takahara, S., *Lancet*, **2**, 1101 (1952).
211 Takahara, S., *in*: Hereditary Disorders of Erythrocyte Metabolism. ed. by Beutler, E. (Grune and Stratton, New York/London, 1968), p. 21.
212 Aebi, H. and Suter, H., *Humangenetik*, **2**, 328 (1966).
213 Aebi, H. and Suter, H., *in*: Biochemical Methods in Red Cell Genetics. ed. by Yunis, J. J. (Academic Press, New York/London, 1969), p. 255.
214 Aebi, H., Bossi, E., Cantz, M., Matsubara, S. and Suter, H., *in*: Hereditary Disorders of Erythrocyte Metabolism, ed. by Beutler, E. (Grune and Stratton, New York/London, 1968), p. 41.
215 Thalhammer, O., Gitzelmann, R. and Panlitschko, M., *Pediatrics*, **42**, 441 (1968).
216 Isselbacher, K. J., Anderson, E. P., Kurahashi, K. and Kalckar, H. M., *Science*, **123**, 635 (1956).
217 Beutler, E. and Mathai, C. K., *in*: Hereditary Disorders of Erythrocyte Metabolism. ed. by Beutler, E. (Grune and Stratton, New York/London, 1968), p. 66.
218 Lesch, M. and Nyhan, W. L., *Amer. J. Med.*, **36**, 561 (1964).

Blood Preservation

C.-H. de VERDIER and L. GARBY

Departments of Clinical Chemistry and Clinical Physiology, University Hospital, Uppsala, Sweden

The conditions for erythrocyte preservation must be chosen with regard to the functions that are considered most important. For that reason the following three functions of the erythrocyte are being discussed: oxygen transport, proton and carbon dioxide transport, and survival after transfusion.

Oxygen transport is dependent on the intracellular concentration of the physiologically active ligands of hemoglobin: protons, carbon dioxide, and 2,3-diphosphoglycerate. After equilibration in the recipient's circulation the remaining effect of storage at $+4°C$ is in most solutions chiefly a decrease of the concentration of the 2,3-diphospoglycerate.

The effect of storage on proton and carbon dioxide transport is also mainly mediated over the concentration of 2,3-diphosphoglycerate. A low concentration of this compound causes the following functional changes:

1. Decrease of oxygen-linked proton binding
2. Increase of oxygen-linked carbamino binding
3. Decrease of erythrocyte-plasma proton gradient

The effect of storage on the posttransfusion survival is mostly mediated over ATP as there exists a good correlation between ATP concentration and viability. Other compounds, *e.g.*, lipids in the membranes, may also be of importance although the degree of correlation is less known.

INTRODUCTION

The importance of finding suitable methods of preservation of whole blood for transfusion purposes has long been recognized. Recent progress in several fields of practical medicine has underlined the necessity of having readily available transfusion blood of high quality. Following the discovery in 1943 of the dramatic effect of an acid-citrate-dextrose medium on the post-transfusion viability of red cells stored in the cold, research during the last 30 years has provided new knowledge for further improvement of the practical procedures. Of fundamental importance for this development has been 1) the realisation by Yoshikawa and his co-workers (Nakao *et al.*, 1959) of the importance of adenine nucleotides for the normal metabolism and function of red cells and 2) the discovery by Chanutin and Curnish (1967) and Benesch and Benesch (1967) of the role of organic phosphates in the oxygen affinity of hemoglobin. It is to these two aspects that the present review will be mainly directed.

A comprehensive and critical review of the literature up to 1971 can be found in a recent textbook by Mollison (1972). Several aspects were treated in the proceedings of an international symposium in Frankfurt, Germany, in 1969, edited by Spielmann and Seidl (1970).

REQUIREMENTS OF ERYTHROCYTE TRANSPORT FUNCTIONS NORMAL PERFORMANCE

The most appropriate tests of the effects of storage on the erythrocyte must always be a direct or indirect investigation of the possibilities for stored erythrocytes to fulfil their function immediately and late after transfusion. In order to estimate the fitness of the erythrocyte, it is important to know their transport functions in relation to the tissue requirements.

The red cells are adapted to perform several specific transport functions of the blood. The most important single molecule transported by the red cells is oxygen. In a variety of conditions, this molecule must be carried from the lungs to the tissues in such a way as to ensure an adequate supply of oxygen at specified tensions. In addition to oxygen transport, the red cells also participate in a critical manner in the transport of carbon dioxide from the tissues to the lungs and of protons from the tissues to the kidneys. Furthermore, the blood has to carry protons from the tissues, where they are formed when the carbon dioxide reaches the capillary blood, and to the lungs, where the protons are taken up when the blood is ventilated in the lungs. Several other metabolites are also transported by the red-cell system. The importance of the red cells for the transport of purines has been emphasized (Brown and Paterson, 1971).

1) Oxygen Transport

a) The Oxygen Consumption of Tissues

An average man consumes at rest 10 m*M* oxygen per min. With a cardiac output of 5 liter blood per min and a maximal oxygen binding capacity of the blood of about 10 m*M* only 20% of the oxygen transported to the tissues is released. This low utilization is due to the

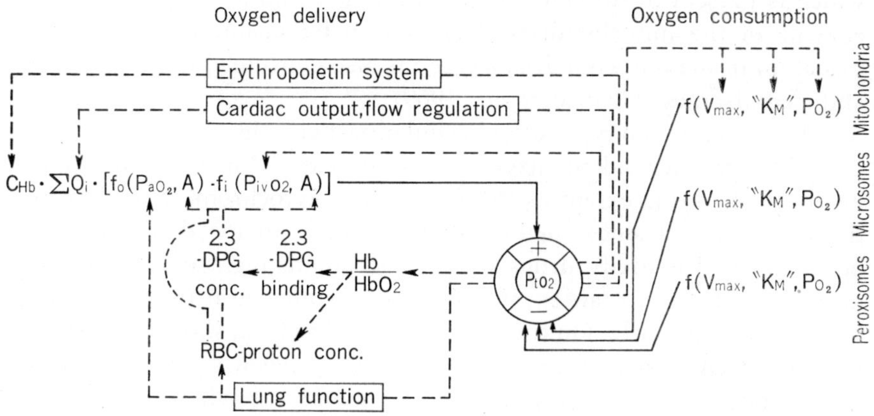

Fig. 1. The left-hand side of the figure illustrates the delivery of oxygen to the tissue and its regulation. All the circulatory loops are considered and the sum of the delivery in all these constitute the total net transport of oxygen from the lungs to the tissues. The arterial and venous blood oxygen saturation is expressed as functions of the oxygen tension (P_{O_2}) and the hemoglobin oxygen affinity (A). Due to different P_{CO_2} and pH in different loops the functions that determines the venous saturation have been given different expressions (f_i).

A general description of the mathematical relation between saturation, oxygen tension and affinity (P_{50}) is given through the Hill equation. The release of oxygen to the tissues is regulated directly through the venous oxygen tension and indirectly through cardiac output, the 2,3-DPG system and erythropoietin. Of these three indirect regulation mechanisms, cardiac output has the most rapid response and erythropoietin the slowest one.

The right-hand side of the figure describes the drain of oxygen through three main types of oxygen-dependent enzyme reactions with different apparent K_M values for oxygen. As the pool of oxygen in the tissues is comparatively small the delivery and the consumption of oxygen are approximately equal over a longer period of time. The tissue oxygen tension (P_{tO_2}) is directly a result of the flows (——) and indirectly a result of the regulation mechanisms (- - - -).

comparatively high oxygen tension required by the tissues. During physical exercise the increased demand for oxygen is covered mainly by increased cardiac output. A decreased oxygen tension in the tissues further increases the oxygen delivery.

Molecular oxygen is consumed in the tissues in enzyme reactions catalyzed by oxygenases and oxidases. Quantitatively, the most important oxygen-reacting enzyme is cytochrome c oxidase. This enzyme which is present in the mitochondrial inner membrane is the terminal enzyme of the mitochondrial electron-transfer chain. In addition to oxidation in the mitochondria, oxygen is also consumed in microsomes and peroxisomes (Chance *et al.*, 1969).

In the latter two types of subcellular particles the continuous function of oxygen-dependent enzymes is not necessary for the maintenance of life to the same extent as the function of cytochrome c oxidase in the mitochondria since their main function is to metabolize steroid hormones and detoxify drugs etc. A continuous high turnover is not needed for these substances; it may thus be sufficient if they are metabolized intermittently. On the other hand, it has been shown that these enzymes need higher oxygen concentrations (oxygen tensions) to oxygenate their substrates properly. Most patients receiving blood transfusions need oxygen for basic oxidative phosphorylation—ATP production and for other oxygen-requiring processes in the parenchymal organs. With the exception of the heart and respiratory muscles, little oxygen is needed for ATP production for muscular work. A patient in immediate need of improved oxygen transport function should consequently be given blood with a low oxygen affinity, *i.e.*, blood that can release much oxygen at a comparatively high oxygen pressure. The right-hand side of Fig. 1 summarizes the oxygen-consuming reactions in the tissues and their effect on the tissue oxygen tension.

b) The Normal Oxygen-Transport Function of the Blood

The supply of oxygen to the tissues can be discussed as the amount of oxygen supplied per unit of time at a fixed average oxygen tension or as the tension developed at a fixed consumption. The relation between the blood flow, the oxygen-binding capacity of the blood and the oxygen affinity of the blood on one hand and the oxygen supply to the tissues on the other hand can conveniently be expressed by the oxygen conservation equation written in the following form.

$$\dot{V}_{O_2} = \dot{Q} \cdot C_{Hb} \cdot (S_a - S_v)$$

where $\dot{V}_{O_2}$ is the oxygen supplied per unit of time, $\dot{Q}$ is the blood flow, C_{Hb} is the hemoglobin content equivalent to the oxygen-binding capacity of the blood and S_a and S_v are the oxygen saturations of the blood at the arterial and venous end, respectively. At fixed oxygen tensions in the arterial and venous blood the values of S_a and S_v depend solely on the oxygen affinity of the blood under the actual conditions. Consequently, in Fig. 1, S_a and S_v have been expressed as functions of the respective oxygen tensions, P_{aO_2} and P_{vO_2}, and the hemoglobin oxygen affinity in the arterial blood.

The affinity of the blood for oxygen is determined by the properties of the hemoglobin molecule and by the activities of the three physiological ligands in the red cells: protons, carbon dioxide and 2,3-DPG. Through direct effects or through allosteric linkage, the binding of oxygen is dependent on the activity of each of the other ligands. The molecular and chemical basis of the reactions between hemoglobin and its four ligands have been elucidated to a considerable degree during the past few years (see Perutz, 1970 and the proceedings from a recent symposium edited by Astrup and Rörth, 1972). Hemoglobin appears to exist in two main conformations with respect to its quarternary structure; a deoxy conformation and an oxy conformation. The deoxy conformation has a high affinity for protons, carbon dioxide and 2,3-DPG and these ligands tend to stabilize the molecule in the deoxy conformation with its low affinity for oxygen. The oxygen-linked protons bind to three specific pairs of residues, two in the α chains and one in the β chains; these are the so-called Bohr protons. Carbon dioxide can react to form carbamino residues with all four N-terminal valines although there is evidence that in the intact red cell only two of the terminals are involved (Garby, Robert and Zaar, 1972). Formation of a carbamino residue is accompanied by the release of 1.3 to 1.7 protons. Formation of an oxygen-heme link is accompanied by the release of 0.4 to 0.8 protons, depending on the oxygen saturation level. 2,3-DPG has one oxygen-linked binding site involving several residues in the central cavity between the two β chains.

The effect of each of these ligands on the oxygen affinity of hemoglobin can be expressed by the relation due to Wyman (1964),

$$\left[\frac{\delta \ln P_{O_2}}{\delta \ln x}\right]\bar{O}_2, \ln y, \ln z = -\left[\frac{\delta \bar{X}}{\delta \bar{O}_2}\right] \ln x, \ln y, \ln z$$

where P_{O_2} is the oxygen tension, O_2 is the number of moles of oxygen bound per mole of hemoglobin, x, y and z are activities of the ligands and $\bar{X}$, $\bar{Y}$ and $\bar{Z}$ are the number of mole of the ligand bound per mole of hemoglobin. A thorough discussion of the numerical values of these coefficients for the conditions in intact red cells is given by Siggaard-Andersen *et al.* (1972). The interactions between oxygen, protons and carbon dioxide lead to an increased capacity of the blood to deliver oxygen in tissues producing the latter two components and to take up oxygen in the lungs. The function of 2,3-DPG is to provide an end point for several feedback loops for the long-term regulation of the oxygen affinity of the blood (Fig. 1).

2) Proton and Carbon Dioxide Transport

Carbon dioxide is transported as dissolved carbon dioxide, carbonic acid, bicarbonate and hemoglobin-bound carbamino residues. The formation of bicarbonate and, as mentioned earlier, of carbamino residues involves the release of protons. Blood has a high proton buffering capacity and hemoglobin is the dominant system, with a buffer value of about 30 m*M* protons per mole hemoglobin tetramer. Under physiological conditions (P_{CO_2}=40 mmHg) the buffering capacity of hemoglobin is augmented by the oxygen-linked proton binding which on an average amounts to 0.5 *M* protons per mole of oxygen bound (Siggaard-Andersen, 1971). More than half of the protons released during carbon dioxide transport are in fact neutralized by this mechanism.

The capacity of hemoglobin to bind carbon dioxide as carbamino residue is limited and the oxygen-linked carbamino binding is only about 0.1 *M* per mole of oxygen bound or about 1 m*M* per litre of whole blood (Garby, Robert and Zaar, 1972). The physiological significance of this binding is not clear. As the binding of carbon dioxide is poor the main purpose may not be to transport carbon dioxide but to decrease the affinity for oxygen.

Both the oxygen-linked proton binding and the oxygen-linked carbamino binding are influenced by the red-cell 2,3-DPG concentration. This effect will be discussed in section 2 (see page 417).

3) The Survival of Red Cells in the Circulation

The great majority of the red cells formed by the bone marrow survive in the normal circulation for 100–130 days. As the cells age, they become smaller and more dense and lose part of their membrane. The loss of membrane may be accompanied by loss of hemoglobin, *i.e.*, erythrocyte fragmentation, but the extent of this mechanism of cell death during normal conditions is not known. The capacity of many enzyme systems decreases with red-cell age and changes in cofactor concentrations and rates have also been described. The following chapter of this book contains a critical review of the problem of establishing age-dependent changes in the metabolism and function of circulating red cells, especially during the last part of red-cell life.

When red cells become depleted of ATP, they become spherical

(Nakao *et al.*, 1960 and 1961) and loose their normal deformability (Weed *et al.*, 1969). This loss of deformability appears to be connected to the state of contractile protein molecules in or immediately under the membrane and is dependent not only on the ATP concentration but also on the calcium concentration. Rigid red cells become trapped in the spleen and there is a good deal of evidence (Weed *et al.*, 1969) that this mechanism of cell removal from the circulation is of major importance in many hemolytic states. Whether this mechanism is of importance for the death of normal cells under normal conditions is not known, partly because the age dependency of the ATP content is still controversial (cf. chapter 19).

Alterations in the structure and function of the red-cell membrane are also important determinants of red-cell viability (See a recent review by Cooper and Shattil, 1971). Present knowledge of the molecular structure and function of the red-cell membrane is however, still at the purely descriptive stage and the alterations described are defined at a low resolution.

EFFECT OF STORAGE ON ERYTHROCYTE POST-TRANSFUSION FUNCTION AND VIABILITY

Red cells stored in liquid media are subject to alterations of many kinds. The low pH and the low temperature slow down the rate of glucose consumption considerably and so makes less energy available to the cells. At the same time however, the reactions consuming ATP and electrons are also slowed down. After one or two weeks of storage the ATP concentration is definitely below normal and this change is believed to act as a trigger for further metabolic and structural derangements. From a practical clinical standpoint, the most important change appear to be those which lead to a decreased post-transfusion viability and those which lead to an increased oxygen affinity.

1) *Changes in the Oxygen Transport Function*

Blood stored in ACD solution exhibits a progressive increase in its affinity to oxygen (Valtis and Kennedy, 1954). When the affinity is expressed as the oxygen tension required to keep half of the hemoglobin saturated with oxygen, P_{50}, the value at a plasma pH of 7.40 and a carbon dioxide tension of 40 mmHg decreases from a normal value of 27 mmHg to a value of 15–20 mmHg after two weeks of storage. This considerable increase in oxygen affinity is due to the fact that the

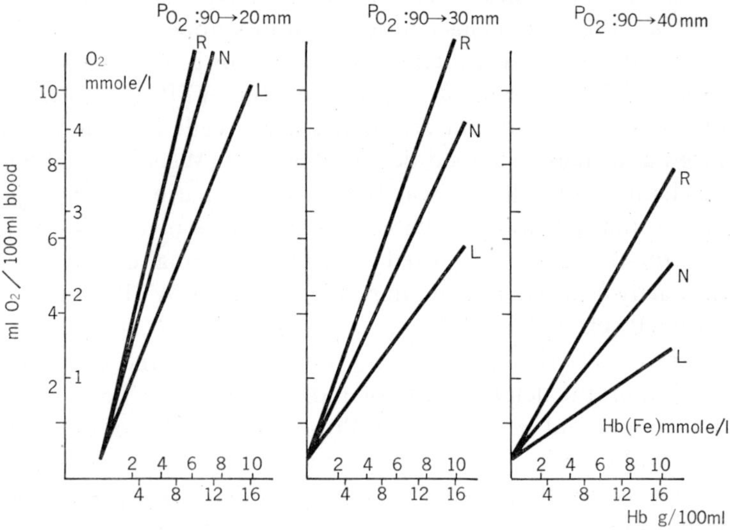

Fig. 2. Release of oxygen from blood with high, normal and low hemoglobin affinity for oxygen. The release at different hemoglobin concentrations is calculated from 3 oxygen dissociation curves which are normal (N) (P_{50}=27 mm Hg), left-shifted (L) (P_{50}=18 mm) or right-shifted (R) (P_{50}=32 mm).

Hemoglobin concentration is expressed both as mmole/l (monomer) and g/100 ml, oxygen release both as mmole/l and ml per 100 ml blood.

red-cell content of organic phosphates, mainly 2,3-DPG, decreases during the first two weeks of storage (Åkerblom *et al.*, 1968; Bunn *et al.*, 1969). The effect of a decreased concentration of 2,3-DPG is due not only to the decrease in the actual ligand activity but also due to the effect of the ligand on the distribution of protons between the extracellular end the intracellular phases. As shown by Duhm (1971), the intracellular pH increases from about 7.23 to about 7.30 when the concentration of 2,3-DPG in the red cells decreased from a normal level of 0.83 mole/mole hemoglobin to zero, and when the plasma pH is kept constant at 7.40. Such an increase in intracellular pH will lower the P_{50} value with about 2 mmHg.

Immediately prior to transfusion, the blood oxygen affinity is low because of the low pH of the medium and in the cells. However, because of the high permeability of the red cells to protons (or hydroxyl ions) (Crandall *et al.*, 1971), the low intracellular pH is restored within minutes after transfusion to the value prescribed by the recipient plasma pH and the Donnan conditions, so that the oxygen affinity of the transfused cells become as high as that mentioned above. The restoration of the 2,3-DPG content in the transfused cells occurs with a half-time of about six hours (Valeri and Hirsch, 1969; Beutler and Wood, 1969) and there is some evidence that cells stored for a period longer than five weeks have a somewhat reduced capacity to restore their 2,3-DPG content (Högman *et al.*, 1971). The oxygen affinity of the transfused cells decreases in parallel with the increase in 2,3-DPG concentration.

The effect on the tissue oxygen supply of the alterations in blood oxygen affinity can be calculated and in Fig. 2 data are presented for blood with high, normal and low affinity, with P_{50} values of 18 (L), 27 (N) and 32 (R) mmHg, respectively. The value for blood with a left-shifted oxygen dissociation curve (L) will rarely be found in the circulation as it corresponds to a complete exchange transfusion with 2,3-DPG depleted red blood cells. In most cases, it will, however, be possible to estimate the P_{50}-value or the 2,3-DPG content of the circulating red cells and thus draw an appropriate line between L and N. The question of which oxygen tension range ($P_{aO_2} \rightarrow P_{vO_2}$) is the most relevant, cannot at present not possibly be answered. As a reference, the following P_{vO_2} values can be given: venous renal blood 53 mmHg, mixed venous blood 38 mmHg and venous hepatic blood 38 mmHg (Marshall and Shepherd, 1968).

2) *Changes in the Proton- and Carbon Dioxide-Transport Function*

The effect of storage on these functions is probably mainly mediated over the effect on 2,3-DPG concentration. A low 2,3-DPG concentration will exert its effect through the following mechanism.

1. Decrease of the oxygen-linked proton binding,
2. Increase of the oxygen-linked carbamino binding,
3. Decrease of the plasma-erythrocyte pH gradient.

1) The oxygen-linked proton binding of whole blood decreases from about 0.32 eq per mole of oxygen bound at a plasma pH of 7.40, a P_{CO_2} of 40 mmHg and a red-cell 2,3-DPG concentration of 5 m*M* to a value of about 0.19 at zero 2,3-DPG concentration (Siggaard-Andersen and Salling, 1971). This phenomenon is, by virtue of Wyman's (1964) reciprocal effects (cp. eq. 1), reflected also in the effect of protons on the oxygen affinity which, at half-saturation and a P_{CO_2} of 40 mm Hg, decreased from a value of—0.37 at a 2,3-DPG concentration of 5 m*M* to a value of —0.30 at a 1 m*M* 2,3-DPG concentration

TABLE I. ATP, post-transfusion viability and 2,3-DPG during storage of blood in various preservatives. Figures, given in percent of initial values, are approximative; large differences may occur in blood from different donors. A similar version of this table has been published earlier (de Verdier *et al.*, 1972).

Preservative	Storage period, weeks																		Ref.
	1			2			3			4			5			6			
	ATP	viab	2,3-DPG	ATP	viab	2,3-DPG	ATP	viab	2,3-DPG	ATP	viab	2,3-DPG	ATP	viab	2,3-DPG	ATP	viab	2,3-DPG	
ACD	90	>90	60	80	85	10	60	80	5	40	65–70	5	30	60	—	25	45		32, 12, 43, 45, 34, 35, 39, 47
ACD- adenine .50 m*M*	110	>90	40	90	>90	10	80	85	5	70	85	5	60	75–80	—	40	70		32, 12, 43, 45, 34, 39, 47
CPD	75		120	70		85	65	80	40	40	70	10	30	55	5	25		—	45, 34, 39, 7, 26, 48
CPD- adenine .25 m*M*	85		110	85		70	80	85	30	65	75–80	10	50	70	5	40		—	48
CPD- adenine .50 m*M*	95		100	90		40	85		10	70		5	60	75–80	—		70		39, 7, 48
ACD-IAG inosine 10 m*M* adenine .5 m*M* guanosine .5 m*M*				80		85	75	85		70	85	30		85		60	75–80	20	7, 15, 28
ACD-AG adenine .5 m*M* guanosine .5 m*M*							100						65	80		55	70		26, 28
ACD-AI adenine .25 m*M* inosine 2.5 m*M*		>90			90			80			80			80			65		35
CPD+PIP phosphate 10 m*M* inosine 5 m*M*	70		150	60		150	55		105	45		35	35		10				47, 46
pyruvate 5 m*M* (+4°C)	PIP-addition on day 14:						80		120	70		100							

(Wranne, Woodson and Detter, 1972). This difference was found to be the same in fresh blood with depleted 2,3-DPG and in blood stored in ACD for three weeks.

2) The oxygen-linked carbamino binding, on the other hand, increases considerably when the 2,3-DPG concentration falls so that the effect of a decreased 2,3-DPG concentration on the classical Bohr effect, *i.e.*, a change in pH due solely to a change in P_{CO_2}, is increased from a value of —0.52 to a value of —0.67. (Wranne, Woodson and Detter, 1972). These data refer to fresh blood with depleted 2,3-DPG.

3) The effect of 2,3-DPG on the intracorpuscular pH has been discussed in the previous section. Apart from the effect on oxygen transport the effect of an increased erythrocyte pH on carbon dioxide and proton transport will be negligible. 2,3-DPG-deficient blood will thus have an increased proton binding in blood passing a capillary where proton release is due mainly to carbon dioxide uptake but a decreased proton binding in blood where proton release is due mainly to lactate uptake. The physiological and clinical significance of these changes in proton and carbamino binding in 2,3-DPG-deficient blood is, however, at the present time not known.

3) Post-Transfusion Viability

When fresh red blood cells are transfused to a compatible recipient they will continue to survive normally, *i.e.*, the number of transfused cells in the circulation will decrease at a rate of about 1% per day. From a practical point of view, post-transfusion survival or viability is usually defined as the percentage of transfused cells still in the circulation after 24 or 48 hr. The decrease in 24 hr post-transfusion viability with storage is shown in Table I. As shown in the table, there is a clear-cut association between the post-transfusion viability and the red-cell ATP content. (Simon and Sugita, 1965; de Verdier *et al.*, 1964; Åkerblom *et al.*, 1967; Dern *et al.*, 1967). This association appears to be causal. The mechanism by which the lowered ATP content leads to diminished viability has been much discussed. The work of Haradin *et al.*, (1969) and of LaCelle (1969) have provided good evidence that the decrease is causally associated with a loss of red-cell deformability due to a loss of red-cell ATP.

Storage of red cells in liquid media is also associated with a decrease in total lipid content with the same decrease in lipid phosphorus and cholesterol (Haradin *et al.*, 1969). When the blood is incubated with adenosine, both the ATP and the viability increase whereas there is no effect on the lipid content. To this extent and as a first approximation, the lipid content or composition does not appear to be a major determinant of red-cell post-transfusion viability.

4) Practical Solutions

Preservation of blood in the frozen state offers theoretically the best solution to the preservation problem since it has been shown that both the viability and the red-cell content of ATP and 2,3-DPG are well-preserved. However, the costs in terms of man-hours, special containers or bags and equipment for freezing and washing have so far prevented the more general use of frozen blood for routine purposes. The problem is well-illustrated by the fact that several different modifications of techniques are at present in use and under development. Several techniques are described and discussed in a review by Valeri (1966) and in the proceedings of the symposium in Frankfurt edited by Spielmann and Seidl (1970).

Preservation in liquid media at a temperature slightly above 0°C is therefore considered to be the most practical method. Two basic media, the acid-citrate-dextrose solution (ACD) and the citrate-phosphate-dextrose solution (CPD), have been extensively studied with respect to their effect on red-cell physiology and, in particular, the effect on post-transfusion viability and erythrocyte content of ATP and 2,3-DPG. As illustrated in Table I, preservation in ACD leads to a fairly rapid fall in the concentration of 2,3-DPG and therefore to a rise in the oxygen affinity. The use of this solution cannot therefore be recommended unless the storage time is less than about 10 days. The CPD solution, because of its higher initial pH, preserves the 2,3-DPG concentration better. The post-transfusion viability of red cells stored in these two solutions decreases continuously and is about 70% at the end of four weeks. Addition of adenine to a final concentration of 0.25–0.5 m*M* leads to a slower decline in the red-cell ATP level and to a better posttransfusion viability. However, the addition of adenine slows down the synthesis of 2,3-DPG so that the 2,3-DPG levels falls more rapidly. This is metabolically explained by the increased adenine nucleotide content, especially ADP, which is caused by adenine. An increase in ADP concentration will convert more 1,3-DPG to 3-PG and less will be left for the alternative metabolic pathway to 2,3-DPG. (Schröter and v. Heyden, 1965). A reasonable compromise between the ATP-elevating and the 2,3-DPG-reducing effects of adenine is obtained through the use of a CPD solution containing adenine at a final concentration of 0.25 m*M*.

Further improvement of both the post-transfusion survival and the oxygen-transport function can be obtained through addition of compounds that stimulate the synthesis of 2,3-DPG and ATP at some time period during the storage. Addition of mixtures of inosine, phosphate and pyruvate has been tested and found to have a strong effect (Table I). It seems to be an advantage if the additions are made later during storage, as this makes it possible to decrease the amounts added. As inosine is metabolized to hypoxanthine and, later in the body, to urace, it is important to decrease the uricosogenic effect by reduction of the administered amount directly or indirectly through washing of the blood before the transfusion.

It should be added that the effects of transfusion of blood with different concentrations of intracorpuscular components on the tissue metabolism are speculative, based on theoretical grounds. Direct measurements of biochemical and physiological parameters in the tissues are largely lacking. Also, there is a need for controlled studies to evaluate the clinical importance of transfusion of blood with suboptimal respiratory function.

ADDENDUM

a) *Recent Reviews*

At the International Blood Transfusion Congress, Washington D. C., September 1972, different aspects of blood preservation were discussed. (Beutler, pp. 285–297 ; de Verdier *et al.*, pp. 299–315 ; Hollán, pp. 317–327; Chaplin, pp. 329–342; Valeri *et al.*, pp. 343–365 in Progress in Transfusion and Transplantation. Ed. P. J. Schmidt Am. Ass. Blood Banks 1972).

The proceedings from a National Academy of Sciences Symposium in June 1972 with the title Preservation of Red Blood Cells (Eds. Chaplin, Jaffé, Lenfant & Valeri ; Natl. Acad. Sciences Washington D. C. 1973) contain several important reports from U.S. investigators.

b) *Physiological Function of the Erythrocytes*

In a recent paper (Elwyn, Launder, Parikh & Wise: *Amer. J. Physiol.*, **222**, 1333, 1972) evidences were given for the rôle of experimental erythrocytes in amino acid transport. During the last years the γ-glutanyl cycle for amino acid transport was described (Meister, A.: *Science*, **180**, 33, 1973). The significance of this transport function of the erythrocytes must be established, however, before it is worthwhile to study the influence of preservation on this function.

c) Effect of Storage on Erythrocyte Metabolism

Minakami (VIIth International Berlin Symposium on Structure and Function of Erythrocytes Berlin, GDR, 1973) has emphasized the effect of the impermeable extracellular citrate ion on the Donnan conditions and the intracellular pH. Intracellular pH is important for the understanding of the changes in metabolite concentrations during storage.

d) Intraindividual Variation of Concentration of Intracorpuscular Components and Possibility to Predict Storageability

This question was discussed in two recent articles (Åkerblom, Andreasson & de Verdier and Andreasson, de Verdier & Åkerblom: VIIth International Berlin Symposium on Structure and Function of Erythrocytes Berlin).

Before and during storage the intraindividual variation for ATP and 2,3-DPG concentration was smaller than the interindividual variation. Intraindividual coefficients of variation for ATP concentration was smaller than for 2,3-DPG.

REFERENCES

1 Astrup, P. and Rörth, M. (eds.), Oxygen affinity of hemoglobin red cell acid-base status. Alfred Benzon Symposium IV. Munksgaard, Copenhagen (1972).

2 Benesch, R. and Benesch, R. E., The effect of organic phosphates from the human erythrocyte on the allosteric properties of hemoglobin. *Biochem. Biophys. Res. Comm.*, **26**, 162 (1967).

3 Beutler, E. and Wood, L., The *in vivo* regeneration of red cell 2,3-diphosphoglyceric acid after transfusion of stored blood. *J. Lab. Clin. Med.*, **74**, 300 (1969).

4 Brown, R. R. and Paterson, A. R. P., Turnover of purine nucleotides in rabbit erythrocytes: Lack of *in vivo* effect of the nucleoside transport inhibitor, *p*-nitrobenzyl-6-thioguanosine. *Canad. J. Biochem.*, **49**, 1251 (1971).

5 Bunn, H. F., May, M. H. and Kocholaty, W. F., Hemoglobin function in stored blood. *J. Clin. Invest*, **48**, 311 (1969).

6 Chance, B., Thurman, R. and Gosalvez, M., Oxygen affinities of cellular respiration. *Försvarsmedicin*, **5**, 235 (1969).

7 Chanutin, A., The effect of the addition of adenine and nucleosides at the beginning of storage on the concentration of phosphates of human erythrocytes during storage in acid-citrate-dextrose and citrate-phosphate-dextrose. *Transfusion*, **7**, 120 (1967).

8 Chanutin, A. and Curnish, R., Effect of organic and inorganic phosphates on the oxygen equilibrium of human erythrocytes. *Acta Biochem. Biophys.*, **121**, 96 (1967).

9 Cooper, R. A. and Shattil, S. J., Mechanisms of hemolysis—the minimal red-cell defect. *New Engl. J. Med.*, **285**, 1514 (1971).

10 Crandall, E. D., Klocke, R. A. and Forster, R. E., Hydroxyl ion movements across the human erythrocyte membrane. *J. Gen. Physiol.*, **57**, 664 (1971).

11 Dern, R. J., Brewer, G. J. and Wiorkowski, J. J., Studies on the preservation of human blood. II. The relationship of erythrocyte adenosine triphosphate levels and other *in vitro* measures to red-cell storageability. *J. Lab. Clin. Med.*, **69**, 968 (1967).

12 de Verdier, C.-H., Garby, L., Hjelm, M., *et al.*, Adenine in blood preservation: Post-transfusion viability and biochemical changes. *Transfusion*, **4**, 331 (1964).

13 de Verdier, C.-H., Åkerblom, O., Arturson, G., Garby, L., Högman, C. F., Kreuger, A. and Westman, M., Maintenance of oxygen-transport function of stored blood. The XIIIth Congress of the International Society of Blood Transfusion (XIIIth Congr. int. Soc. Blood Transf.) Plenary Sessions, Washington, D. C. (1972), in press.

14 Duhm, J., Effects of 2,3-diphosphoglycerate and other organic phosphate compounds on oxygen affinity and intracellular pH of human erythrocytes. *Pflügers Arch.*, **326**, 341 (1971).

15 Fritzsche, W., Siedentopf, H. G. and Spielmann, W., Untersuchungen zur verbesserten Zellkonservierung. IV. Überlebenzeitbestimmungen und klinische Erfahrungen mit IAG-konservierten Blut. *Klin. Wochenschr.*, **43**, 881 (1965).

16 Garby, L., Robert, M. and Zaar, B., Proton- and carbamino-linked oxygen affinity of normal human blood. *Acta Physiol. Scand.*, **84**, 482 (1972)

17 Haradin, A. R., Weed, R. I. and Reed, C. F., Changes in physical properties of stored erythrocytes. *Transfusion*, **9**, 229 (1969).

18 Högman, C. F., Åkerblom, O., de Verdier, C.-H., *et al.*, Optimal use of different storage procedures. *Bibl. Haemat*, **38** (pt 2), 175 (1971).

19 La Celle, P. L., Alteration of deformability of the erythrocyte membrane in stored blood. *Transfusion*, **9**, 238 (1969).

20 Marshall, R. J. and Shephard, J. T., Cardiac function in health and disease, Philadelphia, London, Toronto, Saunders Co., 14 (1968).

21 Mollison, P. L., Blood transfusion in clinical medicine. 5th Ed. Black-

well Oxford (1972).

22 Nakao, M., Nakao, T., Tatibana, M., Yoshikawa, H. and Abe, T., Effect of inosine and adenine on adenosine triphosphate regeneration and shape transformation in long-stored erythrocytes. *Biochim. Biophys. Acta*, **31**, 564 (1959).

23 Nakao, M., Nakao, T. and Yamazoe, S., Adenosine triphosphate and maintenance of shape of the human red cells. *Nature*, **187**, 945 (1960).

24 Nakao, M., Nakao, S., Yamazoe, S. and Yoshikawa, H., Adenosine triphosphate and shape of erythrocytes. *J. Biochem.*, **45**, 487 (1961).

25 Perutz, M., Stereochemistry of cooperative effects in hemoglobin. *Nature*, **228**, 726 (1970).

26 Roigas, H., Strauss, D. and Raderecht, H. J., Verbesserte Blutkonservierung durch Zusätze von Adenin und Guanosin. *Zschr. Inn. Med.*, **24**, 850 (1969).

27 Schröter, W. and von Heyden, H., Kinetik des 2,3-Diphosphoglyceratumsatzes in menschlichen Erythrocyten. *Biochem. Z.*, **341**, 387 (1965).

28 Seidl, S. and Spielmann, W., Comparative studies on the effect of different nucleosides *in* red-cell preservation, *in*; ed. by Spielmann, M. and Seidl, S.: Modern problems of blood preservation, Stuttgart (Gustav Fischer Verlag, 1970), pp. 72–77.

29 Siggaard-Andersen, O., Oxygen-linked hydrogen ion binding of human hemoglobin. Effects of carbon dioxide and 2,3-diphosphoglycerate. I. Studies on erythrolysate. *Scand. J. Clin. Lab. Invest.*, **27**, 351 (1971).

30 Siggaard-Andersen, O. and Salling, N., Oxygen-linked hydrogen ion binding of human hemoglobin. Effects of carbon dioxide and 2,3-diphosphoglycerate. II. Studies on whole blood. *Scand. J. Clin. Lab. Invest.*, **27**, 361 (1971).

31 Siggaard-Andersen, O., Rörth, M., Nörgaard-Pedersen, B., Sparre-Andersen, O. and Johansen, E., Oxygen-linked hydrogen ion binding of human hemoglobin. Effects of carbon dioxide and 2,3-diphosphoglycerate. IV. Thermodynamical relationship between the variables. *Scand. J. Clin. Lab. Invest.* (1972), in press.

32 Simon, E. R. and Sugita, Y., Red-cell preservation; addition of adenine to improve preservation in ACD solution. Proc 10th Congr. Int. Soc. Blood Transf. Stockholm 1964 (Basel/New York, Karger, 1965), pp. 607–615.

33 Spielmann, W. and Seidl, S. (eds.), Modern problems of blood preservation. Gustav Fischer Verlag, Stuttgart (1970).

34 Strumia, P. V. and Strumia, M. H., Preservation of blood in acid-citrate-dextrose anticoagulant solution for more than twenty-one days. *Amer. J. Clin. Path.*, **52**, 671 (1969).

35 Strumia, M. M., Strumia, P. V. and Eusebi, A. J., The preservation of blood for transfusion. VII. Effect of adenine and inosine on the adeno-

sine triphosphate and viability of red cells when added to blood stored from zero to seventy days at 1°C. *J. Lab. Clin. Med.*, **75**, 244 (1970).

36 Valeri, C. R., Frozen blood. *New Engl. J. Med.*, **275**, 365, 425 (1966).

37 Valeri, C. R. and Hirsch, N. M., Restoration *in vivo* of erythrocyte adenosine triphosphate, 2,3-diphosphoglycerate, potassium ion and sodium ion concentration following transfusion of acid citrate-dextrose-stored human red blood cells. *J. Lab. Clin. Med.*, **73**, 722 (1969).

38 Valtis, D. J. and Kennedy, A. C., Defective gas-transport function of stored red blood cells. *Lancet*, **1**, 119 (1954).

39 Warner, W. L., Red cell preservation and survival determinations in anticoagulant systems, *in*; ed. by Spielmann, W. and Seidl, S., Modern problems in blood preservation, Stuttgart (Gustav Fischer Verlag, 1970), pp. 63–71.

40 Weed, R. I., LaCelle, P. L. and Merrill, E. W., Metabolic dependance of red-cell membrane deformability. *J. Clin. Invest.*, **48**, 795 (1969).

41 Wranne, B., Woodson, R. D. and Detter, J. C., The Bohr effect: Interaction between H^+, CO_2 and 2,3-DPG in fresh and stored blood. *J. Appl. Physiol.* (1972), in press.

42 Wyman, J., Linked functions and reciprocal effects in hemoglobin: A second look. *Advanc. Prot. Chem.*, **19**, 223 (1964).

43 Åkerblom, O., de Verdier, C.-H. and Finnson, M., *et al.*, Further studies on the effect of adenine in blood preservation. *Transfusion*, **7**, 1 (1967).

44 Åkerblom, O., de Verdier, C.-H., Garby, L., *et al.*, Restoration of defective oxygen-transport function of stored red blood cells by addition of inosine. *Scand. J. Clin. Lab. Invest.*, **21**, 245 (1968).

45 Åkerblom, O., de Verdier, C.-H., Eriksson, Å., *et al.*, Late addition of inosine to stored ACD-adenine blood: Effects on erythrocyte viability and metabolism. *Folia Haemat.*, **91**, 142 (1969).

46 Åkerblom, O. and Ericson, Å., Effects of inosine, pyruvate and inorganic phosphate on the 2,3-DPG level in fresh and stored erythrocytes. VIth International symposium on the structure and function of erythrocytes (Berlin, 1970).

47 Åkerblom, O., unpublished results.

48 Åkerblom, O. and Kreuger, A., Studies on citrate-phosphate-dextrose (CPD) blood supplemented with adenine (to be published).

Methodological Aspects of Current Procedures to Separate Erythrocytes into Age Groups

M. Hjelm*

Department of Clinical Chemistry University Hospital S-750 14 Uppsala, Sweden

Current methods to fractionate erythrocytes into age groups are reviewed. A fractionation ratio is used to evaluate the degree of separation. Erythrocyte populations with cells varying in age with a few days can only be obtained during the initial and especially not during the final ten per cent of the life span.

There are indirect evidences that pronounced biochemical changes take place during a short period at the end of the life span. Present fractionation procedures have to be improved or new ones developed, if it should be possible to measure these changes and to find the biochemical mechanism behind the cell death.

INTRODUCTION

A great number of biochemical and biophysical variables in circulating human and animal erythrocytes change with cell age (Fornaini, 1967, Danon, 1966). Such changes are accompanied by a decreased capacity of the erythrocytes to deliver oxygen to the tissues (Edwards and Rigas, 1967, Edwards, *et al.*, 1971). The sequence of biochemical and biophysical events behind this phenomenon and the death of the cells, however, is not well-defined at present.

There are several reasons for this fact, *e.g.*, (I) the accuracy of present methods to isolate erythrocytes of a specific age within a cell population of all ages in the life span of the cell species may not be sufficient, (II) conclusions about the magnitude and implications of biochemical and biophysical changes obtained by comparing 'noncomparable' erythrocyte populations, *e.g.*, stress reticulocytes with old erythrocytes from the nonmanipulated healthy subject, may not be valid, and (III) basic knowledge of erythrocyte biochemistry and biophysics is still insufficient for a functional understanding of the ageing processes of the erythrocyte. The area of increased knowledge that is of importance

* Present adress; Department of Clinical Chemistry, University Hospital, 5000 Odense, Denmark.

should be defined by a detailed analysis of biochemical and biophysical events, especially at the end of the life span, a demand that again depends on the possibility of separating erythrocytes into distinct age groups.

Thus an attempt has been made in this review to discuss in some detail the principal methods used to obtain erythrocyte populations of different ages, especially the possibility of separating labeled cells at different ages during the life span. No attempt has been made to review the literature completely, quoted investigations being used to elucidate different aspects of the topic.

The reader is especially referred to Fornaini, 1967, for an extensive review with more than 400 references to the biochemistry, and to Danon, 1966, for a comprehensive lecture on the biophysics of erythrocyte ageing. Leif, 1970, has written a highly relevant article on the density of erythrocytes. Many of the older investigations in the area are quoted by Chalfin, 1956 and van Gastel, 1968, also reviewed methods for studying the *in vivo* ageing of erythrocytes.

PRINCIPLE METHODS TO ISOLATE ERYTHROCYTES ACCORDING TO AGE

Current techniques to isolate circulating erythrocytes of a certain age are summarized in Table I.

TABLE I. Principal methods of preparing erythrocyte populations of different mean age.

1. *In vitro* methods	2. *In vivo* methods
a) Plain centrifugation and centrifugation on density gradients	a) Differential agglutination
b) Serial (graded) osmotic hemolysis	b) Bleeding and induced hemolysis
c) Counter-current distribution	c) Hypertransfusion

1) *Plain Centrifugation and Centrifugation on Density Gradients*

It has long been realized that the density of erythrocytes increases with cell age (Key, 1921). Many procedures, using plain centrifugation and centrifugation on density gradients, some of which are listed in Table II, have been proposed. Apparently they vary considerably with respect to type of anticoagulant used, suspending medium or gradient, gravity force, centrifuging time, temperature, etc.

a) *Effect of Anticoagulants*

The effect of heparin, ACD, oxalate, EDTA, Na_2-EDTA and mechanical defibrination (Table II) on the age fractionation of erythrocytes does not seem to have been systematically investigated. It is likely, however, that the type and concentration of the anticoagulant used is of importance for the efficiency of the fractionating procedure. Increased sedimentation rate and increased rouleaux formation by fibrinogen (Fåhreus, 1921) not precipitated during mechanical defibrination (Piomelli, Lurinsky and Wasserman, 1966), might in principle increase the possibility of obtaining pure fractions of young erythrocytes as reticulocytes having a decreased tendency for rouleaux formation (Stephens, 1940), and might possibly also enrich old erythrocytes if they have an increased tendency for rouleaux formation compared with the young erythrocytes. The effect of heparin on rouleaux formation by young and old erythrocytes might also be of importance (Wintrobe, 1967, Hjelm, 1972), especially in methods using plain centrifugation in heparin plasma.

The possible effects of ACD, oxalate and EDTA on the pH value and the osmolarity of the suspending medium with concomitant changes of erythrocyte volume and density should also be recognized (Piomelli, Lurinsky and Wasserman, 1966, Leif, 1970).

b) *The Suspending Medium or Gradient*

In one systematic investigation (Prentice and Bishop, 1965) using *plain centrifugation*, erythrocytes were almost as efficiently fractionated in heparin plasma as in a Krebs-Ringer-phosphate buffer or solutions of 0.9% NaCl and 5–10% sucrose. Hypertonic (20%) sucrose was also used. Solutions of dextran (Mol. wt. 10,500 and 41,000) and polyvinyl pyrrolidone (Mol. wt. 40,000) in water or saline, induced clumping of the erythrocytes and were considered unsuitable. A 30% albumin solution has also been used (Pranker, 1958).

It should be pointed out that using plain centrifugation, erythrocytes are fractionated into age groups under nonequilibrium conditions (Garby and Hjelm, 1963, Prentice and Bishop, 1965) with a high degree of reproducibility.

Albumin has been used to centrifuge erythrocytes on *continuous* (Leif and Vinograd, 1964, Bishop and Prentice, 1966) and *discontinuous gradients* (Piomelli, Lurinsky and Wasserman, 1966). Discontinuous gradients have also been prepared by methyl phthalate and di-*n*-butyl phthalate (Danon and Marikovsky, 1965, Brook *et al.*, 1966). Dextran,

TABLE II. Plain centrifugation and

Procedure	Type of cells	Anticoagulant
Plain centrifugation		
a) One-step	human	heparin
	,,	,,
	,,	,,
	,,	ACD[3)]
	,,	heparin
	rabbit	,,
	,,	,,
	,,	
	,,[2)]	,,
	,,	mechanical defibrination
	dog	Na_2-EDTA
b) Varied	human	heparin
	,,[2)]	,,
c) Refractionation[1)]	,,	EDTA
	rabbit	heparin
Centrifugation on density gradients		
	human	dilution[4)]
	,,	varied[5)]
		heparin
	rabbit	,,
	,,	mechanical defibrination
	,,	heparin
	rat	,,

1) Top and bottom of refractionated original top and bottom fractions; 2) 4) The original blood sample was immediately diluted in Alsever's solution; 5) vidual results for different anticoagulants used are given; 6) Krebs-Ringer-efficiency, 5, and 20% sucrose was less efficient; Dextran (Mol. wt. 10, 500– Stepwise procedure; 8) 2-step plain centrifugation for both original and re-room temperature through not always stated.

a) Borun, Frigueroa and Perry, 1957, b) Rigas and Koler, 1961, c) Garby and and Bishop, 1965, g) Chalfin, 1956, h) Piomelli, Lurinsky, and Wasserman, m) Leif and Vinograd, 1964. n) Danon and Marikovsky, 1964, o) Brok *et al.*, Batt, 1970.

centrifugation in density gradients.

Suspending medium or gradient	Centrifugal force, g	Centrifugal time, min	Centrifugal temp., +°C	Ref.
plasma	2,000	40	R[10]	a
,,	1,600	120	4	b
,,	67,000	120	4	b
,,	134,000	10, 120	4	c
,,	1–12,000	15–240	20	d
,,	15,000	40	R	e
varied[6]	383–1644	15–60	R	f
plasma	5,000–39,000	30	4	f
,,	20,000	30	R	g
albumin 30%				h
,,	5,900	40	4	i
,,	100+2,000	10+45	R	k
,,	100+2,000	10+45	R	k
albumin 30%	4,000+10,000[8]	10+5	R+ 4	l
plasma	1,600	30		f
albumin continuous	23,500	60	R	m
methyl phtalate	12,000	14	R	n
,,[7]	12,000	14	R	o
,,	12,000	14	R	p
albumin discontinuous	167,000	60	4	h
,,	35,500	15–75	4	q
,,	9)	30	R	r

Reticulocytosis induced by bleeding; 3) Acid-citrate-dextrose (NIH formula B); Defibrinated, heparinized, citrated, oxalated and EDTA-treated blood. No indi- phosphate buffer, 0.9% NaCl, 10% sucrose and plasma had the same separatory 41,000), polyvinyl pyrrolidone (Mol. wt. 40, 000) induced roleaux formation; 7) fractionated cell fractions; 9) 25,000 rpm, radius not stated; 10) R=most likely

Hjelm, 1963, d) O'Connel, Caruso and Sass, 1965, e) Hoffman, 1958, f) Prentice 1966, i) Coopersmith and Ingram, 1968, k) Bernstein, 1959, l) Prankerd, 1958, 1966, p) Danon *et al.*, 1965, q) Bishop and Prentice, 1966, r) Winterbourn and

known to aggregate erythrocytes (Thorsen and Hint, 1950) and found unsuitable by several investigators (Leif and Vinograd, 1964, Bishop and Prentice, 1966, Piomelli, Lurinsky and Wasserman, 1966) has recently been used as a discontinuous gradient to separate erythrocytes according to density (Gross *et al.*, 1972).

By separating erythrocytes on density gradients, a highly reproducible separation of the cells is obtained under equilibrium conditions (Leif, 1970).

c) Force, Time and Temperature of the Centrifugation

On plain centrifugation, the degree of age fractionation increases with rotor speed, the highest values of the fractionation ratio (*vide infra*, degree of age fractionation of erythrocytes) without recentrifugation being obtained by ultracentrifugation (Prentice and Bishop, 1965). If part of the cell column is recentrifuged, an increased degree of fractionation can be achieved at about 2,000–10,000 g (Prankerd, 1958, Prentice and Bishop, 1965). The rotor speed has apparently not been systematically varied when centrifuging erythrocytes on density gradients.

The effect of varying the time of centrifugation on the degree of age fractionation has been investigated to some extent. The fractionation ratio on plain centrifugation did not increase between 10 min and 2 hr at 134,000 g (Garby and Hjelm, 1963), increased between 15 min and 2 hr at 2,000 g (O'Connell, Caruso and Sass, 1965), and increased slightly between 15 and 60 min at 1,644 g (Prentice and Bishop, 1965). Thus the separation of erythrocytes into age groups is probably achieved in a few minutes on plain centrifugation at high rotor speeds, the time necessary to obtain an optimal degree of density distribution of the cells in a certain system possibly being inversely related to the rotor speed at lower g numbers.

Distinct bands of erythrocytes on a discontinuous albumin gradient at 35,000 g were obtained after 45 min and not improved further after 75 min (Bishop and Prentice, 1966).

The effect of temperature on the efficiency of the separatory procedures, though important, as briefly mentioned by Danon, 1966, has not been systematically studied. From a general point of view, biochemical and biophysical investigations on erythrocytes separated at room or at an unspecified temperature (Chalfin, 1956, Borun, 1957, Hoffman, 1958, Prankerd, 1958, Bernstein, 1959, Danon and Marikovsky, 1964, Danon *et al.*, 1965, Brok *et al.*, 1966), may not be valid for *in vivo* conditions as the active metabolism of erythrocytes *in vitro* may

TABLE III. Calculated percentage of erythrocytes labeled with ^{59}Fe and ^{14}C-glycine and maximal theoretical fractionation ratios.

Erythrocytes from	Life span	Erythrocytes labeled with ^{59}Fe or ^{14}C-glycine: Days of labeling after administration of label	Per cent of circulating labeled cells	Maximal theoretical fractionation ratio[1)]
Man	120	4	3.3	30
Dog	100	4	4.0	25
Rabbit	60	4	6.7	15
Rat	60	4	6.7	15

[1)] Maximal theoretical fraction ratio $= \frac{T}{t}$, where t = days during which reticulocytes are labeled and T = the life span of the erythrocyte.

induce various artifacts.

d) The Degree of Age Fractionation of Erythrocytes

The distribution of erythrocytes not older than 2 days in a cell column containing cells of all ages separated according to density, can be evaluated by reticulocyte counts as reticulocytes lose their morphological characteristics after 1 or 2 days (Finch *et al.*, 1949, Stryckmans *et al.*, 1968, Ganzoni, Hillman and Finch, 1969).

^{59}Fe or ^{14}C-glycine has been used to label reticulocytes *in vivo* and to evaluate the possibility of isolating the labeled cells at different times after the labeling. Reticulocytes released into circulation during about 4 days are labeled with ^{59}Fe or ^{14}C-glycine *in vivo* after a single injection of the label and cells not older than about 2 days can be labeled with ^{14}C-glycine *in vitro* (Ferrebee, Gibson and Peacock, 1946, Dreyfus, Schapira and Kruh, 1950, Brok *et al.*, 1966).

A *fractionation ratio*, the radioactivity* of ^{59}Fe or ^{14}C-glycine in different parts of the centrifuged erythrocyte column divided by the radioactivity* of the whole cell population, has been calculated to evaluate the degree of separation of labeled cell obtained. A *maximal theoretical fractionation ratio* that should be obtained in a cell fraction containing only labeled erythrocytes can be calculated from the percentage of labeled cells in the whole cell population*, as in Table III.

In practice the fractionation ratios obtained are lower than the theoretical values, as is evident from Table IV. In this table the de-

* cpm/g of haemoglobin.

TAB

Procedure	Type of cells	Label	Fractionation ratio of	
			Top fraction	Bottom fraction
Plain centrifugation				
a) One-step	human	^{59}Fe	2.5	1.7
	,,	,,	1.9	1.3
	,,	,,	2.3	1.6
	,,	,,	4.2	1.8
	,,	,,	5.9	—
	rabbit	,,	3.2	1.6
	,,	,,	2.0	1.5
	,,	,,	2.1	—
	,,[2)]	Reticulocytes	—	—
	,,	^{59}Fe	3.8	1.3
	dog	,,	6.3	1.3
b) Varied	human	Reticulocytes	—	—
	,,[2)]	,,	—	—
c) Refractionation[1)]	,,	^{59}Fe	9.1	7.1
	rabbit	,,	11.4	—
Centrifugation on density gradients				
	human	,,		
	,,	,,		
		,,	14	—
	rabbit	,,	—	8.0
	,,	^{14}C-glycine	5.5	3.1
	,,	^{59}Fe	5.0	1.7
	,,	,,	8.7	1.6
	rat	^{14}C-glycine	8.7	2.3

1) 2) *Vide* Table II; 3) Calculated according to the formula f × p, where f = the in Table 3; 4) In some cases the fractionation ratio in the cell fraction next to 5) Not possible to calculate from available data; 6) Assuming a hematocrit value part of the cell column has been analysed; 7) References are the same as in

gree of age fractionation has also been calculated as a percentage of labeled erythrocytes in appropriate parts of the cell column (using the fractionation ratios stated and the calculated percentage of labeled cells in the whole erythrocyte population from Table III) to permit comparisons between methods using different cell species.

LE IV.

Calculated percentage of labeled cells[8)] in		Sampling, days after labeling for		Top or bottom fraction in % of total cell column	Ref.[7)]
Top fraction	Bottom[4)] fraction	Top fraction	Bottom fraction		
8.3	5.6	4	120	25	a
6.3	4.3	4	115	33	b
7.6	5.3	4	115	33	b
14	5.9	6	118	11	c
20	—	8	—	6	d
21	11	2	48	20	e
13	10	7	49	13	f
14	—	7	—	13	f
90	—	—	—	5	g
25	8.7	1	45	13	h
25	5.2	5	100	10	i
8.0	—	5	—	10	k
50	—	4	—	10	k
30	23	5	98	6[6)]	l
76	—	5	—	—	f
—[4)]	—[5)]	—	—	—	m
—[4)]	—[5)]	—	—	—	n
26	—	1	—	2	o
—	54	—	25	10	p
37	21	10	60	17	h
33	11	10	60	17	h
58	11	1	49	—	q
58	15	0	55	10	r

actual fractionation ratio obtained and p=calculated percentage of labeled cells the bottom fraction has been used, being larger than for the bottom fraction; of 40% of the original blood sample and that 0.5 ml of the top and bottom Table II.

Reticulocyte counts around 10% and labeled cells corresponding to between 6 and 25% of the total number of labeled cells, are obtained after plain centrifugation and to 26 to 58% after centrifugation on density gradients in the top fraction with erythrocytes from healthy,

TABLE V. Serial (graded)

Type of cells	Washing solution	Temp. during hemolysis	Label
Human	NaCl, 0.85% not buffered	4–37	^{59}Fe
,,	KCl, isotonic buffered by HCO_3^-, pH 7.4	0	,,
,,	NaCl, 0.9% buffered by phosphate, pH 7.4	R	,,

a) Simon and Topper, 1957; b) Marks and Johnson, 1958; c) Sass, Levy and

nonmanipulated subjects.

The percentage of labeled cells in the top fraction increases after recentrifugation (30–76%) and reticulocyte counts close to 100% have been obtained in the top fraction after bleeding the rabbits. (Chalfin, 1956, Bernstein, 1959, see also 2b).

The percentage of labeled old erythrocytes in the bottom fraction of the erythrocyte column is less than the percentage of young erythrocytes in the top fraction. Values between 4.9–11% after plain centrifugation, 11–21-(54)% after centrifugation on density gradients and 33% after recentrifugation of ^{59}Fe-labeled old erythrocytes in the bottom fraction demonstrate the difficulties in obtaining, by these procedures, well-defined age groups at the end of the life span of the erythrocytes.

Labeling of erythrocytes with ^{14}C-glycine indicate, however, that the number of old erythrocytes might be higher than calculated from the distribution of ^{59}Fe in the cell column, the main reason being that ^{59}Fe is continuously reutilized by random destruction of circulating labeled cells. (Berlin, Waldman and Weissman, 1959, van Gastel *et al.*, 1965). This reutilization of ^{59}Fe should explain why the distribution of ^{59}Fe in an erythrocyte population after centrifugation is almost uniform when half the life span of the cells has passed in rabbit (Hoffman, 1958, Prentice and Bishop, 1965, Pionelli, Lurinsky and Wasserman, 1966) and man (Borun, Figueroa and Perry, 1957, Rigas and Koler, 1961, Walter, 1963, Garby and Hjelm, 1963). However, the enrichment of labeled cells in the middle of the erythrocyte column at that time, as judged with ^{14}C-glycine, is also poor. It seems impossible, however, to obtain erythrocyte fractions more than 50% 'pure' and differing in mean age by say 2 days* during the last 10% of the life span using

* cf. Table III.

osmotic hemolysis.

Calculated percentage of labeled cells in		Days after labeling in		Most or least resistant cells in percentage of total cells population	Ref.
most resistant cells	least resistant cells	most resistant cells	least resistant cells		
50	—	3	120	5	a
19	11	5	190	varied	b
11	—	5	—	?	c

Walter, 1963.

differences in density with increasing cell age. Still, such a degree of separation is probably necessary to give an accurate description of the end of the erythrocyte life span.

The percentage of labeled erythrocytes might depend on the relative size of the cell population sampled from the erythrocyte column after centrifugation. There is also a tendency for the percentage of labeled cells to increase with decreasing relative size of top and bottom fractions, as is evident from Table IV. It is probably necessary to improve the sampling technique further to be able to isolate cell fractions containing a few percent of the total cell population, as recent investigations (Brok *et al.*, 1966) have demonstrated that biochemical changes measured in a 2% cell fraction were not demonstrable in a 10% fraction.

The enrichment of reticulocytes might possibly be simplified by using Stephens' observation in 1940, that a mixture of 5 parts of whole blood from nonmanipulated dogs, mixed with 1 part of 3.8% sodium citrate on standing in a tube, shows a stratification with one of the zones containing reticulocytes, 82–96% pure.

2) *Serial (Graded) Osmotic Hemolysis*

By 1938, Dameshek and Schwarz had already clearly shown that reticulocytes do not hemolyse to the same degree as old erythrocytes in certain hypotonic salt solutions. This observation was confirmed by Stephens in 1940, and has later been used to isolate the content of older cells for biochemical investigations and younger cells for biophysical and biochemical measurements (Chalfin, 1956, Simon and Topper, 1957, Marks and Johnson, 1958, Sass, Levy and Walter, 1963, Dannon, 1966). Again, different conditions have been used with respect to washing procedure, temperature of washing and serial osmotic hemolysis, as exemplified in Table V. (see also van Gastel, 1968).

The washing procedure has not been systematically investigated, both buffered and unbuffered solutions as well as NaCl and KCl being used. The temperature has been vaired and it can be noted that inconsistent results were obtained at 4°C, (Simon and Topper, 1957), a temperature used by Marks and Johnson, 1958 to prevent the inactivation of erythrocyte enzymes released, but with a lower degree of separation of labeled erythrocytes.

The highest number of labeled erythrocytes obtained was 50 and 11% in the cell fractions most and least resistant to osmotic hemolysis respectively. This is in accordance with the results obtained after centrifuging erythrocyte populations. Thus the same difficulties in investigating the last period of the life span with serial osmotic hemolysis should be found as with centrifugation. Again there is allo a practical problem in isolating sufficient small cell fractions (see above). A small fraction of reticulocytes in nonmanipulated human subjects seem to consist of cells less resistant to hemolysis. (Simon and Topper, 1957, Sass, Levy and Walter, 1963). These cells may represent 'stress reticulocytes' (1 c, 2 b) also produced under physiological conditions.

3) Counter-Current Distribution of Erythrocytes

A 2-phase system consisting of a mixture of 2 aqueous solutions of different polymers—dextran and polyethylene glycol—developed by Albertsson and Baired in 1962, has been used to separate erythrocytes into age groups (Walter and Selby, 1966). A variant of this method—multiple sedimentation—was published by Walter and Albertsson in 1971. Rat reticulocytes from nonmanipulated animals are enriched to some extent. It can be calculated from figures on the 'relative specific activity ' of ^{59}Fe, that erythrocyte populations are obtained containing 8% reticulocytes. However, the cell population obtained 2 days after labelling with ^{59}Fe is heterogeneous, as 2 populations of labeled cells are obtained, 1 type of cells being reticulocytes which appear at the same place in the counter-current pattern as old cells and the other cell population consisting of young erythrocytes. This finding is in agreement with results reported by Simon and Topper in 1957 and Sass, Levy and Walter in 1963, using serial osmotic hemolysis to isolate erythrocyte populations of different mean age.

In accordance with previous methods discussed, the counter-current technique does not give well-defined age groups or erythrocytes at the end of the life span of the cells (Walter and Albertsson, 1971). Counter-current distribution of erythrocytes has been performed at room temperature, which may limit the applicability of the method for the measurement of at least some erythrocytic variables.

4) In Vivo Methods

a) Differential Agglutination (Ashby, 1919)

This technique to isolate circulating erythrocytes of blood group O in a recipient of another blood group should in principle be an ideal method to study erythrocytes at the end of the life span. The method has also been used to study age-dependent biochemical changes both in human being (Löhr *et al.*, 1958) and in animals (Allison and Burn, 1955). From a practical point of view, however, the problem is, how efficiently donor cells can be isolated from the recipient's cells.

It has been found that about 1 to 2% of the recipient's cells are not agglutinated (Mollison, 1956). If say 700 ml of donor erythrocytes are initially mixed with 2,100 ml of recipient cells, there is approximatelly 1 donor cells in 300 recipient cells 100 days after the blood transfusion. This means, that only 33% of donor cells are present in the isolated cell population already at that time, with 1% of the recipient's cells not being agglutinated. Thus the possibility of obtaining valid information about biochemical and biophysical changes at the end of the life span seems limited with differential agglutination procedure. The effect of time and temperature on biochemical and biophysical variables in the isolated erythrocytes has not been systematically tested but should not be neglected.

b) Induced Hemolysis and Bleeding

A pronounced reticulocytosis has classically been induced in animals by phenylhydrazine, PHZ (Chalfin, 1956) and by repeated bleeding in animals and in man (Plum, 1943, Chalfin, 1956, Chapman and Schaumburg, 1967, Shojania *et al.*, 1968). However, it was early experimentally verified that reticulocytes produced in response to PHZ-induced hemolytical anemia differ in many respects from reticulocytes occurring in the circulation during physiological circumstances (Chalfin, 1956). That macroreticulocytes of 'stress' reticulocytes produced in response both to PHZ and bleeding are not comparable with normocytic reticulocytes and young erythrocytes, has later been substantially verified (Simon and Topper, 1957, Walter and Selby, 1966, Card and Valberg, 1967, Card, Paulson and Valberg, 1968, Card *et al.*,

1969). Thus, biochemical and biophysical investigations on erythrocytes from manipulated subjects may not be valid for the *in vivo* ageing of erythrocytes during physiological conditions as macroreticulocytes and mature erythrocytes of 'stress reticulocytes' could possibly not be directly compared with their corresponding physiological cell types. Investigations of macroreticulocytes and their more mature forms are still valid for the ageing of this type of cell, however, and the ageing of stress reticulocytes should offer an interesting alternative to test the validity of a hypothesis for cell death, as the survival of erythrocytes from macroreticulocytes is shortened compared with normal erythrocytes.

c) *Hypertransfusion in Animal Models*

Recently an experimental model has been proposed to study normal red-cell population in rats. The initial red-cell mass of a large number of in-bred rats was repeatedly transferred into an ever smaller number of animals, making it possible to follow the ageing of the inital cell population by the suppression of erythropoiesis by transfusion-induced polycytaemia (Ganzoni, Oakes and Hillman, 1971). With this experimental model is was possible to follow the initial cell population during 48 days without contamination by new erythrocytes produced in the bone marrow. Extrapolated data into the last period of the life span of the erythrocytes indicate that MCV, MCH and MCHC change almost as drastically during the first and last 15% of the life span. This change was opposite in direction for MCHC during the first and last parts of the life span.

CONCLUDING REMARKS ON THE BIOCHEMISTRY AND BIOPHYSICS OF ERYTHROCYTE AGEING

The biochemistry and biophysics of erythrocyte ageing has been extensively reviewed by Fornaini in 1967 and Danon in 1966, respectively. It is evident from these articles, that certain *trends*, *i.e.*, that the variables increase or decrease over a certain time interval, have been established for many biochemical and biophysical variables during the ageing of the erythrocytes. Such trends seem to be well-established during the initial and middle periods, but are less well-known during the terminal part of the life span. These circumstances could mainly be explained by the isolating of well-defined erythrocyte populations with increasing cell age, as demonstrated in the present survey of actual fractionation methods.

The possibility of obtaining detailed information about the relation between age and erythrocyte biochemistry and biophysics seems restricted using present fractionation methods as here documented. Improved methods should be developed to obtain 'pure' erythrocyte populations, differing in mean age by a few days, especially during (a) the initial part of the life span, as the magnitude and relative change of erythrocyte variables with time during this period probably is a function of the erythrocyte production rate (Card and Valberg, 1967) and (b) the last 10% of erythrocyte life, to establish the functional sequence of biochemical and biophysical events proceeding the death of the erythrocyte.

REFERENCES

1 Albertsson, P. A. and Baird, G. D., Counter-current distribution of cells. *Exptl. Cell Res.*, **28**, 296 (1962).

2 Allison, A. C. and Burn, G. P., Enzyme Activity as a function of age in the human erythrocyte. *Br. J. Haemat.*, **1**, 291 (1955).

3a Ashby, W., The determination of the length of life of transfused blood corpuscles in man. *J. Exp. Med.*, **29**, 267 (1919).

3b Berlin, N. I., Waldmann, T. A. and Weisman, S. M., Life span of red blood cells. *Physiol. Rev.*, **39**, 577 (1959).

4 Bernstein, R. E., Alterations in metabolic energetics and cation transport during ageing of red cells. *J. Clin. Invest.*, **38**, 1572 (1959).

5 Bishop, C. and Prentice, T. C., Separation of rabbit red cells by density in a bovine serum albumin gradient and correlation of red-cell density with cell age after *in vivo* labeling with ^{59}Fe. *J. Cell. Physiol.*, **67**, 197 (1966).

6 Borun, E. R., Figueroa, W. G. and Perry, S. M., The distribution of ^{59}Fe-tagged human erythrocytes in centrifuged specimens as a function of cell age. *J. Clin. Invest.*, **36**, 676 (1957).

7 Brok, F., Ramot, B., Zwang, E. and Danon, D., Enzyme activities in human red blood cells of different age groups, **2**, 291 (1966).

8 Card, R. T. and Valberg, L. S., Characteristics of shortened survival of stress erythrocytes in the rabbit. *Amer. J. Physiol.*, **213**, 566 (1967).

9 Card, R. T., Paulson, E. J. and Valberg, L. S., Autohemolysis and osmotic fragility of macrocytic erythrocytes produced in response to hemolysis. *Amer. J. Physiol.*, **214**, 45 (1968).

10 Card, R. T., McGrath, M. J., Paulson, E. J. and Valberg, L. S., Life-span and autohemolysis of macrocytic erythrocytes produced in response to hemorrhage. *Amer. J. Physiol.*, **216**, 974 (1969).

11 Chalfin, D., Differences between young and mature rabbit erythrocytes. *J. Cell. Comp. Physiol.*, **47**, 215 (1956).
12 Chapman, R. G. and Schaumberg, L., Glycolysis and glycolytic enzyme activity of ageing red cells in man. *Br. J. Haemat.*, **13**, 665 (1967).
13 Coopersmith, A. and Ingram, M., Red-cell volymes and erythropoiesis 1. Age: density: volume relationship of normocytes. *Amer. J. Physiol.*, **215**, 1276 (1968).
14 Dameshek, W., Schwartz, S. O. and Gross, S., Hemolysins as the cause of clinical and experimental hemolytical anemias with particular reference to the nature of spherocytosis and increased fragility. *Amer. J. Med. Sci.*, **196**, 769 (1938).
15 Danon, D. and Marikovsky, Y., Determination of density distribution of red-cell population. *J. Lab. Clin. Med.*, **64**, 668 (1964).
16 Danon, D., Marikovsky, Y., Furedi, A. and Ohad, I., On the separation of old from young erythrocytes in hypotonic bovine serum albumin solutions. *Biochim. Biophys. Acta.*, **104**, 281 (1965).
17 Danon, D., Biophysical aspects of red-cell ageing. *Bibl. Haemat.*, **29**, 178 (1966).
18 Dreyfus, J.C., Schapira, G. and Kruh, J., Fractionnement des hématies selon leur age. Centrifugation d'hématies marquées par le fer radioactif. *Soc. Biol.*, **144**, 792 (1950).
19 Edwards, M. J. and Rigas, D. A., Electrolyte-Labile increase of Oxygen affinity during *in vivo* ageing of hemoglobin. *J. Clin. Invest.*, **46**, 1579 (1967).
20 Edwards, M. J., Canon, B., Albertson, J. and Bigley, R. H., Mean red-cell age as a determinant of blood oxygen affinity. *Nature*, **230**, 583 (1971).
21 Fåhreus, R., The suspension stability of the blood. *Acta Med. Scand.*, **55**, 1 (1921).
22 Ferrebee, J. W., Gibson, J. G. and Peacock, W. E., The age of the erythrocyte invaved by plasmodium vivax. Studies on malarial parasites. *J. Infect. Dis.*, **78**, 180 (1946).
23 Finch, C. A., Wolff, J. A., Rath, C. E. and Fluharty, R. G., Iron metabolism. Erythrocyte iron turnover. *J. Lab. Clin. Med.*, **34**, 1480 (1949).
24 Fornaini, G., Biochemical modifications during the life span of the erythrocyte. *Ital. J. Biochem.*, **16**, 257 (1967).
25 Ganzoni, A., Hillman, R. S. and Finch, C. A., Maturation of the macroreticulocyte. *Br. J. Haemat.*, **16**, 119 (1969).
26 Ganzoni, A. M., Oakes, R. and Hillman, R. S., Red-cell ageing *in vivo*. *J. Clin. Invest.*, **50**, 1373 (1971).
27 Garby, L. and Hjelm, M., Ultracentrifugal fractionation of human erythrocytes with respect to cell age. *Blut. Z. Blutforsch.*, **9**, 1 (1963).
28 van Gastel, C., van den Berg, D., de Gier, J. and van Deenen, L. M.,

Some lipid characteristics of normal red blood cells of different age. *Br. J. Haemat.*, **11**, 193 (1965).

29 van Gastel, C., Methods for studying the *in vivo* ageing of red cells. Blood Information Service 1968 (Library of congress catalog card no 68–9821).

30 Gross, J., Hatwig, A., Staak, R., Rosenthal, D., Grauel, E. I. and Syllm-Rapoport, I., Dichtegradientzentrifugation von Erythrozyten im Dextranmedium: Dichteverteilung im Dextran und in Phthalatestern in Rapoport/Jung (ed.): Structur und Function der Erythrozyten. VI. Internationales Synposium (Akademi-Verlag, Berlin, 1972), p. 529.

31 Hjelm, M., unpublished results (1972).

32 Hoffman, J. F., On the relationship of certain erythrocyte characteristics to their physiological age. *J. Cell. Comp. Physiol.*, **51**, 415 (1958).

33 Key, J. A., Studies on erythrocytes with special reference to reticulum, polychromatophilia and mitochrondria. *Arch. Int. Med.*, **28**, 511 (1921).

34 Leif, R. C. and Vinograd, J., The distribution of buoyant density of human erythrocytes in bovine albumin solutions. *Proc. Nat. Acad. Sci.*, **51**, 520 (1964).

35 Leif, R. C., Buoyant density separation of cells in Wied, ed. by Ba, Automated cell identification and cell sorting (Academic Press, New York and London, 1970), p. 21.

36 Löhr, G. W., Waller, H. D., Karges, O., Schlegel, B. and Miller, A. A., Zur Biochemie der Alterung menschlicher Erythrocyten. *Klin. Wschr.*, **21**, 1008 (1958).

37 Marks, P. A. and Johnson, A. B., Relationship between the age of human erythrocytes and their osmotic resistance: A basis for separating young and old erythrocytes. *J. Clin. Invest.*, **37**, 1542 (1958).

38 Mollison, P. L., Blood transfusion in clinical medicine. Blackwell Scientific Publications Oxford, II. ed. (1956), p. 120.

39 O'Connell, D. J., Caruso, C. J. and Sass, M. D., Separation of Erythrocytes of different ages. *Clin. Chem.*, **11**, 771 (1965).

40 Piomelli, S., Lurinsky, G. and Wasserman, L. R., The mechanism of red-cell ageing. I. Relationship between cell age and specific gravity evaluated by ultracentrifugation in a discontinuous density gradient. *J. Lab. & Clin. Med.*, **69**, 660 (1966).

41 Plum, C. M., Reticulocyte-ripening substances in plasma in animals with increased erythropoiesis. *Acta Physiol. Scand.*, **5**, 175 (1943).

42 Prankerd, T. A. J., The ageing of red cells. *J. Physiol.*, **143**, 325 (1958)

43 Prentice, T. C. and Bishop, C., Separation of rabbit cells by density methods and characteristics of separated layers. *J. Cell. Comp. Physiol.*, **65**, 113 (1965).

44 Rigas, D. A. and Koler, R. D., Ultracentrifugal fractionation of human

erythrocytes on the basis of cell age. *J. Lab. & Clin. Med.*, **58**, 242 (1961).

45 Sass, M. D., Levy, L. M. and Walter, H., Characteristics of erythrocytes of different ages II. Enzyme activity and osmotic fragility. *Canad. J. Biochem. Physiol.*, **41**, 2287 (1963).

46 Shojania, A. M., Israels, L. G. and Zipursky, A., The relationship of adenosine triphospate concentration to erythrocyte ageing. *J. Lab. & Clin. Med.*, **71**, 41 (1968).

47 Simon, E. R. and Topper, Y. J., Fractionation of human erythrocytes on the basis of their age. *Nature*, **4596**, 1211 (1957).

48 Stephens, J. G., Surface and fragility differences between mature and immature red cells. *J. Physiol.*, **99**, 30 (1940).

49 Stryckmans, P. A., Cronkite, E. P., Giacomelli, G., Schiffer, L. M. and Schnappauf, Hp., The maturation and fate of reticulocytes after *in vitro* labeling with tritiated amino acids. *Blood*, **31**, 33 (1968).

50 Thorsen, G. and Hint, H., Aggregation, sedimentation and intravascular sludging of erythrocytes. *Acta Chir. Scand.*, 1950, suppl. 154.

51 Walter, H. and Selby, F. W., Counter-current distribution of red blood cells of slightly different ages. *Biochim. Biophys. Acta.*, **112**, 146 (1966).

52 Walter, H. and Albertsson, P. Å., Fractionation of red blood cells by multiple sedimentation at unit gravity. *Exptl. Cell Res.*, **67**, 218 (1971).

53 Winterbourn, C. C. and Batt, R. D., Lipid composition of human red cells of different ages. *Biochim. Biophys. Acta.*, **202**, 1 (1970).

54 Wintrobe, M., Clinical Hematology, Sixth Edition, Lea & Febiger, Philadelphia (1967), p. 358.

SUBJECT INDEX